WELLNESS

Published by YES! Inc.
1035 31st Street, N.W.
Washington, D.C. 20007

Distributed by Random House

WELLNESS

Cris Popenoe

COVER PHOTOGRAPH: from **A Haiku Journey,** Dennis Stock
and Dorothy Britton. Kodansha International Ltd., 1974.

Table of Contents

HOW TO USE THIS GUIDE 7

ANATOMY & PHYSIOLOGY. 9

BODY WORK 17
    Aikido 20
    The Alexander Technique 22
    Bioenergetics 24
    Dance 29
    Karate 36
    Massage 39
    The Mensendieck System 42
    Running 44
    Tai Chi Chuan 50
    Yoga 53

COLOR & AURA 68

COOKBOOKS 84
    Baby Food 89
    Bread 90
    Macrobiotics 99

DEATH 104

HEALING 116
    Arthritis 120
    Bach Flower Remedies 124
    Cancer 130
    The Digestive System 145
    Fasting 154
    Irisdiagnosis 168

Mental Health 182
Sugar. 201
Vision 209

HERBS 218
Ginseng. 229

HOMOEOPATHY 245
Cell Salts 253

LIFE ENERGIES 274
Franz Mesmer 291
Wilhelm Reich. 295
Nikola Tesla 304

NATURAL CHILDBIRTH 308
Breastfeeding. 312

NUTRITION. 327
Food Pollution 336
Natural Beauty 351
Raw Foods 358
Vegetarianism 364
Vitamins & Minerals 366

ORGANIC GARDENING 375

ORIENTAL MEDICINE 384
Reflexology. 398
Shiatsu & Acupressure. .400

APPENDICES 411
How to Obtain These Books 413
Supplements 416
Publishers' Codes & Addresses. 419
Author Index 429

How To Use This Guide

Books in **Wellness** are arranged into subjects, as listed in the Table of Contents, then alphabetically by author. Subsections contain groups of books about a particular discipline or concept we feel to be of substantial importance to our theme. Subsections appear in the alphabetical order of the subject area to which they pertain, but the books listed alphabetically under subsection headings do not follow the order of general entries. A double rule indicates the end of a subsection.

If you don't find a book you are looking for in the section you expect to find it in and you know the author, turn to the author index at the back. It lists all the pages on which books by that author appear, and you can see where else to try. Our ideas about classification and yours may not agree.

Following the author and title we list the price. If it begins with a *c,* it means the book is in cloth (hardcover); otherwise it is in paper. Our policy is to list the paper edition wherever possible. We sometimes list the cloth edition as well when it is markedly superior or there is a substantial demand for it. The prices are the prices at which we sell the book at this writing. Because many of the books are imported, prices at your local bookstore may be above or below ours from time to time.

Quotations within the reviews are set in italics. At the end of each review is a three letter code for the publisher and two numbers for the date of this edition. The names and addresses of the publishers are given in the list of Publishers' Codes and Addresses. The date we cite is not that of the most recent printing or the paperback edition, but generally represents when the book first came out with this exact text. The idea is to let you know how current the material is.

We have picked out a few books in each section that we particularly recommend. These books have been set in bold face type for easy identification. These are usually introductory books or books suitable for the general reader.

You may wonder how we select these books. Our effort in **Wellness** as in **Books for Inner Development**, the first Yes! Bookshop Guide, reflects the service policy of our bookshop—we want to offer as comprehensive a selection as possible within the subjects we handle. This means we try to include all the books that we feel make a significant contribution to their subjects. On the other hand, we do not include books that we feel are essentially worthless or do not make a positive contribution—no matter how popular.

We're in this business because we love it and we specialize in these fields because they interest us the most. The individual reviews represent our view and our view alone. They have not been influenced by authors or publishers. We appreciate the difficulty of sorting through the vast proliferation of books in many fields. We have tried to make the reviews as useful as possible for those of you who don't have easy access to the actual books. We hope we have succeeded. If we have not, please let us hear from you.

Anatomy & Physiology

The physical body is a masterpiece of some sixty trillion cells, beautifully designed and precisely arranged. Inhabiting this incredible piece of evolved matter is something even more beautiful—the force or energy of life itself which animates the limbs, organs, and all the parts of the body. Like the physical body, this energy has its own subtle anatomy of fields, vortices, and channels.

There are two fundamental modes of exploring the human form: science and mysticism. Generally, the scientists study the body objectively and empirically. When their eyes, ears, nose, or hands cannot unravel the secrets of the body, they employ technical instruments which are far more perceptive than their own gross senses. The information thus gathered must then be verified by other scientists before it is considered fact.

Mystics, on the other hand, take a subjective, experiential approach. They explore their own beings internally with their intuition and inner senses. Instead of devising machines and tools to extend their searches, mystics continually refine and develop themselves. The anatomy discerned by a mystic can only be verified by one going through the same process of refinement and development.

Scientists and mystics alike explore unknown and uncharted realms of human nature. The seemingly contradictory statements of science and mysticism merely indicate that the two disciplines employ different methods and look at different aspects of a human being. Each discipline has its own special applications and values which do not exclude the legitimacy of the other. When both scientific anatomy and mystical anatomy are studied together, they are found to dovetail surprisingly well.

Slowly, a synthesis is emerging which is putting to rest age old controversies between seemingly disparate realms of knowledge and producing exciting new psssibilities for all mankind. By knowing our anatomy and inner self more fully, we can better heal our ills and understand the nature of our life.

—Bud Brainard

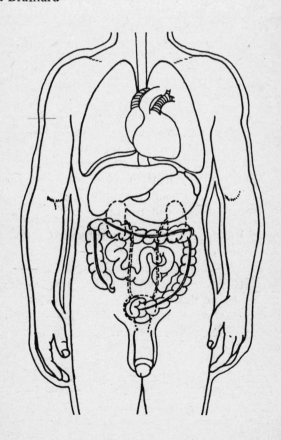

ASIMOV, ISAAC. *THE HUMAN BODY,* 1.50. This is a well written, informative study which explains the structure and operation of the human body utilizing both anatomy and physiology. As usual Asimov makes his subject understandable and exciting to the layman. Illustrations, index, 320pp. NAL 63

ASIMOV, ISAAC. *THE HUMAN BRAIN,* 1.25. A companion volume to Asimov's **The Human Body**, in which Asimov explores the physical structure of the cerebral hemisphere and the functioning of the hormones, pancreas, thyroid, adrenal cortex, gonads, nerves, nervous system, cerebrum, brain stem and spinal cord, senses, ears, eyes, reflexes, and mind—all of which are controlled by the brain. The text is well illustrated with line drawings and the material is explained with the clarity for which Asimov is noted. Index, 357pp. NAL 63

BAKER, DOUGLAS. *ESOTERIC ANATOMY,* 16.00. Dr. Baker is an English physician who is well versed in the esoteric sciences. Many of his observations are derived from theosophy. This study is more interesting than many of his books because it draws heavily on his own experiences and observations. Each part of the human anatomy is explored and graphically illustrated and the esoteric organs are discussed as fully as the exoteric ones. The illustrations are often in color and many of the line drawings are clear and presented in a scientific manner. On the whole the book is less scattered than many of Baker's books. Very fully indexed, 8"x11½", 247pp. Bak 76

CROUCH, JAMES. *INTRODUCTION TO HUMAN ANATOMY,* 7.50. A well organized, comprehensive, and extensively illustrated laboratory manual which is designed for premedical students. The illustrations are large and are very clearly drawn and, while it is designed to be used for dissection, it should be helpful to anyone who wants to learn the details of human anatomy. Extensive descriptive material accompanies the plates. There's also a section of questions. Glossary, index, 8½"x11", 269pp. MPC 73

DUMONT, THERON. *THE SOLAR PLEXUS OR ABDOMINAL BRAIN,* 1.00. Dumont believes that the solar plexus is one of man's four brains (the others being the cerebrum, the cerebellum, and the medulla oblong), ruling man's emotional center and regulating his vitality and health. In this small book he examines the solar plexus,

GRAY, HENRY. *GRAY'S ANATOMY,* 6.95. This is a new edition of this classic work and it includes 780 illustrations, with 172 in color. It is a very comprehensive, dryly written study of every part of the human body. While **Gray's Anatomy** is far from our favorite book on the subject, it is an important text which supplements some of the more recent works. Index, 1257pp. Crn 77

HALL, MANLY P. *MAN: GRAND SYMBOL OF THE MYSTERIES,* c10.00. A new edition of Hall's fascinating essays on occult anatomy, profusely illustrated with woodcuts and line drawings. Includes chapters on *the macrocosm and the microcosm, the story of the cell, the brain and the release of the soul, the heart, the seat of life, the spinal column and the world tree (the tree of life), kundalini, the pineal gland, sight,* and much else. Hall relates his material to the ancient mystery teachings and as usual incorporates a great deal of fascinating philosophy. Extensive index, oversize, 254pp. PRS 72

HALL, MANLY P. *THE OCCULT ANATOMY OF MAN,* 1.50. An interesting treatise based on the ancient mystery teachings. 36pp. PRS 57

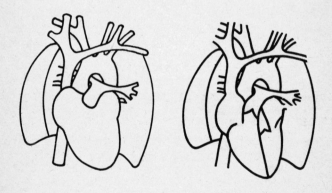

HEIDENSTAM, DAVID, ed. *MAN'S BODY: AN OWNER'S MANUAL,* 6.95. This is an **Our Bodies, Ourselves** for men—although the approach is more traditional than the latter book. **Man's Body** is lavishly illustrated and contains clear information on bodily functions and possible malfunctions, health and fitness, sexuality, life expectancy and aging, and much else. Over 1000 diagrams, drawings, and charts are included. Index, 8½"x11", about 250pp. TWP 76

HEINDEL, MAX. *THE VITAL BODY,* 2.50. An esoteric treatise based on Rosicrucian philosophy. Heindel defines the vital body as follows: *The vital body is made of ether and pervades the visible body as ether permeates all other forms, except that human beings specialize a greater amount of the universal ether than other forms. That ethereal body is our instrument for specializing the vital energy of the Sun.* 198pp. Ros 50

HELINE, CORINNE. *OCCULT ANATOMY AND THE BIBLE,* c6.00. Elaborates upon the idea that the mystery of the universe is expressed through the formation and birth of a child, and extended throughout the physical life of spiritual rebirths. 365pp. NAP 37

KAPP, M.W. *GLANDS: OUR INVISIBLE GUARDIANS,* c5.75. This is an excellent esoteric analysis of the glands based on Rosicrucian philosophy and on the ancient mystery teachings. Each of the glands is discussed at length. Index, 97pp. Amo 58

LEADBEATER, C.W. *THE CHAKRAS,* c4.75/3.45. According to Hindu teachings, there are subtle psychic sense organs in man's body which channel psychic energies and vital force, and are related to the glandular and nervous systems. They are also said to serve as a link between physical, psychic, and super-physical states of consciousness. These centers are called chakras, a Sanskrit term meaning wheels or discs. Leadbeater's book was first published in 1927, and has become a classic in its field. It is handsomely illustrated with ten color plates and many drawings. The material is comprehensive and very clearly illuminated. 132pp. TPH

NILSSON, LENNART. *BEHOLD MAN,* c25.00. Nilsson is a Swedish photographer who has been working on close-ups of the life of living things since the early 1950's, progressing from insects to small sea animals and, finally, to human beings. Many of his photos were published in **Life** magazine. **Behold Man** takes the reader on a remarkable odyssey inside the human body. In 350 photographs, most of them in color, the extraordinary complexity and variety of the body is presented in a way that has never before been seen. Employing newly designed optical devices, powerful electron microscopes, and specially calibrated instruments capable of magnifying minute tissues to thousands of times larger than life size, Nilsson opens up the unseen landscape of our bodies and the processes that sustain them. His pictures reveal the secrets of how our senses work, how the body communicates with itself, and how such crucial cycles as respiration, digestion, and reproduction are carried out. His camera investigates every region of the body, from the structure of a single cell to the most delicately balanced interaction of bodily functions. Supported by a clear, straightforward text, many line drawings and extensive captions, **Behold Man** invites every reader to share its beautiful and mysterious discoveries about the human body and how it works. Indexed, oversize, 254pp. LBC 73

PEARCE, EVELYN. *ANATOMY AND PHYSIOLOGY FOR NURSES,* 4.95. This is far and away the best anatomy book for both the layman and the professional that we know of. Each part of the body is discussed and illustrated and even the smallest areas can be readily viewed. The material is well organized and the explanations are clear and to the point. Excellent line drawings. Glossary, fully indexed, 411pp. Fab 75

RAYNER, CLAIRE, et al. *ATLAS OF THE BODY AND MIND,* c25.00. This is a stunning book which takes the reader on a voyage through the workings of the human body, emphasizing the elaborate interactions of the mind and body. The thorough text—supported by over 400 color paintings, photographs, and cutaway drawings—plus an extensive glossary and complete index, make this an invaluable resource. The text is divided into the following major sections: *evolution of man, framework of the body, energy for the machine, control systems, the senses, the brain, the intellect, defenses of the body, reproduction, span of life,* and *the future.* An amazing book which can be studied over a lifetime. 10¾"x14½", 208pp. RMN 76

RENDEL, PETER. *INTRODUCTION TO THE CHAKRAS,* 1.00. This is a well written, concise study. The first six chapters explain the occult anatomy of man. The magnetic polarities and energy fields are discussed as they relate to the flow of vitality and to the seven chakras. Special emphasis is placed on the brow and the crown chakras. The next chapters deal with the application of these principles in practice through yoga and self training. A final chapter traces the relationship between astrology and the chakras. Rendel emphasizes recognition of the principles involved and the energies which constitute the system, and the control and use of these energies. Includes illustrations throughout. Highly recommended as a basic primer. 64pp. Wei 74

ROSICRUCIAN FELLOWSHIP. *THE MYSTERY OF THE DUCTLESS GLANDS,* 1.25. An examination of the structure, function, and spiritual significance of the seven ductless glands. The spiritual function of the glands is based on information given by Max Heindel and the physiological structure and function is based on a textbook on the ductless glands written by Dr. Louis Berman. 85pp. Ros 40

SCHLOSSBERG, LEON and GEORGE ZUIDEMA. *THE JOHNS HOPKINS ATLAS OF HUMAN FUNCTIONAL ANATOMY,* **6.95.** 148 color illustrations of all systems and organs of the human body drawn by a medical artist from Johns Hopkins University are each accompanied by a descriptive text written by the faculty of Johns Hopkins School of Medicine. The illustrations and descriptions have been carefully prepared to assist an understanding of the physiology and interrelation of body systems. The drawings are as clear as any we've seen and we recommend this book highly to all students of anatomy and physiology. Glossary, index, 8½"x11", 108pp. JHU 77

SCIENCE OF LIFE BOOKS, *GLANDS AND YOUR HEALTH,* 1.35. A simplified treatise which discusses each one of the glands and explains the vital role played by the glands in the human organism. Includes information on weight control, hormone chemistry, feeding the glands, brain function, and the effect of the endocrine and sex glands on personality. 64pp. SLB 75

STANFORD, RAY. *THE SPIRIT UNTO THE CHURCHES,* 8.50. Transcription of a series of readings given through Stanford, a well known psychic. *These readings deal with the physical, mental, and spiritual aspects of the human endocrine glands and their supraphysical counterparts, which yogis referred to in ancient times as "chakras" (Sanskrit for "wheels").* —from the foreword. Each of the glands is discussed in a separate chapter. This new edition also includes a chapter, written by Stanford, on the application of the information given in the readings. There's also a correlation chart of the seven centers. 8½"x11", 223pp. AUM 77

STEEN, EDWIN and ASHLEY MONTAGU. *ANATOMY AND PHYSIOLOGY,* 2.95/each. This is a very complete, well written set. Most of the illustrations are half tones and are very well done. The explanatory material is complete, and not overly complicated. The books are part of Barnes and Noble's College Outline Series. Despite our intellectual prejudice against the idea of a college outline book, they are excellent introductory surveys. Volume I reviews the cells, tissues, integument, skeletal, muscular, and digestive systems, blood, lymph, and circulatory system. Volume II covers the urinary, respiratory, and nervous systems, sensations and sense organs, endocrine and reproductive systems. Each volume is separately indexed and has over 300pp. H&R 59

WALKER, BENJAMIN. *MAN AND THE BEASTS WITHIN,* c12.95. An encyclopedic survey. Over 150 lengthy entries deal with the esoteric anatomy and physiology of the human body, and additional references are given for each entry. Many of the topics are only peripherally related to anatomy and physiology and the book is a bit of a hodgepodge. Nonetheless, it does provide information not readily available elsewhere. Index, 353pp. S&D 77

YOKOCHI, C. *PHOTOGRAPHIC ANATOMY OF THE HUMAN BODY,* c19.50. This is a remarkable book which features vivid full color photographs of actual human cadavers. Every principle organ and body system is illustrated by means of over 200 photographs. These include cutaway and cross-section views of complete torsos and a double-page spread of a torso from which all skin covering has been meticulously removed. Most of the photographs are of freshly prepared sections or organs and not the usual unlifelike specimens from stored cadavers. This is an amazing book which we highly recommend to all who are deeply interested in learning about anatomy. 8½"x11", 100pp. UPP 71

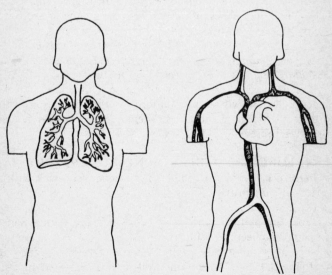

Body Work

A healthy body moves free and easy. It is unencumbered by aches and pains, the dead weight of sluggish organs and tensed muscles. It is light and ready to move, from the moment it opens eagerly to the day, until its comfortable folding down for the night. Perfect health is the birthright of every body. The unity of the healthy body and its parts and functions all cooperate for the achievement of the maintenance and perfection of life.

A healthy body sustains a healthy intellect with zest, energy, enthusiasm, vigor, and courage. The personality we manifest and the way we feel about ourselves are directly related to the freedom the body is given in expressing itself. Through movement a person reveals much of his inner life. A healthy body animates the enjoyment of life.

Growing up need not mean you can no longer expect to "sleep like a baby" or wake up zestfully with a hearty appetite for living. Watch a baby. A healthy infant is a study in motion. Head, arms, legs, lungs, torso—every nerve and muscle vibrates, alternatively pushing out and pulling in, throbbing between tension and release, uninhibited, instinctive and free. These seemingly spasmodic actions express a perfectly coordinated system in which each part is interrelated and interacting. A healthy body is one in which organs, nerves, and muscles cooperate to maintain a symmetry of body rhythms.

None of the suppleness, enthusiasm, or amazing endurance of a baby (it can body-cry for hours without exhaustion) need be lost in adulthood. There are outlets for body motion which should be utilized if you hope to sustain your original gift of health. You cannot stop moving (exercising) or breathe incorrectly and still expect to have a baby's powerful lungs, vibrant diaphragm, elastic intestines, and strong heart. Nor will your nerves be steady enough or your mind clear enough to handle the mental and emotional challenges of adulthood.

Moving through the day with a natural charge of energy, without false stimulation from caffeine, nicotine, or pep pills, is the inherent right of everyone. The type of exhilaration that emanates from a baby should be the native state of a healthy body, regardless of age. Adult good health is a sophisticated version of an infant's agility, charm, and even muscular strength (which is relative, of course, but try pulling your finger away from a baby's grasp). These are not toys to be put away when you grow up—they are gifts inherited for life and, without them, health breaks down.

Internal cleanliness, relaxed and sturdy inner organs working cooperatively together, are the best prevention against disease. A healthy body can tolerate foreign bacteria without breaking down.

The unhealthy body frequently reacts improperly to stress, a stimulus to the emotions that provokes the body to react. Failure to release the body responses generated by stress can cause inhibition—centers of tension resulting in colitis, high blood pressure, nervousness, headaches, ulcers, heart disease, emotional insecurity, and many other ills. Dr. Hans Kraus, an internationally known back specialist, says, . . .*tension, or lack of flexibility, is responsible for more attacks of back pain than any other single cause.*

To understand why this happens we must understand the ancient principles of *fight or flight.* Whatever personal or social restraints we may inflict upon ourselves in response to anger, anxiety, fear, or daily minor and major irritations, our body interprets this age-old message as a biological need for sudden spurts of adrenalin and blood and for tensed muscles—in short, the body must be ready for action.

When no action occurs, when we want to stamp in anger or jump in joy, we freeze or tighten up. The biological responses of our bodies begin to work against us, blood pressure builds, muscles become snagged in tension, and internal juices start consuming devitalized organ tissue. Sooner or later a symptom of disease develops. You go to the doctor and the symptom is treated and (you hope) eliminated. But, unless you deal with stress and tension, you will be back in the doctor's office with the same or a different ill.

Three world-renowned specialists, Dr. Paul Dudley White, the heart specialist, Dr. Hans Selye, and Dr. Hans Kraus, both authorities on the subject of stress, all concur that *lack of exercise combined with constant irritation produces an imbalance, a sickness in our emotional and physical functions.* We are bombarded with different types of stress daily. City dwellers are constantly hit with noise from cars and industry, pollution from water and air. Unless we are careful, much of our food will be loaded with poisons. There is physical and mental stress from overwork producing fatigue and perhaps later disease.

But there are positive aspects of stress. Stress in sports, games, arts, crafts, music, and accomplishment represents a challenge to the human organism, an opportunity to test one's strength and become stronger physically, mentally, and spiritually. As such, it is a healthy part of being alive.

When stress is internalized and not transformed into a form of action or productivity/creativity, the energy flow shuts down. Stress, having no outlet, begins to prey on the body and the mind.

Restoring the body to a healthful level of activity in our society requires the constructive use of tension and stress to buttress the body—to release a positive flow of energy.

19

The achievement of good health needs a certain degree of physical and psychological stress to convert the pressure of daily living into the positive stress of exercise.

—from **The East/West Exercise Book** by David Smith

Aikido

Aikido is literally the road *(do)* to a union *(ai)* with the real substance of the universe *(ki)*. The practice of aikido aims at the refinement of our *ki* and its harmonious union with the *ki* of the universe. As Terry Dobson, an aikido teacher, says: *Many people watching Aikido for the first time are struck by the paradoxes they see. . . .The teacher speaks about harmony, and then throws the student to the ground. The student bows, and thanks the teacher for the experience. Another teacher talks about love, and then turns right around and shows a sword technique. Somebody else says Aikido is a martial art—a way of the warrior—and then stresses relaxation. Many people see these concepts as opposites and it is difficult for them to imagine how they can be resolved. Those of us who study Aikido are happy with our paradoxes. We know that the successful resolution of opposites produces harmony and recognize that opposition lies in the mind of the beholder. . . .Each of us is conditioned by experience to view things and situations in a different light. . . .Aikido is—among other things—a way to re-frame experience. . . .One of the fundamental concepts it helps to re-frame is that of power. Power is commonly held to depend on size and strength. . . .Aikido teaches us that power is connected to spirit, to "ki," to harmony with the universal flow. It teaches us to be open to change, to move with the flow of life. . . .Our training teaches us that by alternately throwing and being thrown, we are expanding our spirit, increasing our ability to both give and receive. As our ability to move with spirit increases, we find we have more control over our lives, more practical power.*

SHIODA, GOZO. *DYNAMIC AIKIDO,* c8.95. Shioda is the chief instructor of the Yoshinka Aikido Dojo. Here he presents the history, basic movements, and fundamental techniques of theoretical and applied aikido. 500 photographs and line drawings. 160pp. Kod 68

TOHEI, KOICHI. *AIKIDO IN DAILY LIFE,* 5.95. This is our most popular book on aikido. In the first section, Tohei teaches how to breathe properly and how to concentrate one's spirit; while in the second part he shows the application of aikido to daily living. Forty-eight illustrations, 220pp. Jap 66

TOHEI, KOICHI. *THE BOOK OF KI,* 5.95. Tohei presents the philosophical framework and specific disciplines by which an individual can attune him or herself with the *ki,* or universal life energy. This book has been long awaited by those who have followed Tohei's work and have read his books on aikido. 150 illustrations, index, oversize, 128pp. Jap 76

TOHEI, KOICHI. *THIS IS AIKIDO,* c15.50. This is the definitive text on aikido as a spiritual discipline and Tohei's first book. The first part discusses the psychology of aikido in detail and includes a glossary. The second and largest section is devoted to techniques all of which are illustrated with step-by-step photographs laid out in the circular format in which an aikido practitioner moves. The descriptive material is clear and excellent and the illustrations are very well done. Over 1000 illustrations, 8½"x12", 180pp. Jap 68

TOHEI, KOICHI. *WHAT IS AIKIDO?* 3.95. This is an illustrated exploration of the basics of aikido, emphasizing aikido's fundamental spirit and including seventy photographs and many line drawings. 118pp. Jap 62

UYESHIBA, KISSHIMARU. *AIKIDO,* c12.95. This is a combined edited version of two earlier Japanese works by aikido master Morihei Uyeshiba's only son, Kisshoman, now Director of Aikido International. Well illustrated, covering both technique and the development of aikido by Uyeshiba, this book presents the master's life experience and as such is essential reading for all aikido and

martial arts aficionados. 190pp. Jap 74

WESTBROOK, A. and O. RATTI. *AIKIDO AND THE DYNAMIC SPHERE,* c12.75. This is an excellent full scale treatment of the art of aikido, in which its goal of neutralizing aggression is pursued through over 1200 illustrations and thirty-three charts and tables. 375pp. Tut 70

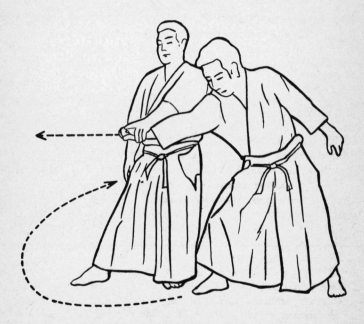

The Alexander Technique

Matthias Alexander was an actor who lived in the first part of the twentieth century. He developed his radical system of body dynamics as a response to a major illness of his own. The system's basic premise is that incorrect alignment of the head, neck, and shoulders (which is unconscious and almost universal in modern man by the age of eleven) sets off imbalances which throw the whole muscular system askew. The Alexander technique is designed to teach people to "use" themselves in a better and more conscious way. In the language of Alexander, "use" refers to the way we do things—how we stand, sit, walk, run, jump, play. Virtually all of us are habitually guilty of misuse, which results in unnecessary strain and tensions, awkwardness, imbalance, discomfort, or even pain—for example in the form of chronic neck and back aches. The major task of an Alexander teacher is to give the student the repeated sensation of good use in both resting states and in the performance of basic physical movements such as sitting down, walking, and lifting objects.

BARLOW, WILFRED. *THE ALEXANDER TECHNIQUE,* c7.95. Dr. Barlow is Alexander's foremost pupil and the Medical Director of the Alexander Institute in London. He draws from his years of experience as well as case histories, charts, and the results of surveys he conducted himself in his presentation. Every aspect of the technique is discussed in this definitive work, including material on practical applications. Indexed, references, 228pp. RaH 73

JONES, FRANK. *BODY AWARENESS IN ACTION: A STUDY OF THE ALEXANDER TECHNIQUE,* c9.95. A vivid introduction to Alexander and his teaching which draws on Alexander's own writings and on the author's own long association with Alexander and with his brother. Jones supplements the Alexanders' findings with his own carefully designed research at Tufts University Institute of Experimental Psychology, where he measured bodily movement in action and thereby provided scientific proof for the discoveries of Alexander. Notes, index, 224pp. ScB 76

MAISEL, EDWARD, ed. *THE RESURRECTION OF THE BODY: THE WRITINGS OF F. MATTHIAS ALEXANDER,* 2.95. This is the most comprehensive edition available of Alexander's writings. Notes on the technique are included along with a variety of case studies. The editor provides an excellent long introduction. Notes, 252pp. UnB 69

BARTAL, LEA and NIRA NE'EMAN. *MOVEMENT, AWARE-NESS AND CREATIVITY,* c7.95. The authors are Israelis who have worked extensively with dancers, actors, drama students, and children. They learned that bodies can be trained to be more effective tools of expression by applying inner discipline, intelligence, and awareness, and that uninhibited use of the body can develop imagination and the creative potential of the individual. This book sets out their approach to movement. It is a complete teaching program, with chapter-by-chapter descriptions of their own techniques. The book should be useful to both professionals and everyone interested in the development of creativity and imagination through movement. Illustrated throughout with photographs and line drawings. 179pp. H&R 75

Bioenergetics

The principles and practices of bioenergetic therapy rest on the functional identity of the mind and body. This means that any real change in a person's thinking and, therefore, in his behavior and feeling, is conditioned upon a change in the functioning of his body. The two functions that are most important in this regard are *breathing* and *movement.* Both of these functions are disturbed in every person who has an emotional conflict by chronic muscular tensions that are the physical counterpart of psychological conflicts. Through these muscular tensions conflicts become structured in the body. When this happens, they cannot be resolved until the tensions are released. To release these muscular tensions one must feel them as a limitation of self-expression. It is not enough to be aware of their pain. And most people are not even aware of that. When a muscular tension becomes chronic, it is removed from consciousness, and one loses an awareness of the tension.

The basic bioenergetic concept is that each chronic muscle tension pattern must be dealt with on three levels: (1) its history or origin in the infantile or childhood situation; (2) its present-day meaning in terms of the individual's character, and (3) its effect on bodily functioning. Only this holistic view of the phenomena of muscle tension can provide those changes in the personality that can have a lasting value.—Alexander Lowen, **Pleasure.**

JOHNSON, LELAND. *BIOENERGETICS,* 3.00. *This monograph has been vibrating in our experience for the past several years as we* [in the Houston Center for Human Potential] *have worked with each other and ourselves in our own growth and expansion. . . .We have drawn on techniques, modes and methods from a variety of sources as we continue to explore what we can become.* The first pages explore energy, both in terms of flows and blockages and include many illustrations and quotations. The rest of the book details specific exercises to increase body awareness and is illustrated with photographs. Bibliography, oversize, 32pp. Esp 74

KELEMAN, STANLEY. *THE HUMAN GROUND: SEXUALITY, SELF AND SURVIVAL,* 4.95. *Stanley Keleman is a teacher of awareness in the classic sense. Out of his own experience he finds words and exercises to evoke insight and learning in others. . . .His essential message is simple: be yourself, experience your bodily life directly. . . .This book is an expanded and revised edition of* **The Human Ground** *and* **Sexuality, Self and Survival,** *which were originally compiled out of a number of weekend workshops. . . .In* **The Human Ground,** *Stanley Keleman talks about the ways in which we take on self-definition. . .and how they may or may not be grounded in one's natural being. In* **Sexuality, Self and Survival,** *using vignettes from workshops, he demonstrates how the central energy of our sexual nature becomes diverted, dissipated, blocked, and warped by conditioned responses that may begin in the cradle or with toilet training.*—from the introduction by Gay Luce. 191pp. S&B 75

KELEMAN, STANLEY. *YOUR BODY SPEAKS ITS MIND,* 1.75. This is Keleman's most complete book on understanding the language of our bodies: "We do not *have* our bodies, we *are* our bodies. . .your body is not only alive, but formative." Using his experiences of working with people, he shows how they achieve formative experiences which put them in touch with the full range of human emotions. Through his program for "grounding" and "experiencing," he tries to provide ways to deal with the anxiety and anger confined through years of denial in a tense musculature and to help people free themselves to express the positive and loving feelings previously unavailable. Keleman writes clearly and directly and the reader can get a good feeling for the bioenergetic experience from his exposition and from the first person accounts he quotes. 189pp. S&S 75

KURTZ, RON and HECTOR PRESTERA. *THE BODY REVEALS*, 4.95/1.95. The structure of your body is a graphic expression of your physical, emotional, and mental state. It reveals past trauma and present personality as well as expressed and unexpressed feelings. The authors of this book are both body therapists, with extensive experience in group and in private body work. Here they present an illustrated primer on reading the body gleaned from a wide variety of disciplines. The opening chapters discuss just what body structure can tell you. In the next section, the authors examine each part of the body and give detailed information on the relationship between body parts and corresponding emotions and attributes. This is followed by five illustrated case studies and instructions for examining your own body structure. Bibliography, 159pp. H&R 76

LOWEN, ALEXANDER. *THE BETRAYAL OF THE BODY*, 1.95. Alexander Lowen is the developer of bioenergetic theory as we know it today. In this book he argues that the schizoid personality is the dominant one in America and is manifested by a split between our feelings and our actions. Here he traces this assertion through many case studies and demonstrates how we can reclaim our bodies and our lives through bioenergetics. 275pp. McM 67

LOWEN, ALEXANDER. *BIOENERGETICS*, 2.50. This is the definitive book on bioenergetic therapy. Lowen presents a full explanation of the principles and techniques and a historical review of their development from the work of Wilhelm Reich. Those involved in bioenergetics believe that "You are your body," and how your body functions energetically determines what you feel, think, and do. Disturbances in the body's vital energetic processes affect both mental and physical health. Dr. Lowen explains why so many people lack energy, pointing out how chronic muscular tensions restrict breathing, limit movement, and reduce a person's effectiveness in dealing with life. The bioenergetic approach leads to an understanding of these tensions as the direct result of the suppression of feeling and their release through direct body work. In addition, Dr. Lowen analyzes a number of common physical disorders such as headaches and lower back pain and shows how they can be overcome by unlocking the muscular tensions that create them. This account is more clearly written than Lowen's earlier work and is illustrated with line drawings of bioenergetic exercises. Index, 352pp. Vik 75

LOWEN, ALEXANDER. *DEPRESSION AND THE BODY*, 2.50. Discusses how we can overcome depression by activating dormant life forces and by training mind and body to respond to each other. 318pp. Vik 74

LOWEN, ALEXANDER. *LANGUAGE OF THE BODY,* 2.95. This is Lowen's first book, originally published as **The Physical Dynamics of Character Structure.** Contains a critique of conventional analysis, followed by extended discussion of various character types such as oral, masochistic, hysterical, phallic, narcissistic, etc. 404pp. McM 58

LOWEN, ALEXANDER. *LOVE AND ORGASM,* 1.95. Explores the physical and psychic effects of orgasm and argues that full orgiastic release is only possible in mature heterosexual love. 319pp. McM 65

LOWEN, ALEXANDER. *PLEASURE,* 1.95. Defining pleasure as a *bodily experience,* Dr. Lowen states that *there is no such thing as pure mental pleasure* and points out that *the capacity for pleasure is also the capacity for creative self-expression.* In most adults, however, the struggle for power competes with the striving for pleasure, undermines creativity, and causes muscular tensions. This book describes a way out of this dilemma through a series of bioenergetic exercises. 251pp. Vik 70

LOWEN, ALEXANDER. *THE WAY TO VIBRANT HEALTH,* 4.95. This is Dr. Lowen's most practical book. Step-by-step illustrations and photographs outline many of the major bioenergetic exercises. A great deal of additional material is also included. This is an essential book for all who are interested in learning about bioenergetics. 176pp. H&R 77

ROSENBERG, JACK. *TOTAL ORGASM,* 3.95. *This book is not a sex manual. . . .I have drawn into it elements from Gestalt awareness training, dance and movement therapies, . . .basic body therapies such as that of Wilhelm Reich and bioenergetic therapy, the struc-*

tural patterning concepts of Ida Rolf and Moshe Feldenkrais, some asanas from hatha yoga, plus my personal experience and experimentation as a therapist. This is a large illustrated volume with exercises which teach the practitioner to use his breathing and certain movements to build energy in the body. 214pp. RaH 73

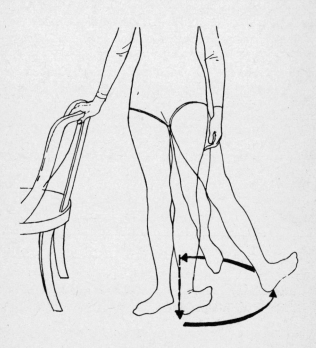

BRISTOW, ROBERT. *ACHES AND PAINS: HOW THE OLDER PERSON CAN FIND RELIEF USING HEAT, MASSAGE, AND EXERCISE,* c8.95. A collection of simple exercises and self-massage techniques for the middle aged and elderly. Each part of the body is discussed individually, and information is included on the ailments most common to that area. The exercises are simple and are concisely presented. Photographs and line drawings throughout. It's not a great book, but we don't know of any other ones that cover the same material. 7¼"x10¼", 123pp. RaH 74

BROOKS, CHARLES. *SENSORY AWARENESS,* c12.95. The term *sensory awareness* was first coined by Charlotte Selver as a name for the work she has been actively developing in the U.S. since 1938. Here Charles Brooks, her husband and collaborator, presents us with a written equivalent of her workshops and an understanding of her lifework—which is not a technique but a practice based on distinguishing what is natural from what is conditioned. The workshops themselves evolve around the close study of the simplest aspects of our functioning—sitting, standing, lying, breathing—and are concerned with breaking down the barriers that have come between our consciousness and the world around us, so that these barriers have a chance of dissolving, thus opening the way to a clearer perception of ourselves as whole beings and to a more authentic sense of the nature of our experience. Many illustrations, 265pp. Vik 74

DA LIU. *TAOIST HEALTH EXERCISE BOOK,* 3.95. See the Oriental Medicine section.

Dance

Dance, dance wherever you may be, I am the Lord of the dance, said he. . . . is the refrain of a popular religious folk song about Jesus. What dance is he speaking of? What do we mean by "the dance"? Let's begin with a flower. . . .

The life of a flower begins with a seed that has fallen to the ground. It cracks open and then there is the slow sending out of roots, downward, sideways, and a stem upward. It forms buds and bursts open into fullness. The petals close in the rain, reopen and turn toward the sun and finally drop to the earth when their time is over. New shapes are disclosed for us by those that remain when the autumn winds blow away the summer coverings. Let me isolate some of the movements for you—a falling, a holding, an opening, a long, slow stretching and reaching horizontally and vertically with many bends, a smallness that is closed and contained, a burst and release, an unfolding and a dropping—and many more.

All of life is in motion from the tiniest atom converging toward another atom to the thoughts of our minds and movements of our spirit. The human being, like the flower, but infinitely more meaningfully, also stretches, reaches out, closes in, bursts into multitudinous activities, rests, falls down, and rises again.

Dance is the celebration of all this movement and therefore of all life. In a unique way we can discover through dance deep insights into who we are in ourselves, and our relationship to others because our whole person is awakened and charged with life—body, soul and spirit. Dance is like a hand that plunges into muddy water, stirring it and scooping it upward into a fine spray under the sun, revealing all its particles and imparting new life.

Dance makes visible the invisible movements of the spirit.
—from **Learning Through Dance** by Carla DeSola

DE SOLA, CARLA. *LEARNING THROUGH DANCE*, 7.95. *This book is written for. . .teachers who want to explore with their students the depths of energy and communication, freedom and understanding, to be released in each one of us through the dance. This is for the teacher who senses, if only in a dim way, how fundamental dance is to the human spirit and who wants assistance for tapping this energy in order to help unify the bodies, minds, and spirits of her students.* The dances are organized according to themes and step-by-step directions are provided along with photographic illustrations of the movements. Oversize, 244pp. Pau 74

HOWARD, BLANCHE. *DANCE OF THE SELF,* c8.95. **Dance of the Self** is the only book we know of that expresses the heart of modern dance—and yet is geared to the non-professional. It opens by reawakening the senses to the concept of man as a primal being composed of earth, fire, water, and air, and it reorients the body in space as a completely interrelated network of energy lines and centers of force. This awareness of the body provides the groundwork for the experience of natural, rhythmic movement. Preliminary exercises concentrate on specific muscle toning and body strengthening, with breathing exercises, stretches, etc., and the fifty-three lesson plans that follow integrate these in harmonious, unrestricted expressions. Many line drawings illustrate the text. Oversize, 157pp. S&S 74

MORRIS, MARGARET. *CREATION IN DANCE AND LIFE,* c7.35. As a pioneer of modern dance techniques, Margaret Morris is comparable to Isadora Duncan and Martha Graham. In this book she describes, with many diagrams and photographs, her choreographical and teaching methods as well as many ways of group improvisation. Ms. Morris is also a trained physiotherapist and has taught eurhythmics and dance movement to the physically handicapped. This volume also includes her therapeutic techniques for the aged and disabled. 125pp. Owe 75

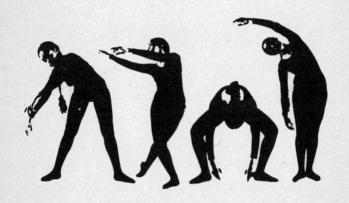

RAFFE, MARJORIE, C. HARWOOD and M. LUNDGREN. *EURYTHMY AND THE IMPULSE OF DANCE,* 2.25. This booklet contains reproductions of the complete series of thirty-five drawings for eurhythmy arising from the collaboration of Rudolf Steiner and Edith Marion. They are preceded by an introduction to eurhythmy, and by a study of the search for renewal of the arts of movement and dance. 63pp. RSP 74

SCHOOP, TRUDI. *WON'T YOU JOIN THE DANCE?* c9.95. Realizing that body image—posture, gesture, movement—is as important to a person's recognition of self as his mental image, Trudi Schoop uses dance as one method of bringing people suffering from schizophrenia back to this world. This book is her personal presentation of the philosophical framework for and practical applications of dance as a healing art. As a basic foundation of her approach, Ms. Schoop believes that schizophrenics should not be viewed as psychiatric cases, but as foreigners who communicate in another language. The challenge to the therapist is to penetrate their customs and to see and feel the world as they do. This book begins with a biographical account of how the author came to be a dance therapist. Following this is a series of practical hints for working with patients and a number of case studies. Illustrations, 216+pp. MPC 74

WOSIEN, MARIE-GABRIELLE. *SACRED DANCE,* 4.95. Creation is movement, and the sacred dance arises from the need to identify with the eternal round of the creative forces in the cosmos. Dancing intensifies awareness, so that the dancer begins to understand how the universe is made up of infinite patterns of motion around a still center. A primordial element of religious tradition all over the world, the dance was a vital part of early Christian worship, and survives in the whirling, orbiting movements of the dervishes of Turkey. In images ranging from Botticelli's dancing angels to the dance patterns of the South Seas, this book evokes one of man's oldest and profoundest impulses—to act out the movements of the powers he senses within himself and within the world. An illuminating introductory text is followed by 142 illustrations, thirty in full color—all described at length. Part of Avon's excellent Art and Cosmos series. Avo 74

DYCHTWALD, KEN. *BODYMIND,* c8.95. Each part of the body relates to the mind in patterns that most of us are unaware of. In this book Dr. Dychtwald, a humanistic psychotherapist, describes how our body reflects our life history and our present state of being. He explores the ways we use the body in our attempts to solve our personal conflicts, thereby creating tensions that disrupt the flow of energy. The book incorporates many eastern and western approaches and offers a variety of therapeutic possibilities and a practical body-mind diagnosis system. Bibliography, index, 320pp. RaH 77

ESHKOL, NOA. *THE HAND BOOK,* 10.75. An in depth study of the detailed notation of hand and finger movements and forms which derives from Ms. Eshkol's study of the sign language of the deaf. The number of active joints in the hands is as great as that of all the rest of the main joints of the body (excluding the separate vertebrae) and an almost infinite number of movements can be expressed and recorded. This presentation is based on the Eshkol-Wachmann Movement Notation system. 9¾"x12¼", 141pp. MNS 71

ESHKOL, NOA. *TWENTY-FIVE LESSONS BY DR. MOSHE FELDENKRAIS,* 16.80. Notated transcriptions of a series of lessons given by Dr. Feldenkrais at the School of Movement, Tel Aviv University. Both the text and the notations have been completely rewritten for this second edition of **Twenty-Five Lessons.** A great deal of explanatory material is included along with the notations. 9½"x11¾", 171pp. MNS 76

ESHKOL, NOA and ABRAHAM WACHMANN. *MOVEMENT NOTATION,* c11.40. This textbook was the first public introduction to the Movement Notation system. The concepts upon which the system is based are explained in detail, and many examples are offered. Movement Notation expresses the spatial relation between the parts of the body in the form of a system of articulated axes. It is possible to write in the notation every visually discernible movement of the human body. This is a technical system which will be of interest only to those who are deeply interested in the physiology of human movement. The authors claim and have theoretically and practically demonstrated that Movement Notation is capable of illustrating any movement sequence or combination of which the human body is capable. 212pp. Wdf 58

FELDENKRAIS, MOSHE. *AWARENESS THROUGH MOVEMENT,* **c6.95. Moshe Feldenkrais is without question one of the most important individuals in the field of body work today. His often revolutionary techniques have helped thousands rethink their relationship with their physical environment. He teaches practical exercises for posture, eyes, and imagination which enable individuals to build better body habits and invoke new dimensions of awareness and self-consciousness. This book is mainly devoted to a presentation of specific exercises and it is illustrated with photographs throughout. We recommend Feldenkrais' work highly. 171pp. H&R 72**

FELDENKRAIS, MOSHE. *BODY AND MATURE BEHAVIOR,* 3.45. An important, technical book, advancing the thesis that study and re-education of muscular behavior patterns are important in understanding and treating emotional problems. The whole self, diet, breathing, sex, muscular and postural habits must be tackled directly and concurrently with emotional re-education, Feldenkrais believes. 167pp. Int 49

FISHER, SEYMOUR. *BODY CONSCIOUSNESS,* 2.45. A scholarly account which probes the way we go about making psychological sense of our bodies. Fisher provides insights into the role body feelings play in the development of our personalities, giving numerous examples, and offering practical suggestions. 176pp. PrH 73

FLUGELMAN, ANDREW, ed. *THE NEW GAMES BOOK,* 4.95. *By all means let us cherish the traditional sports for their many beauties, their unplumbed potential, and for the certainty they afford. But we have signed no long-term contract to suffer their extremes. The time has come to move on, to create new games with new rules more in tune with the times, games in which there are no spectators and no second-string players, games for a whole family and a whole day, games in which aggression fades into laughter.* — George Leonard. This book presents sixty new games, descriptively illustrated with over 250 photographs and extensive commentary. 8¼"x9¼", 193pp. Dou 76

GALLWEY, W. TIMOTHY. *THE INNER GAME OF TENNIS,* c7.95. *It is the thesis of this book that neither mastery nor satisfaction can be found in the playing of any game without giving some attention to the. . .skills of the inner game. . . .The player of the inner game comes to value the art of relaxed concentration above all other skills. . . .He aims at the kind of spontaneous performance which occurs only when the mind is calm and seems at one with the body, which finds its own surprising ways to surpass its own limits again and again. Moreover, while overcoming the common hang-ups of competition, the player of the inner game uncovers a will to win which unlocks all his energy and which is never discouraged by losing. . . .All that is needed is to* un *learn those habits which interfere. . .and then to just* **let it happen.** *To explore the limitless potential within the human body is the quest of the Inner Game; in this book it will be explored through the medium of tennis.* —from the introduction. Gallwey has taught the techniques and ideas he describes in this book and the response has been overwhelmingly good. It's a very popular book and people who buy one often seem to come back for additional copies to give to friends. We haven't read it all, but as tennis aficionados, what we have read sounds like excellent advice both from a spiritual and a technical viewpoint. Oversize, 141pp. RaH 74

GALLWEY, W. TIMOTHY. *INNER TENNIS,* c8.95. Inner tennis is based on the concept that the key to winning tennis lies in every player's head—in his or her ability to concentrate, to trust his body to do what comes naturally, and to let his game just happen. In this book Gallwey presents tested exercises and techniques which are designed to help a player increase her awareness of her body, to concentrate on her muscles, her physical reactions, to improve her relationship to the ball and racket, and much else. Many prefer this book to Gallwey's earlier one, feeling that it contains both deeper insights and more practical information. And many others feel that the two complement each other exceedingly well. The same material is not repeated. 192pp. RaH 76

GLUCK, JAY. *ZEN COMBAT,* 1.75. This is a general book for the beginning student reviewing many of the Japanese arts including karate, aikido, kendo, kongo and jitte, and kyudo. It is illustrated with many small drawings. The most interesting part of the book is the anecdotes about the arts and the masters who developed them. The latter material forms the major part of the book. Bibliography, 218pp. RaH 62

GUNTHER, BERNARD. *SENSE RELAXATION-BELOW YOUR MIND,* 4.95. Techniques developed and used at Esalen which enable you to "turn-on" to your senses—to enhance direct sensory reality in the here and now. These are joyful experiences to have alone, with a lover, or with a group. Beautiful photographs. 8½"x11", 191pp. McM 68

ICHAZO, OSCAR. *PSYCHOCALISTHENICS,* 3.95. Presents a sequence of well tested exercises of the rapid and simultaneous development of mind, body, and spirit. These exercises have been used and refined over the years by thousands of students in the Arica schools. Photographs, 8½"x11". S&S 76

JOHNSON, DON. *THE PROTEAN BODY: A ROLFER'S VIEW OF HUMAN FLEXIBILITY,* 5.95. *This book is based on the assumption that most people experience their bodies as opaque, solid masses that, except for deterioration due to age and accident, are by and large fixed. . . .The body is flexible, a fluid energy field that is in a process of change from the moment of conception until the* *moment of death. The flesh is not a solid dense mass; it is filled with life, consciousness, and energy. . . .A general goal of the first seven sessions of Rolfing is to modify your present body structure: to remove old stress patterns, old postures, old ways of bodily relating to the world.*—Don Johnson. This is a philosophical examination of both the Rolfing experience and the rationale behind it. Illustrated with photographs and anatomical drawings. 8"x8", 154pp. H&R 77

JOHNSON, TOM and TIM MILLER. *THE SAUNA BOOK,* 7.95. This is a beautifully produced volume—everything you want to know about saunas and more! The authors begin with an essay on how to take a sauna and follow with chapters on the sauna tradition and saunas and your body. The final chapters outline construction techniques and discuss all the available factory saunas. Sources are also offered. Delicate line drawings and photographs accompany the text. Index, 8½"x11", 205pp. H&R 77

Karate

In our physical movements, there are those that are natural and others that are not. Through the practice of Karate-do, we can learn to differentiate between the two and also learn to acquire natural movements. We also learn of the power that nature endowed us with and how to use it, for a man has a great deal of hidden power of which he is not aware. . . .He who would follow the way of true karate must seek not only to coexist with his opponent but to achieve unity with him. There is no question of homicide, nor should emphasis ever be placed on winning. When practicing Karate-do, what is important is to be one with your partner, move together, and make progress together. . . .The differences between the karate of today and that of former times extend even to warming-up exercises, for if the way of thinking changes, everything will change. Stress is now placed on suppleness of both mind and body. For those of us who began the practice of karate long ago, the result of making our bodies rigid was to become muscle-bound, and our power was dispersed to many parts of our bodies. The present concept is that the body be relaxed, supple and strong, and the power concentrated in one point. Furthermore, the mind should be clear, that is, without thoughts, and all movements should be made in a natural way. Without a clear, supple mind, the body cannot be supple.—from **The Way of Karate: Beyond Technique** by Shigeru Egami

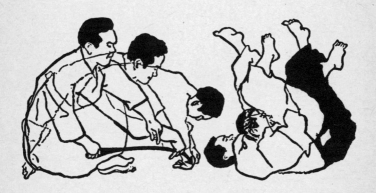

EGAMI, SHIGERU. *THE WAY OF KARATE: BEYOND TECHNIQUE,* c12.95. The martial arts of the East have always been concerned with the development of man's spiritual as well as physical nature. Karate is no different from the other martial arts in this respect. This is the only karate book that we know of that delves deeply into the spiritual aspects of the art. From the method presented here the beginner can learn the basic skills and also develop the discipline that checks the misuse of such skills. The book is oversize and is fully illustrated throughout. Shigeru Egami is president and chief instructor of the Shoto-kan of the Japan Karate-do Shoto-kai. 127pp. Kod 76

HAINES, BRUCE. *KARATE'S HISTORY AND TRADITIONS,* c5.95. In this referenced book, written expressly to counteract the Western trend toward misinformation about Asian martial arts, Haines offers the benefits of his thorough knowledge of Asian history, the origin of karate, and its close connection with Zen Buddhism. 192pp. Tut 68

URBAN, PETER. *THE KARATE DOJO: TRADITIONS AND TALES OF A MARTIAL ART,* c5.95. Discusses in detail the dojo, or school, where karate is taught, with vivid stories from karate's rich history. Tut 67

KIPNIS, CLAUDE. *THE MIME BOOK,* c12.50/6.95. Claude Kipnis has been performing and teaching mime all over the world since 1960. Presently he heads the mime section of the American Academy for Dramatic Arts in New York City. This is a very functional book, specifically concerned with the mechanisms and techniques of mime. The exercises and background material presented here can be very useful to all interested in bodywork. The illustrations are excellent and the material is clearly written. The edge of this oversized book is constructed like a flip-book, so that as you flip its pages, you will see a series of exercises performed. Kipnis defines mime as . . .*the art of recreating the world by moving and positioning the human body* and says that *Left to himself, with nothing and nobody around him, the mime acts in such a way that his audience not only understands but actually sees the world of objects and beings created before him.* This is an excellent presentation, and a beautiful artistic creation. Glossary, 226pp. H&R 74

LEONARD, GEORGE. *THE ULTIMATE ATHLETE,* 2.25. *The athlete that dwells in each of us is more than an abstract ideal. It is a living presence that can change the way we feel and live. Searching for our inner athlete may lead us into sports and regular exercise and thus to the health promised by physical fitness organizations— and that might be justification enough. But what I have in mind goes beyond fitness. It involves entering the realm of music and poetry, of the turning of the planets, of the understanding of death.* Leonard explores all aspects of games and sports—mythology, history, and evolution—as he delves into the true meaning (as he sees it) of athletics: the potentialities of the human body to transcend itself in reaching for the goal of the spirit. Along the way he describes some new games, designed to develop the energy body. An unusual account. Index, 283pp. Avo 75

LERNER, IRA. *DIARY OF THE WAY,* 6.95. A beautifully photographed exploration of the lives and beliefs of three modern masters of aikido, chi kung, and tai chi chuan: Yukiso Yamamoto, Lily Siou, and Andrew Lum. 8½"x10½", 158pp. A&W 76

LUK, CHARLES. *THE SECRETS OF CHINESE MEDICINE,* 3.95. The texts translated here and Luk's commentary provide an excellent survey of the philosophical underpinnings of the Chinese martial arts and especially of tai chi chuan. The emphasis in these texts is on the practice of Chinese meditation and Ch'an, Mahayana, and Taoist techniques are included. Two chapters are devoted to Taoist yoga. Glossary, 231pp. Wei 64

LUK, CHARLES. *TAOIST YOGA,* 2.95. Translations of a comprehensive course of Taoist yoga with instructions by ancient patriarchs and masters—a very clear step-by-step presentation for readers to follow Taoist alchemy. Involves techniques similar to kundalini yoga—whereby the body's sexual energy is retained and thereby transmuted into higher consciousness. Luk provides a good explanatory introduction, an extensive glossary, and many diagrams. 199pp. Wei 70

Massage

Massage is for your mate, your family, and your friends. It is for grandmothers and babies, for pets, for those you love and if you are up to it for those you hate. To do massage is physically to help someone, to take care of them. It is for anyone with whom you feel prepared to share an act of physical caring. Contrary to myth, massage is a healing art and not an advanced sexual technique. . . .The core of massage lies in its unique way of communicating without words. In itself this is not unusual; by touching and hugging, for example, we often let those around us know that we like them, or that we sympathize with them, or that we believe their worth. Massage, however, can transpose this kind of message into a new and different key. When receiving a good massage a person usually falls into a mental-physical state difficult to describe. It is like entering a special room until now locked and hidden away; a room the existence of which is likely to be familiar only to those who practice some form of daily meditation. By itself this state is a gift.

However, he who is giving the massage need not stop there. The more he can tune in to his friend's heightened awareness, the more he can convey something of his own inner self and experience as well. . . .In its essence massage is something simple. It makes us more whole, more fully ourselves. Your hands have the power to give this to others. Learn to trust that power and you will quickly find out better than anyone can tell you what massage is all about.
—George Downing, **The Massage Book**.

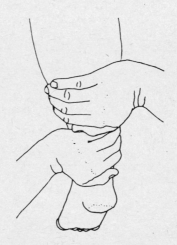

DOWNING, GEORGE. *THE MASSAGE BOOK,* **4.95. This was the first of the massage books and it remains the best one. Downing taught at the Esalen Institute for quite a while and he developed a series of techniques which are well known today. Sensitive line drawings accompany clear step-by-step instructions and a bit of philosophy is interwoven. 8½"x11", 184pp. RaH 72**

DOWNING, GEORGE. *MASSAGE AND MEDITATION,* 1.65. Downing's point of view is that massage and meditation are in key aspects very much alike. In his earlier book he spelled out specific techniques for giving a massage. Here he gives a few general pointers and then quickly moves on to show how massage can have deeper possibilities as a gateway to nonverbal communication between partners and to one's own changing awareness of herself on a bodily level. He first describes a number of short meditative experiments which can be used before, during, or after a massage; next, he presents a number of meditations which one can use to heighten her ability to receive a massage; and finally, he adds a number of meditations which partners can practice together. Illustrations, 85pp. RaH 74

HOFER, JACK. *TOTAL MASSAGE,* 5.95. A step-by-step guide to massage, covering all the basics and clearly illustrated with charcoal drawings. This is certainly an adequate book, but it doesn't have the same high feeling as Downing's book. One nice feature of this book is the author's careful definition of all the terms he uses and his concise explanations. 8½"x11", 223pp. G&D 76

INKELES, GORDON and MURRAY FOOTHORAP. *THE ART OF SENSUAL MASSAGE,* 5.95. Step-by-step instructions with hundreds of beautiful photographs. *There is but one temple in the Universe. . .and that is the human body. Nothing is holier than that form. We touch heaven when we lay our hand on the human body.*—Thomas Carlyle. 161pp. S&S 72

MILLER, ROBERTA. *PSYCHIC MASSAGE,* 3.95. *This book describes a method of healing. It evolved from massage, yet it is more than massage. The addition of psychic awareness makes it possible to heal or balance a person's mind and emotions through his body. Psychic massage cannot be learned by reading. It can only be learned by doing—very much like playing a musical instrument. Therefore, this book is organized in a how to format, so that those who wish may try out the techniques. The primary purpose, however, is to inform rather than to instruct—to present the possibilities and potentialities of a new approach to personal growth.* Illustrated, oversize, 213pp. H&R 75

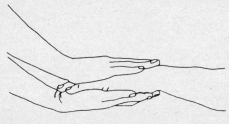

The Mensendieck System

This system was founded by Bess Mensendieck, a sculptor who gave up her career in the early 1900's and became a physician after observing the extreme awkwardness of the bodies of most artist's models. Her desire was to find out exactly what wo/man would have to do to sculpture her own body into a structure s/he could be proud of and which would serve her well. During many years of research she analyzed in detail the individual functions of every bone, joint, and muscle as well as their interactions. She became convinced that the primary exercise anyone needs is the maintenance of correct posture during normal daily activities. Her exercises require little exertion and are suitable even for those suffering from heart ailments. They reflect a deep understanding of anatomy and the mechanics of the body and have been remarkably successful in the treatment of faulty posture and spinal problems. The Mensendieck System has been widely taught in Europe and there is a growing interest in the U.S.

LANGERWERFF, ELLEN and KAREN PERLROTH. *MENSEN-DIECK: YOUR POSTURE AND YOUR PAINS*, c8.95. The authors of this volume are a mother and daughter who have both been certified as Mensendieck specialists and whose combined teaching experience is over forty years. This is a well organized collection of techniques based on the Mensendieck system. The authors begin with exercises which improve posture and basic movements. Next follows a selection of basic techniques which can be applied to everyday activities. A final section offers advanced techniques for selective muscle control and conditioning. Badly drawn, but adequate, line drawings accompany the text. 7¼"x10½", 236pp. Dou 73

MENSENDIECK, BESS. *LOOK BETTER, FEEL BETTER*, c8.95. This is Dr. Mensendieck's own non-technical description of her system. Forty-three movement schemes are outlined and clear explanations tell you which muscles and joints are involved in each movement and the condition each is designed to improve. The instructions are excellent; however, the line drawings accompanying each are not too good. Nonetheless, this is an important book for all who are interested in learning the Mensendieck system. 286pp. H&R 54

MILLER, LOWELL. *META-CALISTHENICS,* 1.75. The author presents a variety of movement techniques designed to produce positive change drawn from Eastern and Western disciplines including Zen and Tibetan Buddhism, yoga, Sufism, Gurdjieff, Arica, and bioenergetics. These all aim at conscious development and Miller has adapted them and added techniques of his own device. A great number are covered and there is little depth to the discussion. Nonetheless we do not know of a similar work which covers so many of these and which gives detailed step-by-step instructions. Unfortunately, there is no apparent organization to the book so the reader has to read through the whole work to find exercises that interest her—although there are general divisions. Also, there are virtually no illustrations. 191pp. S&S 76

MOREHOUSE, LAURENCE and LEONARD GROSS. *TOTAL FITNESS IN 30 MINUTES A WEEK,* 2.95. Dr. Morehouse is a seminal figure in the world of physiology and exercise. He is the author of the standard text on the subject and he is the founding director of the Human Performance Laboratory at UCLA. This book presents his revolutionary techniques to the general public for the first time. The hardcover edition of the book was a best seller and the book is well regarded in all quarters. At the heart of Dr. Morehouse's fitness plan is the concept of effortless exercise which can be incorporated into an individual's daily schedule. The book itself is clearly written and is illustrated with many case studies. 220pp. S&S 75

MUSASHI, MIYAMOTO. *A BOOK OF FIVE RINGS,* 8.95. Born in 1584, Musashi was one of Japan's most renowned warriors. He was a samurai and, by the age of twenty, had fought and won more than sixty contests by killing all of his opponents. Satisfied that he was invincible, Musashi then turned to formulating his philosophy of *the way of the sword,* and it is philosophy which is the heart of this book. **A Book of Five Rings** is also one of the most perceptive psychological guides to strategy ever written, and the philosophy behind it—influenced by Zen, Shinto, and Confucianism—can be

43

applied to many areas of life. This is an extraordinary book which gives the reader a good idea of the ideas which influenced and guided the Japanese civilization for centuries and in which one can often find striking parallels with contemporary Western civilization. This is the first time this classic has appeared in the West, and the book includes many beautiful illustrations. 96pp. OvP 74

NAGAI, HARUKA. *MAKKO-HO: FIVE MINUTES PHYSICAL FITNESS,* 4.50. Presents a complete system of simple exercises which, when practiced over a long period of time, restore and retain physical fitness. The exercises are well illustrated and are quite different from traditional yogic practices. They have been successfully used in Japan for many years. The directions are detailed but quite clear. Practiced correctly, the system does take only five minutes. 83pp. Jap 72

NITOBE, INAZO. *BUSHIDO: THE SOUL OF JAPAN,* c4.95. This neat little volume offers a thoughtful view of the ways and traditions of the Japanese samurai and the intrinsic relationship between the martial virtues of Bushido and the soul of Japan. 203pp. Tut 69

Running

The runner's mind is a drifting stream of consciousness often without formalized thought patterns. The oft-asked question, *why do you run?* is intimately tied to this. When the runner begins to explain his zest for running the explanation is without the essence discovered in the speechless act of the run.

During a run over a number of miles many thoughts pass through the mind. As an individual becomes more fit he spends less time concentrating on the physical activity and has the possibility of transcendence. With optimum fitness altered states of consciousness are possible. The state the mind enters when you are in excellent condition and running freely is similar in some ways to the mental set achieved in meditation.

Heightened awareness in running can be achieved by integrating meditation practices with physical activity. Running thoughts have a certain brilliance from the glow the body enters while running. But environmental distractions and physical fatigue take their toll upon awareness. The quietness achieved in meditation is more serene, but, something of its consciousness can be transferred to the body while running.

What we forget in the haste of the run is that the inner world can be our deliverance. Sometimes a deep joy comes after a long beautiful run which is completed by going inside to affirm the satisfaction. An important realization for me has been that my inner being does not necessarily have to relate to my physical body. Each day can produce a different spirituality as well as physical presence.

The inner world constitutes deliverance for the athlete as well as the person seeking maximum health. By slowing down thoughts the inner journey allows balance, poise, self-understanding; inner world awareness can mean completeness. Physical improvement is only one criteria of personal growth and well-being. Mental awareness and spiritual disciplines are as important in creating a synthesis as are the runner's times.—from **Beyond Jogging: The Innerspaces of Running** by Mike Spino

HENDERSON, JOE. *THE LONG RUN SOLUTION,* 3.95. This is a very personal account of the benefits of running, written in a stream of consciousness vein. The following main topics give a feeling for the material covered: *explaining, addicting, starting, continuing, curing, calming, slowing, breaking, traveling, commuting, waking, seeing, meditating, creating, escaping, talking, testing, training, reflecting, lasting.* The author has been running for over twenty years. 182pp. Wld 76

KOSTRUBALA, THADDEUS. *THE JOY OF RUNNING,* 3.95. The author is a physician who uses running as a central therapeutic technique in his medical practice. In this book he discusses the specific benefits of running and presents a detailed plan. He also includes a variety of exercises to do before running to maximize the benefits and gives suggestions on food and clothing. In addition, Dr. Kostrubala describes the benefits of running and diet for a variety of diseases and includes case studies of his own patients. Bibliography, 159pp. Lip 76

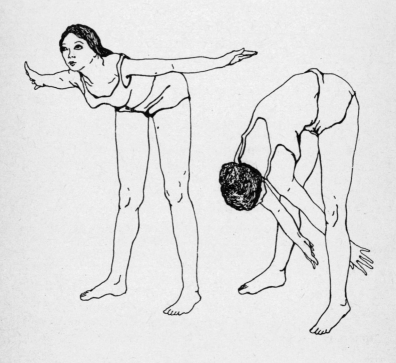

LANCE, KATHRYN. *RUNNING FOR HEALTH AND BEAUTY: A COMPLETE GUIDE FOR WOMEN,* 4.95. Presents a complete program for every level of runner, showing how running can be integrated into everyone's life. Includes tips on getting started, running, women and running, injuries, and much else. Illustrations, index, 207pp. BoM 77

ROHE, FRED. *THE ZEN OF RUNNING,* 3.95. A beautiful photographic study on the joy of running, with poetic hints on what to do and how to be—but always understated and emphasizing the individuality of each being on this planet. What running means to Rohe is clearly stated and what it can mean to anyone else is discussed. 8½"x11". RaH 75

SPINO, MIKE. *BEYOND JOGGING: THE INNERSPACES OF RUNNING,* 3.95/1.25. Mike Spino, physical fitness counselor and director of the Esalen Sports Center in San Francisco, presents individual training programs in this book along with information on his techniques and case studies. *After Mike Spino, running will never be the same. Renouncing the monotonous jog at a single tempo, Spino introduces his students to an imaginative variety of tempos, styles, and visualization techniques that can make running a carnival of delights. His suggestions, ranging from meditation and energy awareness to the methods of Olympic coaches, can benefit beginners and skilled runners alike....* —George Leonard. Illustrations, bibliography, 111pp. CeA 76

ULLYOT, JOAN. *WOMEN'S RUNNING,* 3.95. This is an extremely complete book that tells the reader everything she could possibly want to know about running—and more! Topics covered include training plans, shoes, clothes, diet, physiology, injuries, and treatment. A variety of tables are included. Bibliography, 154pp. Wld 76

RUSH, ANNE KENT. *GETTING CLEAR: BODY WORK FOR WOMEN,* 5.95. An excellent collection of body therapies, verbal therapies, and awareness techniques in use in the Bay Area in California. "This book is written to be experienced and not just read. You can use it by picking sections and subjects interesting to you and trying out some of the exercises. Any of them done over a period of time will become more useful; but even done once, each will have immediate results....I am writing for women because I am a woman and can tell you what tools have been useful to me." Topically arranged, illustrated and highly recommended for all. 8½"x11", 289pp. RaH 73

SIOU, LILY. *CH'I KUNG: THE ART OF MASTERING THE UNSEEN LIFE FORCE,* c14.50. While *Ch'i Kung* is the oldest of the Chinese martial arts, it is not widely practiced today. *Ch'i Kung* calls upon the *Ch'i,* or universal life energy that every person possesses. It directs this energy, stimulates, controls it. In doing so an inner balance is achieved. Primary catalysts of *Ch'i Kung* are slow, disciplined breathing and a series of carefully prescribed movements. Together these set the unseen *Ch'i* force into motion causing it to travel throughout the body providing rejuvenation and relaxation, along with spiritual awareness and well-being. Lily Siou is a master of *Ch'i Kung* and here she gives us a detailed presentation of the philosophy along with step-by-step photographic illustrations of the postures and movements. Oversize, 174pp. Tut 75

SMITH, DAVID. *THE EAST-WEST EXERCISE BOOK,* 7.95. A collection of exercises taken from a wide variety of disciplines, including bioenergetics, yoga, mime, and tai chi. Includes a five-cycle set of exercises and exercises for special problem areas. All of the exercises are illustrated with photographs and include step-by-step instructions. A miscellany of philosophical material is also included. 8½"x11", 221pp. MGH 76

SMITH, ROBERT W. *CHINESE BOXING—MASTERS AND METH-ODS,* c8.95. This is a revealing study of the men and methods Smith encountered in his study and practice of Chinese Boxing. He explores the individual techniques of various masters and in the process describes various types of boxing. Among the men discussed are Hung I-Hsiang, Liao Wu-Ch'ang and Cheng Man-Ch'ing. Includes many illustrations and a glossary, bibliography and notes. 141pp. Kod 74

SMITH, ROBERT W. *HSING-I,* c8.95. Hsing-i is one of the three ancient Chinese internal boxing arts, the other two being tai chi and pa-kua. Like the other two arts, it is essentially moving meditation. Here, for the first time in any Western language, every step is described in detail and fully illustrated with photographs of Hsing-i masters. Smith himself is a well known teacher of the internal arts and he has studied with the leading masters throughout the world. He also includes the advice of masters from Hsing-i's three centuries of scantily recorded history. 112pp. Kod 74

SMITH, ROBERT W. *PA-KUA: CHINESE BOXING FOR FIT-NESS AND SELF-DEFENSE,* c8.95. This is the first book on pa-kua in other than the Chinese language. It offers a complete introduction to the essence of pa-kua circling movements and to the benefits of disciplined study and practice. Using over 400 photographs (many of which show Kuo-Feng-Ch'ih, Smith's teacher in Taiwan) plus many diagrams, Smith demonstrates the flexibility of the self-defense aspects; the accompanying text provides detailed instructions and enlightening insights into the spiritual qualities of this ancient Chinese art. 160pp. Kod 67

SMITH, ROBERT W., ed. *SECRETS OF SHAOLIN TEMPLE BOXING,* c5.95. Shaolin temple boxing is the father of all Chinese boxing forms and the close ancestor of Okinawan and Japanese karate. This is an English presentation of an anonymous Chinese work that Smith found during his study in Taiwan and which he feels presents the fundamental core of shaolin. It is essential reading for those interested in these arts. 71pp. Tut 64

SO, DOSHIN. *SHORINJI KEMPO,* c19.95. Shorinji Kempo is a martial art developed simultaneously with seated Zen meditation by the monks at the temple Shorinji in China in the sixth century. It was taught only to Buddhist priests until recently. Though deeply imbued with the theory of calm in action Shorinji thought maintains that neither of these aspects of the whole can exist independently. This definitive study is written by the present head of the Shorinji and is a thorough introduction which combines detailed photographic explanations of all basic techniques with some of the profound philosophical truths of Shorinji thought. Over 1000 illustrations, 8½"x11", 256pp. Jap 70

SO, DOSHIN. *WHAT IS SHORINJI KEMPO?* 3.95. This is an abridged edition of **Shorinji Kempo,** greatly reduced in size. Many of the techniques are not included and the pictures, being smaller, are much harder to follow. The philosophical explanations are not abridged though. 128pp. Jap 70

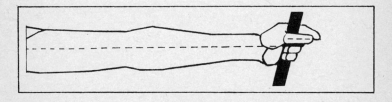

SOLLIER, A. and Z. GYORBIRO. *JAPANESE ARCHERY: ZEN IN ACTION,* c7.00. Archery *(kyudo)* in Japan is more than a sport, it is also a spiritual discipline. The many step-by-step photographs and clear, expert illustrations, and the presentation of *kyudo* terminology in both English and Japanese make the book eminently practical. Includes two introductory chapters, one on Zen and its role in the evolution of judo, karate, and *kyudo,* the other on the development of archery in the West and in the Orient. Glossary, 8½"x11", 94pp. Wea 69

STONE, RANDOLPH. *EASY STRETCHING POSTURES FOR VI-TALITY AND BEAUTY,* 4.00. Dr. Stone suggests a series of squatting exercises based on the natural position of the body during the period of gestation. He feels that these exercises put no special strain on the body and help the energy current flow. Specific directions for each of the twelve exercises are given along with some theoretical material. Illustrations, 52pp. CRC 54

SWEIGARD, LULU. *HUMAN MOVEMENT POTENTIAL,* c14.70. *How does movement proceed, and how can it be performed with greater efficiency? In striving to answer these questions, this book focuses on the interdependence of postural alignment and the performance of movement. It provides an educational method which stresses the inherent capacity of the nervous system to determine the most efficient neuromuscular coordination for each movement. Through this book, I hope to offer my method of teaching body balance and efficient movement—which has been developed during many years of research and training. . . .* This is an incredibly detailed study. Each part of the body is discussed in its own chapter and various specific exercises are offered. The whole work is clearly written and well illustrated. Many anatomical drawings are included. Bibliography, index. H&R 74

Tai Chi Chuan

Centuries old and deeply rooted in the philosophy of Taoism, tai chi chuan is a form of meditation which emphasizes slow movement, relaxation, and calmness of mind. The movements are often circular, and involve a combination of opposites, as, for example, in the shifting of weight that takes place in the change from a solid to an empty step. Wen-Shan Huang describes the movements as *basically slow, continuous, light, gentle, circular, rhythmic, energetic, and graceful. . .capable of developing an intrinsic energy, ready to tune up the body, slow down the aging process, and stretch out the life span of the human being.*

CHENG MAN-CH'ING and ROBERT W. SMITH. *TAI-CHI,* c10.00. Prof. Cheng was a true renowned master of tai chi, an ancient Taoist exercise stressing mind and body relaxation; Robert Smith was a student of Cheng's for thirteen years and is an expert on the martial arts of the Orient. Designed to introduce tai chi for health, sport, and self-defense, this book provides step-by-step directions in Cheng's thirty-seven solo exercise postures with 275 photographs (of Cheng and his associates) and 122 foot weighting diagrams, plus a fold-out diagram of postures. Also contains excellent chapters on Yang Cheng-Fu (Prof. Cheng's teacher), tai chi history, and Tai Chi Ch'uan Classics. This book communicates the philosophy inherent in the practice of this ancient Chinese art. Highly recommended. 112pp. Tut 66

HUANG, AL CHUNG-LIANG. *EMBRACE TIGER, RETURN TO MOUNTAIN—THE ESSENCE OF T'AI CHI,* 3.50. *Huang teaches in a way that is unusual for an Asian master and...for Western masters as well. He begins from the center and not from the fringe. He imparts an understanding of the basic principles of the art before going on to the meticulous details, and he refuses to break down t'ai chi movements into a 1-2-3 drill so as to make the student into a robot.*—from the foreword by Alan Watts. Many illustrations. RPP 73

HUANG, AL and SI CHI KO. *LIVING TAO,* 5.95. *These fleeting moments of my life...have been captured by Ko,...the magician-photographer. We have a book to share with you, glimpses of Tao in practice as a living art....My brush speaks through the dancing cursiveness of Chinese Calligraphy, expressing no-thoughts and be-yond-words....Mostly, I wish to suggest the cyclic balance between meditative stillness and the motions of our vital energy forces.* 8½"x11". CeA 76

HUANG, WEN-SHAN. *FUNDAMENTALS OF TAI CHI CH'UAN,* 12.55. This is essential reading for serious students of tai chi ch'uan. It includes translations of some of the most important classics and is subtitled *An Exposition of its History, Philosophy, Technique, Practice and Application.* Professor Huang is a well known sociologist and has taught at universities in China and the U.S. for many years. The principles of both Chinese philosophy and oriental medicine are incorporated into the text. There is also a section devoted to technical directions for the postures, with photographic illustrations. A fine work in every sense, and a welcome addition to the

51

small number of truly excellent works on the internal arts. Bibliography, index, 569pp. SSk 73

KAUZ, HERMAN. *TAI CHI HANDBOOK,* 3.95. Kauz, a former student of Cheng Men-Ching, has spent most of his life studying the martial arts of the East. With the exception of Prof. Cheng's definitive book on tai chi ch'uan, this is considered by experts to be the best exercise manual. The postures are explained and demonstrated in large clear photographs, and material is included on tai chi as a meditational technique. Includes a section of continuous sequence photographs. Tai chi cannot easily be learned from a book, but the material presented here can be a good introduction for the interested beginner and a good review of techniques and philosophy for the student. 183pp. Dou 74

TANAKA, MINORU, tr. *BUSHIDO: WAY OF THE SAMURAI,* 3.50. This is the first English translation of a Japanese classic, **Hagakure,** which discusses the philosophy of the Samurai. The text is made up of a number of short illustrative stories and aphorisms. 85pp. SnB 75

TODD, MABEL. *THE THINKING BODY,* 8.00. This is an interesting book which combines anatomical line drawings with excellent explanatory material. Ms. Todd orients her study toward an understanding of the fundamental facts underlying the principles of body dynamics. *The basic principles on which the theories are built are discussed at length and these are used to illustrate the final action and control of the body activity, and the influence of unconscious sensations on body control and body action is stressed.*—from the foreword. Bibliography, index, 342pp. DaH 37

WEISS, PAUL. *SPORT: A PHILOSOPHICAL INQUIRY,* 2.95. *The present study makes but a beginning in a new enterprise, the examination of sport in terms of principles which are at once revelatory of the nature of sport and pertinent to other fields—indeed, to the whole of things and knowledge.*—from the preface. This is an interesting inquiry which covers a broad spectrum of sports-related ideas and activities. Bibliography, index, 283pp. SIU 69

Yoga

The name Hatha Yoga goes back to the truth on which this system [Yoga] is founded. Our body is enlivened by positive and negative currents, and when these currents are in complete equilibrium, we enjoy perfect health. In the ancient language of the Orient, the positive current is designated by the letter *Ha* which is equivalent in meaning to *Sun.* The negative current is called *Tha* meaning *Moon.* The word *Yoga* has a double meaning. On the one hand, it is equivalent to *joining* while the second meaning is *yoke.* Thus *Hatha Yoga* signifies the perfect knowledge of the two energies, the positive sun and negative moon energies, their joining in perfect harmony and complete equilibrium, and the ability to control their energies absolutely, that is, to bend them under the yoke of our *Self.*

This system is unique in the entire world, since it consciously perfects the body, compensates for any physical defects, and fills it with glowing life force. Hatha Yoga leads us back to nature, acquaints us with the healing forces dwelling in herbs, trees and roots, teaches us about our own body and the forces acting within it, and leads us to the close harmony of body and soul. The body reacts at the slightest impulses of the mind, and the state of the mind is powerfully influenced by the condition of the body. This reciprocal relationship is utilized by Hatha Yoga, and both mind and body are made healthy. The path to be followed is that of making our body and all its activities conscious. Even the sympathetic nervous system and all those organs whose functioning is usually independent of my consciousness can be made subservient to my will. The incalculable advantage of this is that any malfunctioning can be prevented, and the body can be saved from diseases which originate in functional causes. For example, I can control the activity of my heart and prevent it from palpitations resulting from an external stimulus like fright, bad news, or sudden joy. Thus I can protect my heart from dilation, degeneration of the cardiac muscle, or other diseases. Or if I can control the secretions of my glandular system, I can govern the functions of almost all the organs of my body and thus govern my physical condition.—Selvarajan Yesudian and Elisabeth Haich, **Yoga and Health.**

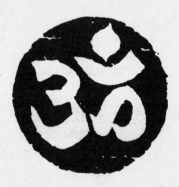

ACHARYA, PUNDIT. *BREATH, SLEEP, THE HEART, AND LIFE,* 3.95. This is a compilation of four books by Pundit Acharya, originally published in the 1950's: **You Haven't Slept, This Precious Heart, Internal Respiration,** and **Breath Is Life.** The presentation is a combination of practical exercises, Acharya's philosophy of life, and examples and analogies showing the human condition. 189pp. DHP 75

BEHANAN, KOVOOR. *YOGA, A SCIENTIFIC EVALUATION,* 3.00. This is a scientific, but nontechnical study of the physiological and philosophical aspects of yoga, written under the auspices of the Institute of Human Relations, Yale University. Dr. Behanan clearly explains and evaluates fundamental concepts of Hindu thought and relates these ideas to familiar Western philosophical conceptions. This is the best book of its type available. Glossary, 281pp. Dov 37

BERNARD, THEOS. *HATHA YOGA,* 3.50. A good philosophical discussion of various aspects of yoga: asanas, purification, pranayama (breathing), mudras (gestures), and samadhi. The text is extensively annotated and is accompanied by photographs of many of the asanas (postures) and a bibliography. 104pp. Wei nd

BRENA, STEVEN. *YOGA AND MEDICINE,* 2.45. This book contends that the average human has far too little control over his own mental and physical health. With this in mind, Dr. Brena, an American physician, reviews both the medical and the yogic concepts of anatomy, physiology, nutrition, respiration, sexual activity, pathology and pain. In each case, he makes a comparative analysis, stressing the many similarities as well as the fundamental differences. Illustrations, notes, 179pp. Pen 72

CARR, RACHEL. *BE A FROG, A BIRD, OR A TREE,* c5.95. Subtitled *Creative Yoga Exercises for Children,* this is a delightful addition to the proliferating books on yoga. The thirty exercises presented here are different from traditional yogic poses. Ms. Carr has made use of every child's most creative tool—his or her imagination—in developing the techniques. The children pretended to be a jumping frog, a shooting arrow, a sturdy tree growing in the forest, and much else. The instructions for each exercise are written in the form of children's verse, the model pictured is a child, and the print is large enough for the child to read it him/herself. There's also a section of background notes for parents or teachers. Oversize, 96pp. Dou 73

CARR, RACHEL. *YOGA FOR ALL AGES,* 3.95. Rachel Carr has devised a six stage yoga course which she feels should enable everyone to enjoy the benefits of yoga with less than thirty minutes of practice a day. Progressing from simple movements to the more complex in stages, these exercises aim at physical conditioning, easing of tensions, and the promotion of physical, mental, and emotional well-being. Very clear instructions, well illustrated with photographs. Index, oversize, 160pp. S&S 72

CARR, RACHEL. *THE YOGA WAY TO RELEASE TENSION,* 2.25. Subtitled *Rachel Carr's Techniques for Relaxation and Mind Control,* this is a combination of a variety of exercises illustrated with line drawings. Included is information on breathing and on muscles and how they work along with exercises for different parts of the body and exercises to increase stamina and muscular action. 147pp. H&R 74

CHRISTENSEN, ALICE and DAVID RANKIN. *"EASY DOES IT"–YOGA FOR PEOPLE OVER 60,* 3.50. This is an excellent manual, based on the authors' extensive work with older people. An elderly woman is the model for the illustrations and they are presented in a step-by-step format. There's also a fair amount of background and introductory material as well as a series of cautions and hints. Included also are breathing exercises and instructions and meditation instruction. A six-week daily routine is also presented. Spiral bound, 8½"x11", 56pp. Sar 76

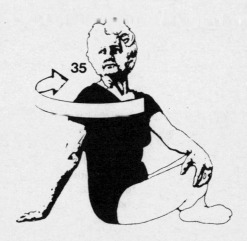

CHRISTENSEN, ALICE and **DAVID RANKIN**. *THE LIGHT OF YOGA BEGINNER'S MANUAL,* 2.95. This oversize manual is especially designed to visually illustrate and clearly explain yoga for beginners. The spiral binding allows the manual to remain flat on the floor, and the student therefore can easily refer to it while doing the exercises. Each pose is illustrated (drawn) step-by-step and the presentation is the clearest we have seen. The descriptive and philosophical material is also good. Highly recommended as an instruction book. 61pp. S&S 73

CRISP, TONY. *YOGA AND CHILDBIRTH,* 1.75. See the Natural Childbirth section.

DECHANET, J.M. *YOGA IN 10 LESSONS,* 1.95. An introductory book for those who do not wish to be overburdened with yogic theory and simply desire instruction in the postures. Each lesson begins with a section on the necessary theory and is followed with clear instructions for the exercises. Fifty-two exercises are described, along with information on the therapeutic effects and the attendant dangers, if any. 174pp. S&S nd

DEVI, INDRA. *FOREVER YOUNG FOREVER HEALTHY,* 1.50. "This book is not intended as a treatise, but as a practical guide to a better, healthier and longer life. It will tell you how to breathe correctly; how and what to eat; how to relax and exercise your body and mind. . . ."–Indra Devi. Ms. Devi spent twelve years in India studying and has taught the techniques all over the U.S. to many prominent personalities. Topics include breathing, relaxation, correct posture, fasting, insomnia, headaches, arthritis, asthma, and much else. Her books are very well written and clear, with many anecdotes and illustrations of the postures. Recommended as a good general introduction to the practicalities. Bibliography, 171pp. Arc 53

DEVI, INDRA. *RENEW YOUR LIFE THROUGH YOGA,* 1.50. A good presentation of yogic and non-yogic relaxation techniques. Includes philosophical material on tension, a long discussion of the art of relaxation with practical suggestions; the science of breathing; yoga postures illustrated for relieving tensions and inducing relaxation; a section on the essence of yoga, and an excellent discussion of nutrition and diet. 256pp. War

DEVI, INDRA. *YOGA FOR AMERICANS,* 1.50. A complete, six week course in hatha yoga with diets, recipes, exercises, and special guides for overweight, arthritis and asthmatics. Profusely illustrated. NAL

DISKIN, EVE. *YOGA FOR CHILDREN,* 4.95. A graded, illustrated guide. The book is attractively designed and the instructional material is clear. In addition, there is a series of hints for parents and teachers. We like Rachel Carr's book better, but this volume contains more exercises, and different ones than Carr's. Index, oversize, 206pp. War 76

DUNNE, DESMOND. *YOGA MADE EASY,* 1.35. This general introductory survey begins with basic information of the theory of yoga and on its physiological benefits. The bulk of the book is devoted to a discussion of yogic practice and is divided into chapters on pranayama, deep relaxation, concentration, meditation, and asanas. Diet suggestions are also offered. This is not a textbook, as each chapter is far too short to fully explain anything. Nonetheless, it presents an adequate overview. Dunne runs a yoga school in Great Britain. Index, 190pp. May 61

GARDE, R.K. *PRINCIPLES AND PRACTICE OF YOGA THER-APY*, 5.00. Dr. Garde is an Indian physician. In this book he clearly shows which diseases can be helped by yoga asanas in conjunction with the help of other yoga adjuncts such as correct breathing. He also includes information on homeopathy and the cell salts, massage, music, the correct diet, and even prayers. This is a very detailed, illustrated account. Excellent glossary. 132pp. Tar nd

GOSWAMI, SHYAM SUNDAR. *HATHA-YOGA*, c12.00. Special features in this book: (1) both the dynamic and static aspects of each exercise have been explained as well as correct techniques in breathing, (2) exercise plans containing the right combinations to suit different ages, sex, conditions of health, etc., (3) breath control exercises explained in a clear and practical manner. The expositions of the exercises are the most detailed we've ever seen. The tone of the book is oriented toward the health aspects of yoga rather than the philosophy. Includes several exercise plans and diets. It is subtitled *An Advanced Method*, and indeed it is. 221pp. Fow nd

HANEY, ERENE and RUTH RICHARDS. *YOGA FOR CHILD-REN*, c5.95. A hand drawn simple instruction manual which teaches some of the most basic positions. The book is clearly written for children and the language is simple. The illustrations are not the best we have seen, but they are adequate. Sixteen exercises are presented in all. 7¼"x9¼". BoM 73

HITTLEMAN, RICHARD. *BE YOUNG WITH YOGA*, 1.95. Hittleman is quite probably the most prolific writer on yoga in America today. He has had frequent television instruction programs and he is very well known. His emphasis is on yoga as a form of exercise, rather than on the spiritual benefits, although he does get into the philosophy somewhat. He presents his material clearly and writes well. Many thousands have used his books as their introduction to yogic practices and exercises. This book presents a seven week program of exercises along with a series of exercises for special ailments. The instructions are very complete and a variety of special hints are also offered. Photographs illustrate the text. Index, 239pp. War 62

HITTLEMAN, RICHARD. *GUIDE TO YOGA MEDITATION*, 1.50. The largest section deals with the essence of yoga philosophy and meditation. It includes various meditational exercises, many illustrated with photographs and diagrams. A smaller section illustrates various yoga asanas. Very clearly written. A good book for the beginning student who wants practical information. 192pp. Ban 69

HITTLEMAN, RICHARD. *INTRODUCTION TO YOGA*, 1.75. A general presentation, with some basic postures and philosophy along with diet suggestions. 192pp. Ban 69

HITTLEMAN, RICHARD. *WEIGHT CONTROL THROUGH YOGA*, 1.50. 108pp. Ban 71

HITTLEMAN, RICHARD. *YOGA: THE EIGHT STEPS TO HEALTH AND PEACE*, 2.25. Hittleman's newest and most in depth book on yogic philosophy and practice. He surveys the different types of yoga and discusses how the techniques of the six major systems of yoga can be applied. Fully illustrated throughout. 217pp. Ban 75

HITTLEMAN, RICHARD. *YOGA FOR HEALTH*, 2.35/each. These three books present a very simplified series of yogic postures, with instructions and background material. The postures are illustrated with line drawings and various hints are included. Book Three presents information on the principles of nutrition along with sample menus and recipes. Oversize, about 40pp. each. YFH 62

HITTLEMAN, RICHARD. *YOGA FOR LIFE RECORD ALBUMS*, 8.75/each. A somewhat commercial presentation of a yoga program developed by Richard Hittleman, one of the best known popularizers of yoga in the U.S. today. Each album is a two record set. The first set includes a short introduction, suggestions on how to best work with the albums, and the beginning postures. The second set consists of instructions in more advanced postures. The instructions are clear and easy to follow. A book of photographs illustrating the postures is included with each album. YFH

HITTLEMAN, RICHARD. *YOGA FOR PHYSICAL FITNESS*, 1.50. A collection of fifty-eight exercises for various ailments and parts of the body are explained and illustrated with photographs. This book is a good supplement to Hittleman's exercise plans. 255pp. War 67

HITTLEMAN, RICHARD. *YOGA FOR SPECIAL PROBLEMS*, 3.75. An illustrated collection of exercises for weight control, arthritis, tension, loss of muscle tone, poor blood circulation, and respiratory problems. 8½"x11", 49pp. YFH 76

HITTLEMAN, RICHARD. *YOGA PHILOSOPHY AND MEDITA-TION,* 2.35. Here Hittleman attempts to distill the essence of Indian philosophy, especially as it relates to yoga. He does so adequately and manages to cover, albeit briefly, all the essentials. 37pp. YFH 64

HITTLEMAN, RICHARD. *YOGA TWENTY-EIGHT DAY EXER-CISE PLAN,* 4.95/1.95. Presents a detailed four week exercise plan. Very good material for a self-teaching program. Also some philosophy. The $4.95 edition has much larger pictures and text. Recommended as the best step-by-step, day-by-day instruction book. 320pp. WPC 69

HITTLEMAN, RICHARD. *THE YOGA WAY TO FIGURE AND FACIAL BEAUTY,* 1.50. A collection of simple postures to firm and tighten various parts of your body. The text is illustrated with step-by-step photographs which are little more than adequate and detailed instructions. Hittleman also includes diet suggestions and information on natural foods. 205pp. Avo 68

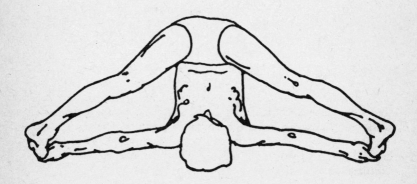

IYENGAR, B.K.S. *LIGHT ON YOGA,* c12.50/4.95. "Probably the most complete Hatha Yoga book."—*Whole Earth Catalog.* 600 pictures and an incredible amount of detailed descriptive text as well as philosophy. The purpose is to describe as simply as possible the asanas (postures) and pranayama (breathing exercises) in the light of our own era, its knowledge and its requirements. Includes detailed primary, intermediate, and advanced asana courses, a table that correlates asanas with the plates that illustrate them, and a detailed glossary. Iyengar's school of yoga is probably the best known in India today and his techniques have been very influential with yoga teachers throughout the world. The $12.50 edition is fully revised and photographs illustrating the exercises appear right next to the descriptions (in the earlier edition the photographs were appended). We highly recommend this book and feel that the revised edition is far superior to the earlier one. 544pp. ScB 77

JOHN, BUBBA FREE. *CONSCIOUS EXERCISE AND THE TRANSCENDENTAL SUN,* 1.95. A compilation from some of Bubba's oral and written instructions. There's some philosophy, but basically the book is a collection of exercises. Included is the famous **Surya Namaskar** (or welcome of the sun). The illustrations are poorly drawn and the reader would find it hard to learn from them. 83pp. DHP 74

KENT, HOWARD. *MY FUN WITH YOGA,* c5.50. A nicely produced, attractively illustrated, collection of simple exercises for young children. The text is written in language designed to appeal to young children and is accompanied by both color drawings and color photographs. The book is a delight to look at and quite a bit of useful philosophical information is included. Children we know love this book. 9¼"x12½", 45pp. Ham 75

KIRSCHNER, M.J. *YOGA FOR HEALTH AND VITALITY,* 4.70. M.J. Kirschner is one of Europe's leading yoga teachers, specializing in yogic exercises for the infirm, the elderly, and those with special problems. In this book he discusses his remedial yoga techniques and carefully explains how to do a variety of specific exercises. The book is illustrated throughout. There are only a few yoga books devoted to healing and this is one of the best we've seen. Index, 175pp. A&U 77

KISS, MICHAELINE. *YOGA FOR YOUNG PEOPLE,* c4.95. Ms. Kiss, the Director of Richard Hittleman's popular Yoga for Health Center in New York, has been teaching yoga for many years. The instructions are detailed and clear and there is information on both going into and coming out of the positions along with a number of practical hints. Only a few postures are introduced, so each is discussed quite thoroughly. However, the book is inadequately illustrated with tiny line drawings that do little more than show what each posture looks like. The book itself does not seem to be partic-

MAJUMDAR, S.K. *INTRODUCTION TO YOGA,* 4.95. "In the following pages, I have tried to give the substance of yoga, its principles and practices, as they have come down to us from an immemorial past. . . .It is my wish to present yoga as a living tradition, not as a system of fixed formulas, to be found in books or schools. Yoga is not a special religion or a particular philosophical doctrine. It is the wisdom of life. It is experience." This is an excellent book, with a long section on principles and perspective; an illustrated practical section; a good chapter on meditation; a selection of quotations from 5000 years of yogic literature; and a glossary. Recommended as an excellent overall introduction. 318pp. UnB nd

MEDVIN, JEANNINE. *PRENATAL YOGA,* 3.50. See the Natural Childbirth section.

MOORE, MARCIA and MARK DOUGLAS. *DIET, SEX AND YOGA,* c6.95. *This book discusses attitudes about the body and presents ways of gaining increased physical control by means of diet, exercise, deep breathing, relaxation, and creative visualization. . . .Essentially, we are talking not only about diet, sex, and yoga, but about your life and what you can do about it.* This is a very clearly written account, fully indexed. 283pp. ArB 66

MOORE, MARCIA and MARK DOUGLAS. *YOGA: SCIENCE OF THE SELF,* c6.95. This is quite a successful attempt at a Westernization of yogic philosophy. Few Sanskrit terms are used, and even these are defined in the glossary. The philosophical material is clearly written and good. Topics include a general discussion of yoga as an ancient wisdom, emphasizing the hatha and raja disciplines; a long section on yoga and psychic development, psychoanalysis, and philosophy; and a presentation of esoteric yoga. There is a section of asanas, but the pictures are inadequate. Good bibliography. 288pp. ArB 67

NARAYANANANDA, SWAMI. *THE SECRETS OF PRANA, PRANAYAMA AND YOGA-ASANAS,* c4.55. A series of practical lessons on pranayama divided into two sections: pranayama for gaining health and happiness and pranayama for higher spiritual attainments. Illustrated with very poor photographs. 118pp. NUY 74

OKI, MASAHIRO. *PRACTICAL YOGA: A PICTORIAL APPROACH,* 4.50. A Zen Buddhist approach to yoga. The first section

ularly oriented to young people, although the instructions are unusually clear. 7¾"x9¼", 89pp. BoM 71

KRIYANANDA, SWAMI. *YOGA POSTURES FOR SELF-AWARENESS,* 2.95. Swami Kriyananda was a direct disciple of Yogananda. He is the founder of Ananda Cooperative Village in California. Stress is placed in this book on the usefulness of yoga postures for spiritual development and for achieving a harmony of mind and soul as well as of body. Many postures are illustrated and discussed and there is additional background material. 85pp. AnP 67

KUVALAYANANDA, SWAMI. *POPULAR YOGA ASANAS,* c7.95. This definitive work explains the yamas, nyamas (mental exercises) and the asanas (physical exercises) from the view of yoga-sastra. Yamas, freely translated, mean inoffensiveness, truthfulness, and continence. Nyamas represent purification, contentment, mortification, study, and complete self-surrender to the Lord. Yoga-sastra holds that the influence of the mind on the body is most important, although asanas have a very definite place in the book. This is an excellent serious study—recommended as the next step after some of the introductory yoga books. Over eighty illustrations, detailed glossary, and many notes. 213pp. Tut 31

KUVALAYANANDA, SWAMI. *PRANAYAMA,* c5.00. A comprehensive, practical text which outlines eight varieties of pranayama advocated by noted hatha yoga teachers through the ages and four varieties taught by Patanjali. The pertinent texts are summarized and many translations are included. Step-by-step instructions for each exercise are also given. Some illustrations, though they are not very good. Glossary, 168pp. PPr 66

LYSEBETH, ANDRE VON. *YOGA SELF TAUGHT,* 2.95. This is the most detailed, comprehensive yoga book we've seen. The photographs show all the intermediate stages of each asana and there is excellent background material for each one including information on the technique, variants, duration, the order in which a series of asanas should follow each other, the method of breathing, how and where to concentrate the mind, the effects of the exercise, and so on. The philosophical chapters are also excellent, and even here much of the material is practical. The whole book is well organized and illustrated and we recommend it highly for both the beginning student and the more advanced one (advanced variations of the postures are also given). 264pp. H&R 68 covers the nature of yoga, health, nourishment, fasting, sex. The latter half gives practical instructions and over 400 step-by-step photographic analyses of yoga poses, corrective exercises, and emotion and breath control. A large, easy to follow book for both the novice and the regular practitioner. 80pp. Jap 71

OKI, MASAHIRO. *YOGA THERAPY,* 5.95. See the Healing section.

PHELAN, NANCY. *A BEGINNER'S GUIDE TO YOGA,* 2.00. An introductory survey. Ms. Phelan describes the principles behind the exercises—both mental and physical—and explains how daily practice can lead to a healthier, more complete life. The postures are fully described, but the photographs are inadequate. 160pp. SBL 73

PHELAN, NANCY and MICHAEL VOLIN. *YOGA FOR WOMEN,* 1.50. Provides a good overview. Presents the philosophy and the practice, with some illustrations—but not enough to learn in any depth. 155pp. H&R 63

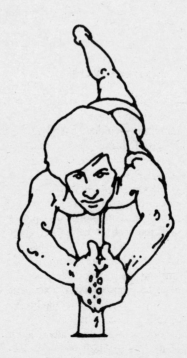

RAMA, SWAMI. _JOINTS AND GLANDS EXERCISES,_ 1.75. A series of exercises, illustrated with line drawings. 46pp. Him 74

SATCHIDANANDA, SWAMI. _INTEGRAL YOGA HATHA,_ 5.95. A pictorial guide to hatha yoga asanas, including bodily postures, deep relaxation methods, breath control, cleansing processes, and systems of mental concentration. The pictures are large and the technical instruction comprehensive. However only the final position is pictured, not the intermediate steps. This book is well regarded. 8½"x11", 189pp. HRW 70

SIMONS, ESTELLE. _YOGA USA A CLASS FOR BEGINNERS,_ 3.98. _It has been my privilege to study Hatha Yoga with many of the finest instructors of our day. . . .Now, in retrospect, I realize that of all these dedicated servers, no one has been of greater personal assistance to me than Estelle Simons. I am, therefore, delighted that this recording will make it possible for students everywhere to hear Estelle's compelling, but also soothing voice and to profit by her supremely competent guidance. I wholeheartedly recommend her system and her unique presentation to all who aspire to tread the path of Yoga to a more vital and wholesome way of life._—Marcia Moore. Photographs of the postures are included. SQN

SIMONS, ESTELLE. _YOGA USA INTERMEDIATE CLASS,_ 3.98. Ms. Simons teaches the following postures: sun pose, shoulder stand, fish, head/knee pose, plough, cobra, locust, bow, moon pose, relaxation pose. Photographs are included. SQN

SIVANANDA, SWAMI. _YOGA PRACTICE,_ c2.40. This book presents a regime of yogic exercises developed especially for Western man. Sivananda describes the method of doing each asana, and explains its effect on the body, the physical defects it can remedy and includes an illustration of each asana. Includes additional practical advice. 64pp. TSC nd

SIVANANDA, SWAMI. _YOGIC HOME EXERCISES,_ 1.50. This is a more detailed presentation of asanas, including the same type of information as in **Yoga Practice,** as well as many pages of theoretical material. Drawings illustrate the text. 101pp. TSC 65

SLATER, WALLACE. _HATHA YOGA,_ 1.25. Presents a very simplified basic course of hatha yoga postures, including meditation and mind control exercises, and advice on personal hygiene and diet. 65pp. TPH nd

STEARN, JESS. *YOGA, YOUTH, AND REINCARNATION,* 1.75. A personal, anecdotal account of Stearn's initiation into yogic practices as a student of Marcia Moore. In the process he discourses on astrology, reincarnation, and diet and health. The appendix details yoga warm-ups, routines, and breathing and this material is illustrated. Glossary, 344pp. Ban 65

THOMPSON, JUDI. *HEALTHY PREGNANCY THE YOGA WAY,* 3.95. See the Natural Childbirth section.

URBANOWSKI, FERRIS. *YOGA FOR NEW PARENTS,* 6.95. See the Natural Childbirth section.

VISHNUDEVANANDA, SWAMI. *COMPLETE ILLUSTRATED BOOK OF YOGA,* c5.95/1.95. All the essential knowledge of the mental science of yoga is contained in this handbook: asanas, breathing exercises, concentration, meditation, diet, and philosophy. Swami Vishnudevananda, teacher of hatha and raja yoga, explains and instructs in clear and direct language the means to the conquest of old age, disease and death through the development and understanding of timeless yogic wisdom. This is one of our most popular yoga books, and we recommend it highly. The $5.95 edition is an especially good value; it has excellent large photographs. 415pp. S&S 60

VOLIN, MICHAEL and NANCY PHELAN. *YOGA OVER FORTY,* 1.75. This book begins with a number of essays under the general rubric of *Yoga and Ageing* which discuss physical and mental conditions common in middle age, diet, and care of the body. The second half of the book is devoted to practical advice and exercises. The instructions for each exercise are fully given along with background information. A series of sketchy line drawings and photographs accompany the text. Index, 158pp. SBL 65

YESUDIAN, SELVARAJAN. *YOGA WEEK BY WEEK,* c6.95. A presentation of fifty-two weeks of exercises which provides a carefully graded, step-by-step course in yoga. The line drawings illustrating the postures could not be worse and the explanations are adequate, but hardly more. Much of the material is discussed at greater length in **Yoga and Health**, so this volume can only be seen as a complement to the earlier one and cannot stand by itself. Inspiring quotations and line drawings of nature scenes are interspersed. 243pp. H&R 75

YESUDIAN, SELVARAJAN and ELISABETH HAICH. *YOGA AND HEALTH,* 1.50. Explains the achievement of physical and mental well being by means of yoga. From a general discussion of principles the authors move on to "practical" hatha yoga, and in this section describe carefully the three essential factors to be combined: control of consciousness, breath control, and physical postures. The text is well illustrated and the exposition is excellent. This is the best work of this type that we've seen. 184pp. H&R 53

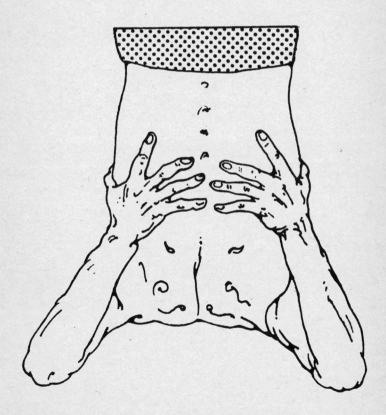

Color & Aura

We cannot live without color. This essence of the life force is all about us. It can make chills run up and down the spine or quicken the soul. If we step into an air-conditioned room which has been painted gray we will undoubtedly complain because it is too cold; yet if the color is orange we will feel most comfortable. Psychologists say that tasks which require muscular effort will be best performed in an environment of warm colors which stimulate and speed up the pulse. If a task involves mental concentration, the calm atmosphere of tranquil blues and green will serve best.

We can separate the color spectrum into two basic groups: the exciting, vibrant red-orange-yellow group; and the passive, calm blue-green group. Individuals who favor the first group are more likely to be extroverts—easily influenced, impressionable and social. There is a great possibility that those who favor the second group will have an attitude of detachment, showing greater interest in themselves than in the world about them. Naturally quiet, they will probably be deliberate and introspective.

Blue is preferred more often by introverts and conservative people, red by extroverts. Yellow is the choice of the intellectual, while well-balanced individuals choose green. Artistic persons usually thrive on purple.

We react to color at an unconscious level and acknowledge color symbolism in the idioms of our language. Some people paint the town red, become entangled in red tape, must read only red-hot news and may turn purple with rage if they can't find a red cent in their pockets.

Color is undoubtedly one of the most dominating influences in our day-to-day existence and yet it is an influence we take very much for granted.

Scientists tell us that we receive all knowledge of the universe through electromagnetic radiation. What we see with the eye alone—visible light—comprises only a very narrow band of that electromagnetic spectrum. There is a dual property to that nature of light: it acts in a pattern of long and short waves and in a particulate or corpuscular form.

Generally, there is a very close relationship between electromagnetic radiation and the atomic structure of matter. The atom is made up of a series of electrons revolving about a central nucleus. Now and then one of these orbiting electrons is released, or there is a radical alteration of the nucleus itself, thereby creating waves of energy. The direction of this electromagnetic radiation, or light, which fills the vacuum of space, is affected by powerful gravitational fields. It is also capable of being bent or refracted.

When visible light—that almost infinitesimal segment of energy waves out of the total spectrum of electromagnetic radiation—is passed through a prism, or is refracted (bent) or is reflected from a grating which has been marked with a series of fine lines, it is spread into rainbow-like colors— a spectrum sequence ranging from short wavelengths to long wavelengths: violet, indigo, blue, green, yellow, orange and red.

This field of energy is all about us. What we perceive as a result of this energy is illusion—only the energy itself is real. Color does not exist in actuality. It is only a sensation in our consciousness. In other words, what we see with our eyes is not the object itself but is a series of various wavelengths of light, traveling at the same rate of speed, being reflected from the object. The object itself is colorless. Some wavelengths are absorbed by the object while others are reflected. The atomic and molecular structure of a yellow object, for instance, is such that it absorbs all wavelengths except yellow, which is reflected to the eye. We are affected by these wavelengths of light, or color, as the vibration is passed on to the brain or to that portion of the cerebral cortex at the back of the head that is known as the striate area.

The only colors recognized as "real" for three centuries have been those that Sir Isaac Newton saw and reported in 1672 when he passed a narrow stream of sunlight through a prism. Since then each of the seven spectral colors he saw, from violet to red, has been assigned to a definite segment of the spectrum, whose wavelength is commonly measured in millimicrons.

Newton identified and called what he saw the seven *homogeneal* colors: violet, indigo, blue, green, yellow, orange and red. Newton went on to show that objects appear to be colored because they absorb certain wavelengths and reflect others, and that it is the reflected rays that reach the eye, indicating shape, form and color. He demonstrated further that there is a complementary color for each color and that the approximation of white light could be achieved through the combination of any two complementary colors. Newton, himself, was unable to produce a pure white, but others who continued to experiment with his theories were able to do so.

By mixing the light from any two colors in his spectrum, Newton was able to produce a color which was intermediate, i.e., yellow, by mixing red and green light; cyan (blue-green) from blue and green light; and purple (a color not thought to be in the spectrum at all) by mixing red and blue light.

Man is not only surrounded with color but also has a love for it. He expresses his emotions through color and has made it an almost commonplace aspect of his life. Whether he realizes it or not, contemporary man has assimilated, with historical consistency, the character and whim of color as it relates to both divine and human meaning, mysticism, the riddles of life and death and the puzzling ways of creation.

There is little, if any, doubt that all living things are affect-ed by visible light and color in one way or another. We all know from simple observation that visible light is necessary for the growth of plant life, and numerous experiments in-dicate that growth is restrained by ultraviolet and infrared wavelengths. Most medical scientists, on the other hand, may not admit that wavelengths or vibrations visible to the human eye have any useful purpose to the human organism other than sight, although they do make use of infrared and ultraviolet radiation in the treatment of certain physiological conditions.

Many theories have been expounded on the subject of color and its use in healing, in personality identification, and in the effective use of color harmony in our wearing apparel and surroundings. As has already been stated, we cannot live without color. It is the essence of the life force all about us. Take away the motion of light or color and we would have no awareness at all of the appearance of matter.

Each atom within the physical body is emitting wavelengths of color and tone constantly. These wavelengths of energy, or color, are in such combinations within each endocrine gland as to set up individual, or unique, vibrations for each. Each of these spiritual centers, however, must vibrate har-moniously with each other if there is to be harmony and health within the total physical, mental and spiritual body. If the vibration at any one center is out of harmony with itself it would be safe to assume that disease or disharmony exists. Consequently, each of the other of the seven glands would have to work harder to compensate for the inhar-monious gland, thereby increasing the possibility of the disruption of total body forces.

To compensate for such possibilities, the Creative Forces give us a continuous source of energy through light. We may think that light and color are given to us purely for beauty but that is not the case. Rather these vibrations are beautiful to us because something within tells us that we need this light in order to be in harmony with ourselves and with others, and so that we may grow and evolve into that which we must.

The pituitary gland transforms the colors of the light rays into revitalizing energies to rebuild those centers that are lacking in energy and to reinforce the energies being created within each gland. For example, an individual whose adrenal gland is disturbed or out of balance will subconsciously reach out for yellow or red. This will be evident in the individual's color preferences, even though the preferred color might be manifested in an impure shade.

To aid in the healing process, the individual should surround himself with pure yellows and reds, whether these colors are pale or strong, in order to supply reinforcing vibrations to the adrenal glands. If the individual applies himself physically, mentally and spiritually through the meditative process to the Creative Forces, healing will be possible.

We must develop a constant awareness that conditions, thoughts and activities are things and that their vibrations, whether color or sound, are felt by others. These vibrations do have an effect upon other entities and things about us.

To be creative we must think about our color schemes in order to put meaning into whatever we do with color. We need to apply our own creative forces in those channels which will give light, life and abundance. If we use the harmony of color, its beauty, in the expression of the soul-self, the spirit may flow through and bring healing influences and helpful forces to others.

Color combinations in clothing may have a greater effect upon others than upon ourselves. In putting together a color combination in wearing apparel, we should consider the emotional impact it will have on those with whom we come in contact. Will it antagonize them? Will it drive them away? Or will it pacify and inspire them? A dominant red will stir things up and may even cause anger; it certainly creates the feeling of energy. Too much bold blue may tell the world that we impose *our* wills. Softer shades of blue pacify and calm troubled minds. Adding a little green can produce healing effects.

Selecting colors for the home follows the same basic pattern, though here larger masses of color are used. In this case, we are creating an atmosphere for ourselves and our families as well as for those we invite into our homes. Yellow may stimulate thought, a touch of orange brings warmth, pale blues cool and calm. We should use our imaginations and follow our intuitions to create the color harmonies we want.

—from **Color and the Edgar Cayce Readings** by Roger Lewis

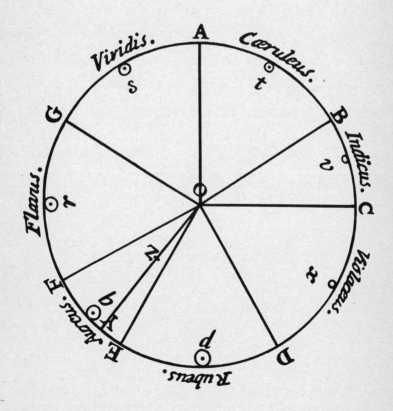

ANDERSON, MARY. *COLOUR HEALING,* 1.50. This is an excellent booklet summarizing many aspects of color healing. Ms. Anderson writes very clearly and incorporates historical, practical, and descriptive material. She includes discussions of the auras, chakras, and subtle bodies, the seven major rays, diagnosis and treatment by color, colors specific to certain diseases, and general material on the scientific background of color research. Recommended for all seeking a general review. 62pp. Wei 75

ANONYMOUS. *THE AURA AND WHAT IT MEANS TO YOU,* 5.50. Summarizes information about the aura as given by many different individuals at different periods of time from their own personal knowledge and experience. No attempt has been made to comment on the material reported and the names of the individuals whose observations are recorded are not given. Topics include physical properties of the aura, science looks at the aura, where does the aura come from, what does it look like, what is it made of, how thought and emotion affect the aura, meaning of the colors, and much else. This is the most comprehensive study available. Index, 8½"x11", 108pp. HeR 55

ANONYMOUS. *COLOR HEALING,* 5.50. This is an exhaustive compilation from the works of leading practitioners of chromotherapy. Includes articles by Edwin Babbitt, Corinne Heline, Roland Hunt, Walter Kilner, Oliver Reiser, George Starr White, and Gladys Mayer. Topics include chromo-therapeutics, colors and their effect on health, the alchemy of light and color, lectures to physicians, and much else. 8½"x11", 177pp. HeR 56

AURA GOGGLES, 13.25. Sturdily made goggles, developed along the guidelines set out by Dr. Kilner, with exchangeable coal-tar dicyanine filters and ventilating frame. MRG

BAGNALL, OSCAR. *THE ORIGIN AND PROPERTIES OF THE HUMAN AURA,* 2.95. Except for Kilner's pioneering efforts, this is the only major work of the aura. It is a generally more readable work than Kilner's and incorporates newer research. Bagnall describes how to construct apparatus for viewing the aura, and gives a clear scientific explanation of the phenomenon, based upon accepted biological and physiological principles. Illustrations, 160pp. Wei 70

BEESLEY, R.P. *THE ROBE OF MANY COLOURS,* 1.50. This is the most illuminating philosophical discussion of the human aura and the energy it represents that we have read. Beesley is a British healer who incorporates auric diagnosis into his technique. Unlike most accounts Beesley does not simply list a series of colors and discuss their meaning. He surveys the aura holistically. There's a Christian flavor to the presentation. 44pp. CPT 68

BESANT, ANNIE and C.W. LEADBEATER. *THOUGHT FORMS,* 3.95. Two clairvoyant Theosophists present their observations of thought and the forms which it creates. Includes material on the meaning of colors and the effects of various forms. The book includes over 50 color plates of illustrative thought forms created by emotions, music, meditation, and various kinds of feelings. An excellent presentation. 77pp. TPH 25

BIRREN, FABER. *COLOR—A SURVEY IN WORDS AND PICTURES,* c15.00. A comprehensive survey of color, explored through many fields of learning including history, anthropology, archaeology, geology, religion, mythology, mysticism, art, literature, culture, tradition, symbolism, astrology, alchemy, science, natural history, and much else. A fascinating, profusely illustrated account. 223pp. UnB 63

BIRREN, FABER. *COLOR IN YOUR WORLD,* 1.25. Birren, the most influential modern color consultant, sets forth his theories of the interrelation of color preferences and personality and presents some fascinating points about color and the human psyche in this detailed introductory analysis. 121pp. McM 62

BIRREN, FABER. *COLOR PERCEPTION IN ART,* 7.95. This book is divided into three sections. The first traces the history of nineteenth and twentieth century color expression from Turner through impressionism to Op Art. Next the parallel history of color theory is covered, beginning with a reliance on the physics of vision and optics and shifting gradually to psychological perception. Earlier color theory focused on simultaneous contrast, afterimages, additive colors, and visual color mixtures; current theory emphasizes illumination, color constancy, adaptation and the law of field size. The aesthetic implications of this change in theory is the subject of the last section. Many black and white and twelve color plates are included. Index, 8"x8", 75pp. Lit 76

BIRREN, FABER. *COLOR PSYCHOLOGY AND THERAPY,* c8.95. Birren presents his most comprehensive analysis of the historical, scientific, and biological aspects of the influence of color on human life. He includes the most recent findings as well as quotations from many older works. He cites these sources not for the theoretical material they present but rather for their possible practical applications. Birren makes his living by prescribing color to the government, to educational institutions, to the armed forces, to industry, and to architects and designers. This is a clearly written, informative book. Good bibliography, index, 302pp. UnB 61

BIRREN, FABER. *PRINCIPLES OF COLOR,* c10.00. An elementary book on color dealing with traditional principles of harmony as well as advanced principles deriving from modern studies of the psychology of perception. Many color plates and illustrations. 96pp. VNR 69

BOOS-HAMBURGER, HILDE. *THE CREATIVE POWER OF COLOR,* 6.95. A collection of exercises and affirmations based on Rudolf Steiner's approach to color in art. The sixty-six exercises are illustrated in full color. Topics include the basis for color experience, and the creative aspects of color—including an analysis of each individual color. This is the most spiritually-oriented of all the works on color and the only one with supplementary exercises. Also contains an extensive bibliography. 8½"x11", 63+pp. NKB 73

BUTLER, W.E. *HOW TO READ THE AURA,* 1.25. The aura is a luminous atmosphere consisting of an electro-magnetic field which surrounds every living thing. This is an excellent introduction which covers the nature of the aura, its structure, the circuit of force, and the emotional-mental aspects of the aura. Also includes instructions on developing auric sight. 64pp. Wei 71

CAYCE, EDGAR. *AURAS,* .75. This booklet is one of the few things that Edgar Cayce ever wrote. The countless books that often bear his name are merely transcriptions of his psychic readings. Cayce was without question the greatest psychic America has ever produced. He gave thousands of health readings while he was in a trance like state. He had finely developed intuitive powers including the gift of being able to see auras easily. **Auras** was written in the last month of his life and it sums up his observations in an unusually clear manner. Each of the primary colors is discussed individually and the value of auric sight is touched on. There's also a summary color chart. 20pp. ARE 45

CLARK, LINDA. *COLOR THERAPY,* c6.95. Linda Clark is a reporter who has written on many aspects of natural healing and nutrition. This book is the result of twenty years of research into the subject, and it is both the newest and the most comprehensive review that we know of. Topics include the effects of light, how light and color work, the psychological impact of color, color and physical health, color and nutrition, color therapy for eye problems, how to apply color therapy, properties of individual colors, gem therapy, auras, and breathing color. The book is well written and organized. Bibliography, 145pp. DAC 75

CLARK, LINDA and **YVONNE MARTINE.** *HEALTH, YOUTH AND BEAUTY THROUGH COLOR BREATHING,* 4.50. While working on her book on color therapy Linda Clark heard about Yvonne Martine's remarkable techniques for using colors to rejuvenate and to heal. This book presents a survey of a variety of Ms. Martine's color breathing techniques. A number of specific treatments are outlined and many case studies are cited. The book is written in the *you can do it, too* vein. Bibliography, notes, index, 95pp. CeA 76

COLVILLE, W.J. *THE HUMAN AURA AND THE SIGNIFICANCE OF COLOR,* 1.50. A collection of three spiritually oriented lectures on the force of color, including analyses of individual colors and a great deal of material on color and the aura in Eastern thought. 70pp. HeR 70

COMPLETE AURA RESEARCH KIT, 45.00. Contains the following tools: a set of aura goggles with fitted 2X filters, soft face fitting of foam rubber, and screw rims; six pairs of color filters for study of inner aura striations; inner aura; outer aura; three pairs, basic set filters (graded diminishing shades); extra dark filters; spare frames. The kit is made by The Metaphysical Research Group in England to the specifications established by Kilner. MRG

COWEN, KITTIE. *COLOR: ITS MANIFESTATION AND VALUE,* 1.75. A series of fifteen esoteric lessons on the manifestations of color based on ancient teachings and incorporating some aspects of inspirational Christianity. Multilithed and stapled, 41pp. BSR nd

CRABB, RILEY. *COLOR–THE BRIDGE TO THE NEW AGE,* 1.50. An analysis of new developments in color research, especially as they apply to life energies. Also includes some clairvoyant interpretations of color. Multilithed and stapled, 29pp. BSR nd

FINCH, ELIZABETH and W.J. *PHOTOCHROMOTHERAPY,* 2.00. An analysis of the technique developed by the authors for using color in healing. Includes chapters on the history of color healing, on what photochromotherapy is, on how it works (how to apply the colors and the effects they have), on the properties of the colors, and also some case histories. 52pp. EsP 72

GOETHE, JOHANN. *THEORY OF COLORS,* 5.95. Goethe, as artist and scientist, probed the phenomenon of color to its origins in the interplay of light and darkness. His investigation of the moral qualities evoked in human feeling by color laid the foundation for an aesthetic of color and the theories he presents in this volume have been very influential up to the present day—although not among the more traditional scientists. Goethe felt that a knowledge of physics was an actual hindrance to understanding and he based his conclusions exclusively upon exhaustive personal observation of the phenomenon of color. Using simple equipment—vessels, prisms, lenses, and the like—the reader is led through a demonstration course not only in subjectively produced colors, but also in the observable physical phenomenon of color. The material here is fascinating, but not recommended to the casual reader. It's slow going. Notes, 485pp. MIT 70

HALL, MANLY P. *THE SYMBOLISM OF LIGHT AND COLOR,* 1.25. A philosophical survey which includes an analysis of historical and religious references to light and color and a summary of Hall's ideas on the subject. 32pp. PRS 76

HELINE, CORINNE. *COLOR AND MUSIC IN THE NEW AGE,* 2.95. This volume includes chapters on the color significance of the zodiacal signs, the presence and absence of color, color therapy, the cosmic aspects of color, the psychology of color in everyday living, color and music correlated with the seasons and the time of day, and occult effects of music. 139pp. NAP 64

HELINE, CORINNE. *HEALING AND REGENERATION THROUGH COLOR,* 1.95. An inspirational, esoteric discussion. 69pp. NAP nd

HILLS, CHRISTOPHER. *NUCLEAR EVOLUTION,* 4.00. See the Life Energies section.

HUNT, ROLAND. *THE EIGHTH KEY TO COLOR: THE MASTER KEY TO THE PREVIOUS SEVEN,* c5.35. A companion volume to **The Seven Keys,** written twenty-two years later. Sets out and analyzes the attributes of the rays in an effort to arrive at a do-it-yourself technique that students can use. Clearly presented and well-illustrated. 101pp. Fow 65

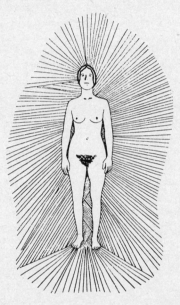

HUNT, ROLAND. *FRAGRANT AND RADIANT HEALING SYMPHONY,* 3.50. Subtitled *An inquiry into the wondrous correlation of the healing virtues of COLOUR, SOUND, and PERFUME and a consideration of their influence and purpose.* The book is badly written and should be read only by those who are deeply interested in esoteric teachings. 160pp. Whi 37

HUNT, ROLAND. *THE SEVEN KEYS TO COLOR HEALING,* c5.40. A correlation of all the known methods and many new and essentially practical techniques for diagnosis and treatment through the radiancy of color. Analyzes each color individually. 124pp. Dan 71

ITTEN, JOHANNES. *THE ELEMENTS OF COLOR,* c9.95. A condensed version of **The Art of Color,** edited and evaluated by Faber Birren. Itten examines both the subjective experience and the objective rationale of color and develops an important color theory. Illustrations (some in color), 96pp. VNR 75

JAEGERS, BEVERLY. *THE HUMAN AURA,* 2.00. Subtitled *How I teach my students to see it* [the aura]. This is a simplified, rather general study of the attributes of the aura and includes experiments designed to help an individual see the aura. Bibliography, 55pp. LuP 71

JOHNSON, KENDALL. *THE LIVING AURA,* c15.00. Kendall was the first American to discover the process known generally as Kirlian photography. He has worked closely with Thelma Moss. Here he details his research and discoveries. This is the most comprehensive modern study of the aura. Illustrated with over 125 black and white photographs and eight pages of color plates. Oversize, 256pp. Haw 76

KILNER, WALTER. *THE AURA,* 2.95. In 1908 Kilner, an English physician, conceived the idea that the human aura might be made visible if viewed through a suitable substance, and he experimented with dicyanin, a coal-tar dye. This dye appeared to have a definite effect upon eyesight, making the observer temporarily short-sighted and therefore more readily able to perceive radiation in the ultra-violet band. After many experiments Kilner published his findings in a book entitled **The Human Atmosphere** (this is the study, with a new title). He described techniques for viewing the aura, which he claimed had inner and outer components. The inner aura followed the body outlines, while the outer aura was more nebulous. Kilner said that there were marked changes in the appearance of the aura in states of health and sickness, and that his viewing screen could be used for diagnosis. 329pp. Wei 75

KILNER, WALTER. *THE HUMAN AURA,* 5.95. A completely revised edition, published nine years after the pioneering work and containing many additional observations and inferences. 318pp. UnB 65

KRIPPNER, STANLEY and DANIEL RUBIN, eds. *THE KIRLIAN AURA,* 3.95. This is the most important study yet done of material related to the recent scientific research and experimentation on the human aura. The material presented is generally technically written and the sources are usually cited. The following are among the selections presented: *Photography by Means of High-Frequency Currents*, by the Kirlians, *Bioplasma or Corona Discharge?* by Thelma Moss and Kendall Johnson, *Some Energy Field Observations of Man and Nature*, by William Tiller, *Chinese Acupuncture and Kirlian Photography*, by Jack Worsley, *Phenomena of Skin Electricity*, by Viktor Adamenko, and *The Art of the Aura*, by Ingo Swan. Also includes a good bibliography and many photographs and line drawings. Index, 208pp. Dou 74

KUPPERS, HAROLD. *COLOR: ORIGIN, SYSTEM, USES*, c22.50. Kuppers provides a new and comprehensive approach to color. He begins with a discussion on the origins of color and its physical characteristics. He then explains the physiological process of sight and the problems such an approach raises in relation to the everyday acceptance of color, and more particularly the need to define the ways in which a color is affected by different circumstances. Such questions in turn affect the attitude to color mixing. Kuppers proposes a new model for color mixing—the Rhombehedral System—and illustrates how to use it. The model explains the laws of color mixing and the relationships between the colors themselves. This text includes many beautiful color diagrams, with explanatory notes. It's designed for those with a great deal of interest and some previous background. Bibliography, oversize, 155pp. VNR 73

LANE, EARLE, ed. *ELECTROPHOTOGRAPHY*, 4.95. This is a handbook on psychoenergetics developed for the generalist who is interested in building and using a Kirlian electrophotographic generator. Complete instructions are given (with schematics) and addresses for buying parts are also listed, along with various suggestions. There are also selections on electro-acupuncture and biofeedback—explanations, charts, and techniques—as well as a bibliography and addresses for additional information. A high point of the text is the eighteen pages of full color Kirlian photographs. The text is certainly not excellent, but with the paucity of material in the field all efforts are welcome, and the photographs are beautiful. 8"x12", 57pp. AOP 75

LEADBEATER, C.W. *MAN, VISIBLE AND INVISIBLE*, c5.25/4.50. A very detailed analysis which records the observations of a clairvoyant investigator who described different auras as he saw them and endeavored to illustrate them with the aid of an artist. Contains material on all aspects of consciousness. Many beautiful color plates. 126pp. TPH 02

LEWIS, ROGER. *COLOR AND THE EDGAR CAYCE READINGS,* 1.50. Lewis is an artist who has studied the Cayce material on color at great length. First, he sets the stage with the scientific examination of color. Then, using the Cayce booklet, **Auras,** he shows how Cayce interpreted various colors when they appeared in the emanation of light around an individual. Because the Cayce readings associated various colors with the seven spiritual centers in the body, Lewis traces the colors on the path of the kundalini, describing the influences of the endocrine glands. Finally he looks at color from the point of view of the color psychologist. Includes many quotations from the Cayce readings. Bibliography, 48pp. ARE 73

LUSCHER, MAX. *THE LUSCHER COLOR TEST,* 1.95. The principle of the Luscher test is that accurate psychological information can be gained about a person through his choices and rejections of colors. This book explains how to take the test and interpret it and includes color cards. 188pp. S&S 48

MAYER, GLADYS. *COLOUR AND HEALING,* 1.90. A spiritual essay by an English anthroposophist. 63pp. NKB 60

OUSELEY, S.G.J. *COLOUR MEDITATIONS, WITH A GUIDE TO COLOR HEALING,* 2.00. Meditations which explain how the different wavelengths of color function in the body, soul, and spirit, and how they can be utilized. The healing section outlines the system of chromotherapy. Fow 49

OUSELEY, S.G.J. *THE POWER OF THE RAYS: THE SCIENCE OF COLOR HEALING,* 2.00. A sequel to **Color Meditations** which explains the methods of using the *cosmic color rays* in the treatment of disease. Ouseley also discusses the aura, the etheric body and the physical body. Fow 51

OUSELEY, S.G.J. *THE SCIENCE OF THE AURA,* 1.10. An introduction to the study of the human aura including the scientific basis, color aspects of the aura, and developing auric sight. 32pp. Fow 49

PANCHADASI, SWAMI. *THE HUMAN AURA,* 1.00. A very nice introduction to the aura, especially its spiritual aspects. YPS 72

SCHINDLER, MARIA. *GOETHE'S THEORY OF COLOR,* c12.90. Discusses the secrets of color and their living spiritual reality. Colors as real forces which speak to our sensations and feelings and imprint their dynamic qualities on our inner life. Includes discussion of physiological colors, combinations, the balanced color circle, moral effects of color, Goethe's theory of color as image of world evolution. A valuable text book with graduated exercises leading the student directly into the living realm of color. Forty-one color plates, 210pp. NKB 64

SHARPE, DEBORAH. *THE PSYCHOLOGY OF COLOR AND DESIGN,* 2.95. A concise study of the psychology of color. Dr. Sharpe is a well known color consultant. A great deal of practical information is imparted here. Notes, indices, 174pp. LtA 75

STANFORD, RAY. *WHAT YOUR AURA TELLS ME,* c6.95. Stanford, a well known psychic describes and explains his ability to see human auras. He tells of how he learned the meaning of auric radiations and relates the psychological and parapsychological testing he has undergone. Many anecdotes and case histories are included. Dou 77

STURZAKER, JAMES. *THE TWELVE RAYS,* 1.50. Although colors are generally seen on only the physical level they have a profound influence on every other level of being—emotional, mental, and spiritual. This book analyzes the main characteristics of colors and the value of color in diagnosing illness in a person's aura before it manifests in the physical body. 64pp. Wei 76

WHITE, GEORGE STARR. *THE STORY OF THE HUMAN AURA,* 7.50. This is a very detailed study of the research done by Dr. White in the early part of the twentieth century. It includes much scientific material not found elsewhere on the aura as a manifestation of the life force, and many case studies of healing specific ailments using the energy of the aura. This is not a terribly readable study, but the material presented here has been the basis of much of the later work. Illustrations (with some color), index, 215pp. HeR 69

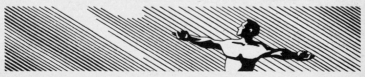

Cookbooks

F ood should have food value: this is the basic principle of good nutrition. How simple and yet how
easily forgotten! It is not enough for food to look
and taste good; it should be nourishing too. If we can only
remember this fact amidst the barrage of advertising and
the clamor of old habits, we will have gone a long way towards better health through healthier eating. The mass
media may din into our ears the taste appeal and convenience of the numerous products of the food industry,
but in selecting our daily bread the essential thing to look
for is nourishment. That doesn't mean that we shouldn't
enjoy what we eat—quite the opposite. But we must reeducate our tastes and rethink many of our old eating
habits if we are to enjoy genuine well-being in body and
mind. If it is used for nourishment, food *will* help bring
the sense of well-being that we are looking for. But in
order to use food for nourishment, we need a basic understanding of the body's needs.

Many people have little knowledge of how their body
works, so it is not unnatural that as they go down the aisle
at the supermarket they have no firm criterion for food
selection. But why remain in the dark about such an important topic? The basic principles of good nourishment
are not complicated, and they can be learned by anyone
who wants to experiment with their application.

Health, from this point of view, is not just an absence of
disease. It is a dynamic, positive state in which we function
at our best, physically and mentally. We can help our bodies
become healthy, strong, and beautiful by eating the right

84

kind of food, in the right amount, at the right time, and in the right company. Translated into daily life, this means eating wholesome, nourishing food in moderate amounts, in the relaxed company of family or friends. It doesn't take long for the entire body to begin to feel better and look better for such care, and soon our old ways of eating begin to lose their appeal. There may still be an occasional desire for banana cream pie or french-fried potatoes, but by and large we would just rather now eat what is really good for the body. In fact, we may find even these old favorites giving us up one day—suddenly we discover that the old habits have simply disappeared for good.

Wise choices in eating depend upon understanding the basic principles of good nourishment. There are three principles which can give a firm foundation to all our experimentation: variety, whole foods, and moderation. Keeping these three in mind makes it possible to avoid food faddism on the one hand and simply sliding back into our old habits on the other.

No one food or food family supplies all the nutrients we need to maintain good health. Variety assures you not only of good-quality, balanced protein in a meatless diet, but also of elusive nutrients like vitamins and trace minerals. Trace minerals, for example, are needed only in small quantities, and the amount of them in foods varies greatly from one food to another. It is impossible to know how well the carrots we had for dinner last night met our trace mineral needs. But if we eat a variety of vegetables, each one will have taken up different nutrients from the soil, and whatever might have been left out of the diet on one day will very likely show up the day after.

Great concern over getting all the subtle trace nutrients has led many people to vitamin pills and a frantic study of nutrient charts. Actually, the most successful way to plan for these vitamin and mineral needs is simply diversity in the diet.

The second principle of good nourishment, relying on

whole foods, has been sorely neglected for the last two decades. Many of us have only vague notions about what our food was like in its fresh and natural state. Between the fresh, natural, whole food and its refined, fractioned commercial product there is an abyss of lost nourishment, even when the refined food has been enriched. In whole foods there is a balance between calories and other nutrients, a certain density of nourishment that is lacking in many refined foods. The basic requirements of human nutrition are water, carbohydrate, protein, a broad range of vitamins and minerals, and a little fat or oil. Whole foods contribute to many of these needs at once; refined foods often contribute to only one or two.

Wheat is a perfect example of how nature has packed the nutrients carefully into our food. The whole kernel's interior, or endosperm, contains starch and a protein called gluten, which find their way into white flour, bread, and pastries. The vitamins and minerals found in the germ—B-1, niacin, B-6, iron, and zinc—are all needed by the body before it can utilize this starch and protein to produce energy and repair tissues, but all are lost in the process of refinement. Also lost in the wheat germ by refinement is the amino acid lysine, without which the gluten protein is severely imbalanced. The hull of the wheat, also removed in processing, contains valuable fiber, a nutrient which is now receiving new respect for its apparent role in keeping the digestive system healthy.

The soybean is another example of a food which Americans commonly eat in its fractioned form. We take the oil out and use it in large amounts as margarine, then buy the protein concentrate to supplement our diet. When the oil is extracted, the fat-soluble nutrients are lost; when the carbohydrate is washed from the protein, the water-soluble nutrients go too. And of the trace minerals present in foods in sometimes microscopic quantities but absolutely essential for health, it is impossible to say how many are missing from the artificially enriched protein concentrate we finally eat. The sum of the parts never quite adds up to the whole.

It is much better to eat corn than corn syrup, whole grain flour than milled flour, whole beans and seeds than their separated oils and protein concentrates. Cultivating what is whole, fresh, and natural in eating is a skill that leads to a simple but extremely satisfying diet.

We have become conditioned to consume things in the hope that they can make us feel better: more vitamins, more herbs, more drugs, more food. Often, however, what we refrain from putting in is as important as what we put in. The third principle of good nourishment, therefore, is moderation—moderation both in the total amount of food we eat and in individual foods.

Most of us do not need as much food as we think. One of the finer points of eating is to stop just when we find that everything is so good we'd like to have just a little more. Instead we usually decide that we might as well stay on at the table for five minutes more—forgetting that those five minutes will probably be followed by five hours of stomachache at night. Real gourmet judgment lies in stopping just short of a stomachache.

Eating slowly makes moderation easier because it gives us a chance to know when we have had enough. There is a physiological basis for this. Normally, the sugar products of digestion enter the blood during the course of a meal and flow through a center in the brain which sends a signal of satiety when the body's needs have been filled. When we eat too fast, we get ahead of the digestive process and may eat too much before the signal is even sent. Eating slowly and peacefully allows time to know when this subtle signal comes, and feel satisfied.

Moderation applies to single foods too. A small amount of sugar taken on a special occasion does no harm, but in large, frequent amounts, it can upset the body's energy cycle and may even precipitate diabetes.

For us and many of our friends, changing our orientation towards food has accompanied a simplification of our lifestyle on many fronts. Breadmaking, for example, requires time—and that may mean withdrawing from other activities, doing fewer things better instead of many things superficially. The time we take to be thoughtful about how we live is extra time for living better. And as our kitchen experiment grows, the principles of good nourishment grow wider in their application, for they are to be tested for their validity in our own experience.

—from **Laurel's Kitchen** by Laurel Robertson, Carol Flinders, and Bronwen Godfrey

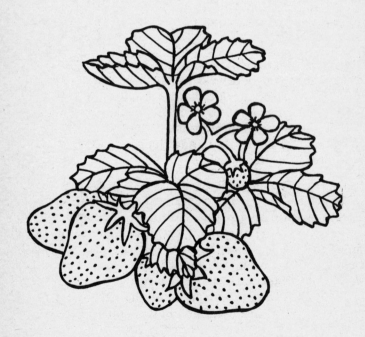

ALTH, MAX. *MAKING YOUR OWN CHEESE AND YOGURT,* c7.95. This is the most complete book of its type that we know of. The directions are clear and some illustrations are included. All aspects are discussed and there are some recipes. Bibliography, 239pp. Cro 73

Baby Food

Our current system of processed baby food is based on insufficient knowledge of infants' nutritional requirements. As reported in **Food Technology**, 1971, researchers have found that *Although the amount of data on nutrient intakes of infants is inadequate for sweeping generalizations, available reports suggest that appreciable percentages of infants are poorly nourished and infants from high socio-economic groups may receive less adequate diets than those from low socio-economic groups.* Until recently most parents took baby feeding for granted and, unless there were special problems, they assumed that the processed baby foods they bought were generally safe and nutritious. Today people are becoming more and more sceptical about the quality of the foods they buy and are looking for alternatives. The alternatives are right in your kitchen. Many foods can be easily blended to provide nutritious meals for babies. The cookbooks for babies give many recipes and general suggestions—and the meals they suggest are often not much harder than opening up a bottle.

KENDA, MARGARET and PHYLLIS WILLIAMS. *THE NATURAL BABY FOOD COOKBOOK*, 1.50. This is the most popular of the baby food cookbooks and also the most complete. Many of the recipes include meat so we're not completely turned on by it. Nonetheless a lot of useful information and nutritious foods are included throughout. Many hints on preparing food are also included along with recipes for special diets. Index, 168pp. Avo 72

TURNER, MARY and JAMES. *MAKING YOUR OWN BABY FOOD*, 1.50. This is our favorite baby food cookbook. All the recipes are clearly presented and the authors have come up with a number of unusual ideas. Ban 70

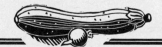

BOULDING, ELISE. *FROM A MONASTERY KITCHEN,* 6.95. A beautifully produced book printed in earth tones on tan paper. The recipes are not always as pure as we like, but the lovely graphics and abundance of quotations on each page make the book very special. The recipes are organized by seasons. Index, 10"x9", 128pp. H&R 76

Bread

Home-baked bread is perhaps the most important part of our diet. It struck us only recently that the real solution to the terrible problem of excessive sugar consumption— the solution, at least, that has worked beautifully for us— is baking our own bread. Bread isn't a dessert at all. It abounds in vitamins, minerals, and protein, and it contains little or no sugar. Yet, for all its nutritional worth, a warm, fragrant loaf of bread is far more satisfying than any number of sugary desserts.

If you have children, try to involve them in breadmaking. It's a great way to spend time together, and once they get the hang of it, they can be a big help. Share with them the beauty of the whole process: the clever ways of the fabled yeasties, the transformation of the dough, as you knead it, into liveliness and resilience, and the very distinctive qualities that the different flours bring to a loaf. Children can start by greasing the cans, shaping the loaves, and forming cinnamon buns with extra dough. In time, they may want to be in charge of a whole baking. Hopefully, an early initiation will lead to a lifelong habit.

Freshly baked bread has a mysterious power to cause friends to drop in unexpectedly. Friends you may not have seen for months will appear at exactly the right moment. Fresh, whole-grain bread, baked with love, is such good food, such *whole* food, that it is a source of real satisfaction to share it around, hot from the oven: so our first piece of advice is just to be sure you bake twice as much as you think you'll need!—from **Laurel's Kitchen** by Laurel Robertson, Carol Flinders, and Bronwen Godfrey

BRAUE, JOHN. *UNCLE JOHN'S ORIGINAL BREAD BOOK,* 1.25. A collection of over 200 unusual bread, biscuit, and muffin recipes. Many of the recipes seem to be variations on traditional German breads. The ingredients are not strictly natural, but they are pretty generally healthful. Good, clear instructions. Well illustrated. Index, 8"x5", 192pp. Pyr 65

BROWN, EDWARD. *TASSAJARA BREAD BOOK,* **3.95. This is practically everybody's favorite bread book. The instructions for basic whole wheat bread are the best we have seen anywhere and they are illustrated with line drawings. The author tries to be as clear as possible and every possible aspect of bread making is reviewed. Many variations are included. Brown also includes recipes for yeasted pastries and yeasted breads as well as unyeasted breads, sourdough bread and pancakes, muffins and quickbreads, and deserts. The book itself is beautifully produced and we recommend it highly. 145pp. ShP 70**

DWORKIN, FLOSS and STAN. *BAKE YOUR OWN BREAD,* 1.50. This is a good bread book containing a wide variety of recipes. The Dworkins begin with general instructions on bread baking and suggest some new method breads. This is followed by clear, detailed instructions on making kneaded breads. A number of different whole wheat recipes are offered and variations are suggested. Other sections include sourdough, spiral breads, rye breads and pumpernickel, challah and brioches, pizza and pitta, and batter breads. Very clear instructions. Index, 211pp. NAL 72

HUNTER, BEATRICE. *WHOLE GRAIN BAKING SAMPLER,* 2.25. Ms. Hunter provides a wide variety of recipes. She emphasizes unusual breads and desserts and over half the book is devoted to cookies and pastries. The instructions are clear and easy to follow and all natural ingredients are used. Many hints are offered for the beginner. The recipes we have tried have turned out great. Glossary, index, 312pp. Kea 72

ROSENVALL, VERNICE, MABEL MILLER, and DORA FLACK. *THE CLASSIC WHEAT FOR MAN COOKBOOK*, 3.95. This book was written by a group of Mormons who hoped to turn their community on to natural foods and especially to natural grain baking. It is far from purist and both meat and sugar are included in some of the recipes. But the recipes are clearly presented and the cakes and cookies are especially good. It also includes good recipes for quick breads and muffins. Index, 9"x6", 162pp. WoP 75

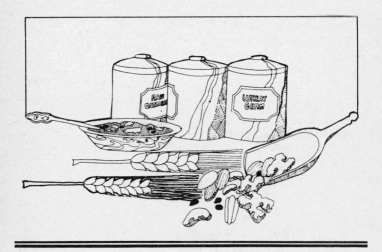

BROWN, EDUARD. *THE TASSAJARA COOKBOOK,* 4.95. This is a beautifully produced book which contains simple-to-prepare recipes. Many of the recipes give tips for substitutions to add to the variety and the instructions are clear and easy to follow. Directions on cutting and cooking are also given and there are illustrations throughout. Some of the recipes are for raw items. Index, 255pp. ShP 73

CADWALLADER, SHARON. *COOKING ADVENTURES FOR KIDS,* 4.95. A collection of simple, basic recipes of foods that kids both like to eat and can make fairly easily, with some supervision. Basic information on terms and weights and measures is also included and there are illustrations throughout. Index, 8½"x8¼", 101pp. HMC 74

CADWALLADER, SHARON. *WHOLE EARTH COOKBOOK NO. 2,* 4.95. A second collection of recipes. This one emphasizes soups and stews and casseroles and is not strictly vegetarian. Spiral bound, index, 123pp. HMC 75

CADWALLADER, SHARON and JUDI OHR. *WHOLE EARTH COOKBOOK,* 4.95/1.95. This was one of the first natural foods cookbooks to come out and it remains a favorite for many people. The dishes are varied and the recipes are easy to follow and not overly complicated. Also includes suggestions for converting old recipes. The $4.95 edition is spiral bound. HMC 71

COURTER, GAY. *THE BEANSPROUT BOOK,* c2.95. Complete directions for sprouting and discussions of the major grains and seeds that are sproutable. Some recipes are included too. This is the most popular of the sprouting guides. Illustrations, bibliography, 96pp. S&S 73

DAVIS, ADELLE. *LET'S COOK IT RIGHT,* 2.25. A very complete cookbook, emphasizing healthful (but not necessarily tasty) recipes. Not vegetarian and not very purist (sugar and additives are often included). Definitely not one of our favorites, but a classic nonetheless. Detailed instructions. Index, 573pp. NAL 70

DUQUETTE, SUSAN. *SUNBURST FARM FAMILY COOKBOOK,* 4.95. A nice collection of recipes emphasizing heavy entrees and including a section of fish recipes. The recipes themselves are fairly simple, and salads and dessert recipes are also included. Not an outstanding cookbook, but certainly more than adequate. The ingredients are all pure. Index, 304pp. WoP 76

DWORKIN, STAN and FLOSS. *BLEND IT SPLENDID,* 1.50. Over 200 blender recipes of every type imaginable. Clear instructions. Index, 230pp. Ban 73

DWORKIN, STAN and FLOSS. *THE GOOD GOODIES,* 4.95. This is the best all around natural food dessert book that we know of. The recipes are imaginative and the instructions are clear. Many other baked items (such as pizza) are also included. Oversize. Rod 74

EWALD, ELLEN. *RECIPES FOR A SMALL PLANET,* 5.95/1.95. This is one of our favorite cookbooks. Not many recipes are included, but all of the ones that we have tried have come out very well. The recipes are simple and they follow the principles of grain combining outlined by Frances Moore Lappe in *Diet for a Small Planet*—although they are far tastier than the recipes in the latter book. All types of recipes are included. The $5.95 edition is spiral bound. RaH 73

FORD, MARJORIE, SUSAN HILLYARD and **MARY KOOCK.** *DEAF SMITH COUNTRY COOKBOOK—NATURAL FOODS FOR FAMILY KITCHENS*, 4.95. This is an excellent overall cookbook and is one of the best natural foods cookbooks to buy if you only want to buy one. It includes descriptions of natural food staples and directions for their care and storage as well as information on sprouting and sample menus. Special sections present recipes for Mexican foods, baby and children's foods, and breads and desserts. The recipes are good and the directions are clear and easy to follow. McM 73

FRIEDLANDER, BARBARA. *THE FINDHORN COOKBOOK*, 7.95. This is the only natural food cookbook that we know of which contains recipes for large groups. Over 200 vegetarian recipes, for 10, 25, 50, or 100 people are presented. Suggestions are also offered for converting standard recipes. All the recipes are drawn from the Findhorn community in Scotland where the author spent time as a cook. A miscellany of other information is also included. Bibliography, index, 264pp. G&D 76

GERRAS, CHARLES, ed. *NATURAL COOKING, THE PREVENTION WAY*, 4.95. A collection of over 800 recipes from the pages of **Prevention Magazine**, the U.S.'s leading nutritional magazine. Most were sent in by readers, so the quality is somewhat uneven. Some non-vegetarian dishes are included. Index, 357pp. NAL 72

GOODWIN, MARY and **GERRY POLLEN.** *CREATIVE FOOD EXPERIENCES FOR CHILDREN*, 4.00. More than a cookbook, this book is designed to turn kids on to natural foods and get them involved in the experience of making the foods themselves. Some useful suggestions are offered, although the book is not entirely successful. 8½"x11". CFS 73

GOULART, FRANCES. *THE ECOLOGICAL ECLAIR*, 3.50. A variety of recipes for "sugarless treats," with very complete directions. Descriptions of major natural sweeteners and home-made sweeteners are given. The tone of the book is a little too cutesie for our taste.

Index, 196pp. McM 75

HANNAFORD, KATHRYN. *COSMIC COOKERY,* 4.95. This is a very useful collection of recipes and general information on making natural foods. The recipes are not very unusual, but they all come out well and are simple to follow. The book itself is beautifully produced. All the basic areas are covered and special features include a glossary, sample menus, and descriptions of basic utensils and basic procedures. Index, oversize, 264pp. Srm 74

HEINDEL, MAX. *NEW AGE VEGETARIAN COOKBOOK,* c6.75/ **4.50. This is probably the oldest vegetarian cookbook that is still generally available and it remains one of the best. The presentation is exceedingly simple and the recipes all work. The book begins with some information on basic foods and vitamins and then presents a long table of food values. This is followed by many menu suggestions and then there's a topically organized collection of recipes—probably the most comprehensive collection available anywhere. There are also sections on high altitude cooking and on canning and preserving. A final section discusses herbs. Fully indexed, 492pp. Ros 68**

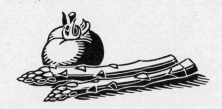

HERTZBERG, RUTH, BEATRICE VAUGHAN and JANET GREENE. *PUTTING FOOD BY,* 4.95. This is an excellent volume which includes step-by-step procedures and clear explanations of the reasons for canning and preserving foods. Illustrations, index, 493pp. GrP 75

HEWITT, JEAN. *THE NEW YORK TIMES NATURAL FOOD COOKBOOK,* 4.95. The best feature of this book is the variety of recipes it offers. We do not know of another book that has such a wide variety. Most of the recipes we have tried are easy to follow and come out well and often there are variations that can be tried. Every conceivable area is covered in depth. Bibliography, index, 434pp. Avo 71

HITTLEMAN, RICHARD. *YOGA NATURAL FOODS COOK-BOOK,* 1.50. This is a simple collection of healthy, pure recipes and a smattering of information about various food types. Index, 160pp. Ban 70

HOBSON, PHYLLIS. *HOME DRYING VEGETABLES, FRUITS AND HERBS,* 2.95. Practical instructions, presented in summary form. Index, 59pp. Gar 75

HOBSON, PHYLLIS. *MAKING HOMEMADE CHEESE AND BUT-TER,* 2.95. Simple directions for making a wide variety of cheeses. Also includes ways of making yogurt and butter. Index, 45pp. Gar 73

HOOKER, ALAN. *VEGETARIAN GOURMET COOKERY,* 4.95. As the title suggests, this is a beautifully produced book which gives detailed directions for the preparation of a number of gourmet dishes. The recipes are complicated and the dishes tend to be heavy —but they are delicious if you like this kind of food. Very clearly presented. Entrees, salads, soups, vegetables, sauces, and desserts are included. Index, oversize, 191pp. One 75

HUNTER, BEATRICE. *FAVORITE NATURAL FOODS,* c7.95. A collection of recipes and tips for better eating by one of America's best known advocates of natural foods. The discussion is topically organized according to item discussed. 219pp. S&S 74

HUNTER, BEATRICE. *THE NATURAL FOODS COOKBOOK,* 2.95/1.25. This has long been considered one of the basic natural foods cookbooks. Over 2000 recipes are included and, while Ms. Hunter often goes overboard on including healthy items (brewer's yeast is a staple feature of her recipes!), she gives excellent instructions and the recipes we have tried have come out fine. Not vegetarian. Very fully indexed, 312pp. S&S 61

HURD, FRANK and ROSALIE. *A GOOD COOK—TEN TALENTS,* 7.95. This is a unique, excellent cookbook. None of the recipes use milk or any milk product and all are thoroughly explained. There's also a profusion of nutritional information and tables and many raw recipes. All those who are seriously interested in natural food cooking should own or have access to this book. Spiral bound, index, 353pp. Hur 68

JENSEN, BERNARD. *BLENDING MAGIC,* 4.40. 650 unusual recipes combined with a review of the importance of raw food and drinks in digestion and in healing. Many food items are critiqued and the principles of general nutrition are reviewed. 235pp. Jen nd

JENSEN, BERNARD. *VITAL FOODS FOR TOTAL HEALTH,* 5.50. An unusual cookbook which combines basic facts about nutrition with a series of recipes. Over half the book is devoted to Jensen's exposition of *food chemistry and body chemistry*—detailing the effects of various foods on the body. Many raw recipes are included along with sample menus. Spiral bound. Index, 382pp. Jen 66

JORDAN, JULIE. *THE WINGS OF LIFE,* 5.95. A nice collection of simple, easy to prepare recipes. Many cooking hints are incorporated into the text. There's nothing outstanding about this book, but it does complement other cookbooks and would be a good primer for those who are not into natural foods and want to try some basic recipes. We've tried several and they have all come out well. The directions are clear and more than adequate. Index, 256pp. Css 76

KINDERLEHRER, JANE. *COOKING WITH LOVE AND WHEAT GERM,* c9.95. Jane Kinderlehrer is a senior editor of **Prevention** Magazine and this book reveals her knowledge of and concern for a whole range of nutrition and diet issues. Thus it is much more than a cookbook, offering helpful advice on how to get started with natural foods, how to survive the college dining hall, or how to keep the cholesterol down. Different sections deal with cooking for children, teenagers, two persons, or oneself alone. One useful and so far unique feature in cookbooks: every recipe contains metric conversions for measures and cooking temperatures. Index, 355pp. Rod 77

LAPPE, FRANCES MOORE. *DIET FOR A SMALL PLANET,* 5.95/1.95. When this book first came out in 1971 it created a stir throughout the country. It was the first scientific study of vegetarianism and of the economic benefits of grains over meat that had been produced in recent times. Over half the book presents Ms. Lappe's arguments for non-meat protein. The recipes themselves often tend to be heavy, and we like those in Ewald's **Recipes** better. But as a document it is must reading for all those who are interested in natural foods. Newly revised. The $5.95 edition is spiral bound. Bibliography, notes, index, 411pp. RaH 75

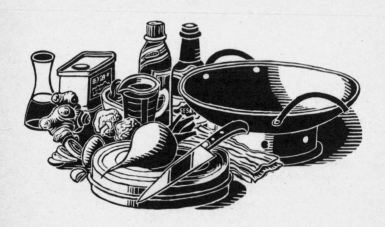

LEE, GARY. *THE CHINESE VEGETARIAN COOKBOOK,* 3.95. This is a beautifully presented book which begins with a discussion of Chinese cooking and also examines the utensils. Each of the vegetables is then discussed individually and recipes are suggested. The recipes themselves are not terribly imaginative, but they cover the essentials and you can improvise from there. Index, 5¼"x8", 181pp. Nit 72

LEE, GARY. *THE WOK COOKBOOK,* 3.95. This is a lovely illustrated book which begins with a detailed discussion of Chinese cooking—including information on the utensils and on the special foods and condiments. There's also a glossary. Most of the recipes call for meat—but this can be left out if desired. The instructions are extensive and more than adequate. This is the most popular book on Chinese cooking. 8½"x5¼", 162pp. Nit 70

LO, KENNETH. *CHINESE VEGETARIAN COOKING,* 3.95. This is our personal favorite among the Chinese cookbooks. All of the recipes that we have tried have come out very well. The directions are more than adequate and all aspects of Chinese food are covered. The recipes tend to be fairly mundane, but it's easy to improvise once you get the general idea. All the terms are defined. Index, 182pp. RaH 74

LOEWENFELD, CLAIRE and BACK. *HERBS, HEALTH AND COOKERY,* 1.95. See the Herbs section.

MCCLURE, JOY, et al. *COOKING FOR CONSCIOUSNESS,* 5.00. It's almost impossible to describe a cookbook in words. This one is subtitled *A Handbook for the Spiritually Minded Vegetarian* and has been put together by members of Ananda Marga. It is attractively put together and seems to be fairly comprehensive. We've tried a few of the recipes and they are well explained and taste good. The recipes tend to be simple and there's an abundance of extra explanatory information about natural foods throughout the book. Some of the recipes are quite unusual and if you are into buying cookbooks we think you will like this one. In addition to the recipes and background information, there is an adequate survey of basic nutrition. Indices, 279pp. AMP 76

Macrobiotics

Translated literally from the Greek, "Macrobiotics" means great life. Macro refers to the macrocosmic universe, the infinite womb out of which springs the Bios, or biological evolution. Macro-bios implies the law that knits the entire universe into a oneness. Living according to this law (expressed as *yin* and *yang*) is the way to achieve health, happiness and fulfillment. Practical macrobiotics is the attempt to grasp this elusive order in nature and to enable every man and woman to administer and use it in everyday life. By so doing we strive to create a civilization of free and happy people in harmony with the environment around them. We understand man to be nourished by sunlight, air, water and earth, in addition to the vegetal forms absorbed directly through the digestive system. We stress the importance of choosing and eating foods that are native to our terrain and climate, those that grow within a radius of 500 miles of our homes.—from **The Art of Just Cooking** by Lima Ohsawa

ABEHSERA, MICHAEL. *COOKING FOR LIFE,* 3.95. This is the most popular of all the macrobiotic cookbooks. Much of the book is devoted to an exploration of macrobiotic philosophy and hundreds of clearly explained recipes are offered. Index, 364pp. Avo 72

ABEHSERA, MICHAEL. *ZEN MACROBIOTIC COOKING,* 1.75. Thoughts on the macrobiotic diet combined with a collection of recipes, a glossary, and cooking tips. Index, 223pp. Avo 68

KUSHI, MICHIO. *ACUPUNCTURE: ANCIENT AND FUTURE WORLDS,* 10.00. A transcription of two of Kushi's seminars. The first is a detailed study of acupuncture which includes information on the philosophical basis of the technique and its relation to the order of the universe. The second seminar is more disjointed. Here Kushi surveys ancient teachings and cosmologies and discusses future global patterns. 136pp. EWF 73

KUSHI, MICHIO. *THE BOOK OF MACROBIOTICS,* 6.95. A basic survey of the philosophical underpinnings of the macrobiotic diet and the macrobiotic way of life. A great deal of practical information is also included. One hundred illustrations, oversize, 176pp. Jap 76

KUSHI, MICHIO. *MACROBIOTIC SEMINARS OF MICHIO KUSHI,* 10.00. Transcription of a series of seminars given in 1972. Most of the information is related to bodily sickness. Illustrations, 152pp. EWF 72

KUSHI, MICHIO. *THE TEACHINGS OF MICHIO KUSHI, VOL. I,* 3.95. A disjointed collection of Kushi's teachings, selected and summarized from a large number of seminars. Many topics are covered and there are illustrations throughout. 112pp. EWF 72

KUSHI, MICHIO. *THE TEACHINGS OF MICHIO KUSHI, VOL. II,* 4.95. Transcriptions of the following lectures: *The Traditional Food of Man, Be Your Own Doctor, Why Did We Become People?, How Did We Become People?, Waves and Particles, Life and/or Death,* and *Apocalyptical Remarks.* 139pp. EWF 71

OHSAWA, LIMA. *THE ART OF JUST COOKING,* 6.50. This delicately illustrated book by the widow of George Ohsawa both explains the macrobiotic philosophy of food and contains over 400 recipes. The recipes are based on over thirty-five years of practical experience cooking and teaching cooking classes. The instructions are very complete and a number of practical hints are offered. Bibliography, index, 215pp. Aut 74

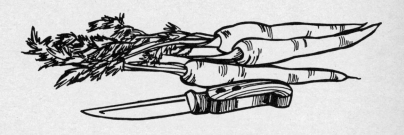

MAYER, PAUL. *VEGETABLE COOKBOOK,* 3.95. A beautifully produced book, filled with simple recipes and background hints and printed in two colors on rice paper. Index, 8¼"x5¼", 182pp. Nit 75

ROBERTSON, LAUREL, CAROL FLINDERS and BRONWEN GODFREY. *LAUREL'S KITCHEN,* c13.95. This is a handsomely produced book which is as comprehensive as any we know of. All the information that someone just getting into natural foods needs to know is here including an excellent section on basic nutrition. The recipes come out well and are easy to follow and, in addition, they are accompanied by extensive background material and beautiful woodblock prints throughout. We highly recommend this book. If you just want to buy one cookbook, this one has everything you need. The authors are members of a California spiritual community and their experiences are incorporated into the tone of the book. 508pp. Nil 76

SACHAROFF, SHANTA. *FLAVORS OF INDIA—RECIPES FROM THE VEGETARIAN HINDU CUISINE,* 4.95. This is a wonderful cookbook. Not only does it offer a number of excellent Indian recipes, but it also gives detailed instructions on preparing the unusual items in the Indian menu. The reader is taken step-by-step through the preparation and everything we have tried has been both authentic and successful. Beautifully illustrated and produced. Oversize. One 74

SANTA MARIA, JACK. *INDIAN VEGETARIAN COOKERY,* 2.95. Hundreds of excellent recipes, but only useful as a supplement to the Sacharoff book—or for someone who is familiar with Indian cooking. Preparation instructions for basic Indian foodstuffs are not included. Wei 74

SHURTLEFF, WILLIAM and AKIKO AOYAGI. *THE BOOK OF MISO,* 6.95. Miso is one of Asia's most important traditional soybean foods. A fermented, high-protein seasoning, it is very flavorful and is one of the major elements in Japanese cuisine. This oversized book contains over 400 miso recipes, easy-to-follow instructions for making miso at home, and an analysis of miso's nutritional benefits. Over 300 illustrations, glossary, bibliography, index, 254pp. Aut 76

SHURTLEFF, WILLIAM and AKIKO AOYAGI. *THE BOOK OF TOFU,* 7.95. Tofu is the most widely used protein in oriental cuisine. It is made from soybeans and is extremely versatile. This beautifully produced book presents over 500 tofu recipes along with easy to follow instructions for making seven varieties of tofu at home and on a community scale. Over 300 illustrations accompany the text. Index, 8¼"x11". 336pp. Aut 75

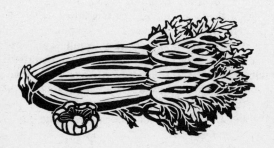

THOMAS, ANNA. *THE VEGETARIAN EPICURE,* c10.00/4.95. This is one of the most popular vegetarian cookbooks. It is beautifully produced and contains gourmet recipes. People seem to enjoy it even if they are not into natural foods. A perfect gift for those whom you want to turn on to natural foods. Some of the recipes include sugar, so it is not entirely purist. Index, 317pp. RaH 72

WEINER, JOAN. *VICTORY THROUGH VEGETABLES,* 2.95. This is a very satisfactory collection of vegetarian recipes, all of which are easy to prepare. The recipes are not entirely pure and contain some additives and sugar. Index, 163pp. HRW 70

WHYTE, KAREN. *THE COMPLETE SPROUTING COOKBOOK,* 3.95. Provides techniques for sprouting twenty-five varieties of seeds and grains and gives 125 nutritional recipes for their use. The directions are simple and the 8¼"x8¼" book is nicely produced. 120pp. Tro 75

WHYTE, KAREN. *THE COMPLETE YOGURT COOKBOOK,* 3.95. Ms. Whyte discusses the history of yogurt, its nutritional importance, how it is made commercially, and how it can be made at home. Over 250 recipes utilizing yogurt are included. 8¼"x8¼", 120pp. Tro 75

WHYTE, KAREN. *ORIGINAL DIET: RAW VEGETARIAN GUIDE AND RECIPE BOOK,* 3.95. Ms. Whyte tells the story of our dietary origins and shows why eating raw foods is best. She includes over 150 recipes. 8¼"x8¼", 120pp. Tro 77

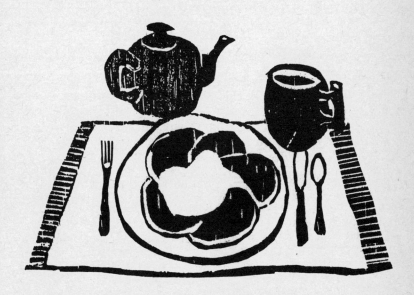

Death

Death is a subject that is evaded, ignored, and denied by our youth-worshipping, progress-oriented society. It is almost as if we have taken on death as just another disease to be conquered. But the fact is that death is inevitable. We will all die; it is only a matter of time. Death is as much a part of human existence, of human growth and development, as being born. It is one of the few things in life we can count on, that we can be assured will occur. Death is not an enemy to be conquered or a prison to be escaped. It is an integral part of our lives that gives meaning to human existence. It sets a limit on our time in this life, urging us on to do something productive with that time as long as it is ours to use. . . .

All that you are and all that you've done and been is culminated in your death. When you're dying, if you're fortunate enough to have some prior warning (other than that we all have all the time if we come to terms with our finiteness), you get your final chance to grow, to become more truly who you really are, to become more fully human. But you don't need to nor should you wait until death is at your doorstep before you start to really live. If you can begin to see death as an invisible, but friendly, companion on your life's journey—gently reminding you not to wait until tomorrow to do what you mean to do—then you can learn to *live* your life rather than simply passing through it.

Whether you die at a young age or when you are older is less important than whether you have fully lived the years you have had. One person may live more in eighteen years than another does in eighty. By living, we do not mean frantically accumulating a range and quantity of experience valued in fantasy by others. Rather, we mean living each day as if it is the only one you have. We mean finding a sense of peace and strength to deal with life's disappointments and pain while always striving to discover vehicles to make more accessible, increase, and sustain the joys and delights of life. One such vehicle is learning to focus on some of the things you have learned to tune out—to notice and take joy in the budding of new leaves in the spring, to wonder at the beauty of the sun rising each morning and setting each night, to take comfort in the smile or touch of another person, to watch with amazement the growth of a child, and to share in children's wonderfully "uncomplexed," enthusiastic, and trusting approach to living. To live.

To rejoice at the opportunity of experiencing each new day is to prepare for one's ultimate acceptance of death. For it is those who have not really lived—who have left issues unsettled, dreams unfulfilled, hopes shattered, and who have let the real things in life (loving and being loved by others, contributing in a positive way to other people's happiness and welfare, finding out what things are *really you*) pass them by—who are most reluctant to die. It is never too late to start living and growing. . . .Growing is the human way of living, and death is the final stage in the development of human beings. For life to be valued every day, not simply near to the time of anticipated death, one's own inevitable death must be faced and accepted. We must allow death to provide a context for our lives, for in it lies the meaning of life and the key to our growth.

—from **Death, The Final Stage of Growth** by Elisabeth Kubler-Ross

BECKER, ERNEST. *THE DENIAL OF DEATH,* 2.95... *.a brilliant and desperately needed synthesis of the most important disciplines in man's life. It puts together what others have torn in pieces and rendered useless. It is one of those rare masterpieces that will stimulate your thoughts, your intellectual curiosity, and last, but not least, your soul....* —Elisabeth Kubler-Ross. This book was a Pulitzer Prize winner in 1974. Notes, index, 329pp. McM 73

BUDGE, E.A. WALLIS. *THE EGYPTIAN BOOK OF THE DEAD,* 4.95. This is a copy of the **Egyptian Book of the Dead**, written about 1500 BC for Ani, Royal Scribe of Thebes. The text embodies a ritual to be performed for the dead, with detailed instructions for the behavior of the disembodied spirit in the *Land of the Gods.* This work, like the **Tibetan Book of the Dead**, is considered a guidebook to initiatory practices rather than death and it served as the most important repository of religious authority for over 3000 years. Reproduced in full here are a clear copy of the Egyptian hieroglyphs, an interlinear transliteration of their sounds, a word-for-word translation, a more flowing transcreation, and a detailed 150 page introduction. 527pp. Dov 67

CHAMPDOR, ALBERT. *THE BOOK OF THE DEAD,* c10.00. A very readable translation, based on the same texts as Budge's but done by a Frenchman who was considerably more learned in the esoteric aspects of the ancient text. Champdor also introduces new material, discovered since Budge's classic 1898 translation. Includes interpretive and descriptive material and over sixty pages of beautifully reproduced illustrations as well as many illustrations in the text itself. If you can afford it we recommend this text rather than Budge's. Translated from the French by Faubion Bowers. 180pp. G&P 66

CORNISH, JOHN. *ABOUT DEATH AND AFTER,* .90. A spiritual inquiry based on the teachings of Rudolf Steiner. 16pp. NKB 75

DEMPSEY, DAVID. *THE WAY WE DIE,* 3.95. In this provocative book Dempsey examines the new science of thanatology—the approach to dying and death that seeks to make the last stages of life as rewarding and meaningful as youth and middle age. Sensitive to the emotional and psychological needs of the dying and their families and friends, Dempsey is also interested in the immediate decisions that surround this experience. He realizes that, for the survivor the experience of death does not end with the final heartbeat.

He examines the lost art of grieving and the illness that comes from not knowing how to mourn, the evidence of survival after death, and the efforts of psychologists and scientists to communicate with the dead. Finally, Dempsey discusses the pioneering work being done by some doctors and hospitals to make death more natural and dignified. Bibliography, notes, index, 288pp. MGH 77

DRAKE, STANLEY. *THOUGH YOU DIE,* 4.80. **Though You Die** *...endeavors to show that there is more that is knowable about death than many people think. There are experiences of the brink of death which are not much spoken about. There are sources of knowledge which are not very widely known, and, above all, there is the central Christian mystery of Christ's overcoming of death.* —from the introduction. Drake is an anthroposophist. 102pp. CCP 62

EVANS-WENTZ, W.Y. *THE TIBETAN BOOK OF THE DEAD,* 2.95. Evans-Wentz is one of the best known Tibetan scholars. This volume, originally published in 1927, was the first book that brought Tibetan Buddhism to the general Western public. This volume, known as the **Bardo Thodol,** is a basic sourcebook for the teachings concerning the Clear Light, the Void, and other major features of the religion. Although the book is used in Tibet as a breviary, and read or recited on the occasion of death, it was originally conceived as a guidebook for initiates who must *die in order to be reborn.* All the basic material is here for an understanding of the inner meaning of Tibetan Buddhism, and Evans-Wentz' scholarship is excellent—however, the book is often hard to read and the translation is not as flowing as we would like. Carl Jung has contributed a Psychological Commentary to this edition and Evans-Wentz himself has written a number of prefaces. Notes, index, 333pp. Oxf 60

FEIFEL, HERMAN, ed. *NEW MEANINGS OF DEATH,* c11.95. Dr. Feifel is a psychologist whose pioneering work on the meaning of death helped lay the foundation for new ways of helping the dying and bereaved. He believes that *in the last analysis all human behavior of consequence is a response to the problems of death.* This volume includes contributions by a distinguished group of scientists, clinicians, and educators. It covers the treatment of the dying person and his or her family, discusses teaching children about death, the role of grief in mental health, the care of the suicidal, and much else. Index, 384pp. MGH 77

FORTUNE, DION. *THROUGH THE GATES OF DEATH,* 2.50. A survey of ancient esoteric teachings which show that death is not something to be feared. 94pp. Wei 68

FREMANTLE, FRANCESCA and CHOGYAM TRUNGPA. *THE TIBETAN BOOK OF THE DEAD,* c12.50/3.95. Ms. Fremantle is thoroughly familiar with the Tibetan language and with this text and Chogyam Trungpa first received a transmission containing the **Bardo Thotrol,** or **Book of the Dead,** at the age of eight. The translators have attempted to both make the translation as faithful to the original as possible and to make it applicable to contemporary society. The text itself concerns the nature of the mind and its projections—beautiful or terrible, peaceful or wrathful—which seem to exist objectively and inhabit the external world. In particular it describes these projections as they appear immediately after death, when they are overwhelming since the consciousness is no longer grounded and shielded by its connection with a physical body. The text teaches how to recognize these forms and, through recognition, attain a state of enlightenment. A thorough commentary is provided by the translators. Illustrations, glossary, bibliography, index, 140pp. ShP 75

GOLD, E.J. *THE AMERICAN BOOK OF THE DEAD,* 4.95. A modern restatement of the ancient esoteric teachings on death, and on dying to this life and being reborn. AOP 74

GROF, STANISLAV and JOAN HALIFAX. *THE HUMAN EN-COUNTER WITH DEATH,* c8.95. Dr. Grof is the most experienced LSD researcher in the U.S. and Ms. Halifax is a medical anthropologist. In this volume they report on a project involving psychotherapy with terminal cancer patients to whom LSD was administered under carefully supervised conditions. For most, LSD-assisted counseling brought alleviation of fear, anxiety, and even physical pain as death came to be understood as a transitional process. Many patients experienced a symbolic confrontation with death and rebirth. Some made contact with spirits of departed relatives or archetypal entities, others linked their malignancy to deep seated feelings of guilt and self hatred. The authors link their findings to reports of those who have experienced clinical death or near death situations, and to myths and rituals of many cultures. Notes, index, 240pp. Dut 77

GROLLMAN, EARL. *TALKING ABOUT DEATH: A DIALOGUE BETWEEN PARENT AND CHILD,* 3.95. A sensitive and helpful dialogue about death which thousands of parents have used to explain the meaning and reality of death to their children. In this new edition the beautifully illustrated dialogue between parent and child is accompanied by a greatly expanded *Parent's Guide* which suggests a variety of ways for parents to use this book, and helps parents themselves to come to terms with the sorrow of death. Also included is a fully annotated listing of resources for those seeking further help. 111pp. Bea 76

HAMPTON, CHARLES. *THE TRANSITION CALLED DEATH,* c3.00. A theosophical treatise. 106pp. TPH 43

HENDERSON, JOSEPH and MAUD OAKES. *THE WISDOM OF THE SERPENT,* 1.95. A Jungian psychiatrist and an anthropologist explore the meanings and manifestations of death through ritual, religion, and myth. They feel that the knowledge that man must die is the force that drives man to create. The tribal initiation of the shaman and the archetype of the serpent exist universally in man's experience, exemplifying the death of the Self and a rebirth into a transcendant, *unknowable* life. The authors trace the images and patterns of psychic liberation through personal encounter, the cycles of nature, spiritual teachings, religious texts, myths of resurrection, poems, and epics. This is a fascinating study, extensively illustrated, with notes and an index. 314pp. McM 63

HICK, JOHN. *DEATH AND ETERNAL LIFE,* c15.00. Dr. Hick is an English Professor of Theology and this is about as theological a presentation of the subject of death as we can imagine. He begins with a survey of the history of belief in the afterlife. He then discusses the contemporary situation in depth, the viewpoints of modern philosophers, and the contributions of parapsychology. Next, he restates the humanist response to death and the problem of evil, finding it ultimately inadequate. This, he maintains, indicates a basic religious argument for immortality. In the final section he surveys various religious viewpoints on immortality. Bibliography, notes, index, 495pp. H&R 76

JURY, MARK and DAN. *GRAMP,* 5.95. A graphic photographic portrayal of an elderly man's last year and of his family's reaction to his decline. This moving portrait was put together by the man's grandson and includes portions of the grandson's diary and verbatim transcriptions of dialogues between gramp and various members of his family. 152pp. Vik 76

KAPLEAU, P. *THE WHEEL OF DEATH: A COLLECTION OF WRITINGS FROM ZEN BUDDHIST AND OTHER SOURCES ON DEATH-REBIRTH-DYING,* 2.95. An anthology which enables the reader to view death through the eyes of great Buddhist, Taoist, Hindu, and Western masters. The sections on rebirth and karma deal succinctly with those complex and often misunderstood doctrines. Glossary, 110pp. H&R 71

KELEMAN, STANLEY. *LIVING YOUR DYING,* 3.95. "A warm and wise book. It will do much to strip away the superfluous terror and helplessness we feel in the presence of death. Keleman shows how our styles of dying are linked to our styles of living and how this makes dying an activity that can be lived creatively rather than an accident that merely happens to us. But the book is more than a handbook for dying. It is a guide to dealing with loss, anger, pain, excitement, grief and endings."—Sam Keen. Kelemen explores all aspects of being fully alive, expanding, and dying to the old in this well written evocative account. Keleman runs The Center for Energetic Studies, which explores the human condition from the perspective of how we inhabit our bodies and embody our emotions. He is the leading West Coast bioenergetic practitioner. 162pp. RaH 74

KOESTENBAUM, PETER. *IS THERE AN ANSWER TO DEATH,* 3.75. A philosophical work which explores ways in which a positive confrontation with death can be a personally liberating experience. Koestenbaum feels that in facing death we face life, and that to come to terms with death early in life is the only way to find our own personal meaning in an alienated world. Case studies and practical exercises are included. Index, 212pp. PrH 76

KUBLER-ROSS, ELISABETH. *DEATH,* 2.95. Ours is a death-denying society. We hide it behind the sterile walls of the hospital and the cosmetic mask in the funeral home. But death is inevitable and we must face the question of how to deal with it. Why do we treat death as a taboo? What are the sources of our fears? How do we express our grief and accept the death of a person close to us? How can we prepare for our own death? From her own personal views and experiences and from comparisons with how our culture and other ones view death and dying, Dr. Kubler-Ross provides some answers to these and other questions by offering a spectrum of viewpoints from ministers and rabbis, doctors, nurses, sociologists, and personal accounts of those near death and their survivors. She shows how through an acceptance of our finiteness, we can grow; for death provides a key to the meaning of human existence. A provocative, evocative book, written by a psychiatrist who has made an extensive study of death. Bibliography, index, 203pp. PrH 75

KUBLER-ROSS, ELISABETH. *ON DEATH AND DYING,* 2.45. *I have worked with dying patients for the past two and a half years and this book will tell about the beginning of this experiment, which turned out to be a meaningful and instructive experience for all participants. It is not meant to be a textbook on how to manage dying patients, nor is it intended as a complete study of the psychology of dying. It is simply an account of a new and challenging opportunity to refocus on the patient as a human being, to include him in dialogues, to learn from him the strengths and weaknesses of our hospital management of the patient. . . .I am simply telling the stories of my patients who shared their agonies, their expectations, and their frustrations with us.*—from the preface. Bibliography, 299pp. McM 69

KUBLER-ROSS, ELISABETH. *QUESTIONS AND ANSWERS ON DEATH AND DYING,* 1.75. This sequel to Dr. Kubler-Ross' earlier book consists of the most frequently asked questions and her answers. Introduction, index, 189pp. McM 74

LESHAN, EDA. *LEARNING TO SAY GOOD-BY: WHEN A PARENT DIES,* c5.95. *Many a hurt family will be thankful for the help that this helpful, honest and practical book has to give. Its message is that children should be allowed to see and share our grief at death, and should have the privilege of expressing their own grief in their own way and at their own time. This sincere, sensitive and supportive book can help many a family through its hardest time. It seems certain to become a classic.*—Louise Ames, Co-director, Gesell Institute of Family Therapy. The writing style is geared toward older children and many case studies accompany the exposition. Illustrations, bibliography, 85pp. McM 76

LIFTON, JAY and ERIC OLSON. *LIVING AND DYING,* 1.95. *Robert Jay Lifton and Eric Olson have produced one of those monumental usable and reusable, readable and re-readable works which promises to produce major shifts in all thinking and teaching* *about the care of the dying.*—**Omega.** Bibliography, index, 155pp. Ban 74

MATSON, ARCHIE. *AFTERLIFE: REPORTS FROM THE THRESHOLD OF DEATH,* 2.95. Almost dying is not an uncommon experience, particularly on the operating table. Many people who have returned from the edge have told extraordinary tales about what they saw—extraordinary, that is, when judged by conventional scientific and religious theories. Here Reverend Matson presents a varied collection of these descriptions drawn from his acquaintances, from parapsychological sources, from medical eyewitness accounts, and from literature. Originally published as **The Waiting World.** Notes, 151pp. H&R 75

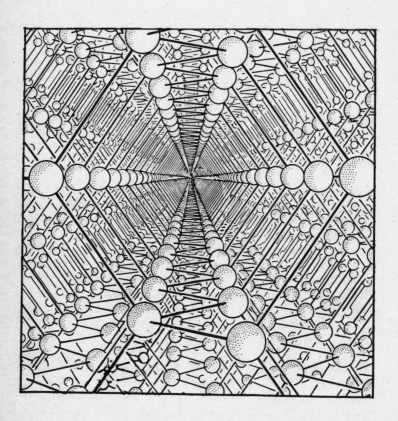

MOODY, RAYMOND. *LIFE AFTER LIFE,* 1.95. This book has created a sensation. Elisabeth Kubler-Ross feels that it is one of the most important documents on death that has ever been published and countless readers agree. It presents a series of case studies of people who have come back from the dead—individuals who almost died and were saved and brought back to this world. In addition to the case studies, the author discusses the meaning of death and cites the impressions of the individuals whose cases are discussed. Bibliography, 187pp. Ban 75

PATTISON, E. MANSELL, et al. *THE EXPERIENCE OF DYING,* 4.95. A collection of portraits of the death experience. The essays illustrate why we fear death and explain why it is often natural to both hate and love the dying person. They also show how death affects the family structure, and explore the source of guilt feelings survivors often experience. All of the selections are based on actual death experiences and all the authors are physicians and psychiatrists. Bibliography, 335pp. PrH 77

PELGRIN, MARK. *AND A TIME TO DIE,* 2.95. This is a moving account of the meditations of a man whose wife has died of cancer and who then learns that he too is suffering from the disease and has only eight months to live. It tells of his search for meaning in his own life and his thoughts as he approaches death. 173pp. TPH 62

PINCUS, LILLY. *DEATH AND THE FAMILY,* 2.95. Death has long been the last remaining taboo in Western society. Now, with new psychological and medical explorations into dying and the acceptance of death, the personal meaning of death has become an area of public concern. In this book a therapist examines the experience of coping with life after a loved one has died. Through detailed case histories of her patients, her friends, and her own life, Ms. Pincus shows how ways of grieving are related to ways of loving and to the nature of the relationship that is mourned. Notes, 289pp. RaH 74

RODMAN, ROBERT. *NOT DYING,* c7.95. A psychoanalyst's moving memoir of his wife's death. Dr. Rodman writes with extraordinary honesty and feeling. Trained to assess emotions and reactions, he observes his own responses and his gradual realization that each person faces death in his or her own way, and that that way must be respected. 216pp. RaH 77

SEGERBERG, OSBORN. *LIVING WITH DEATH,* c7.50. This is a journalistic study which draws on much of the modern research and includes a variety of case studies. Segerberg amplifies his discussion with citations from classical literature. Much of the book is devoted to suggestions of ways for coping with death. Bibliography, index, 140pp. Dut 76

SHEPARD, MARTIN. *SOMEONE YOU LOVE IS DYING,* c7.95. This is a practical guidebook which discusses how to cope with the mixed emotions of anxiety, resentfulness, guilt, despondency, aversion, and helplessness which are a natural reaction to death. Dr. Shepard, a well known psychiatrist, offers specific suggestions on the everyday details involved in preparing for death—including ways of minimizing fear and grief. He also presents a number of case studies and includes information on realistic alternatives to the traditional ways in which we treat individuals who are dying. Bibliography, 220pp. Crn 75

WATSON, LYALL. *THE ROMEO ERROR,* 1.95. Watson discusses the biology of life, the problem of deciding when death occurs, psychological and social attitudes toward death. He also presents the idea that life and death may be indistinguishable, with death merely being a change of state, often temporary and sometimes even curable. Bibliography, index, 275pp. Del 75

WEISS, JESS E. *THE VESTIBULE,* 1.25. Presents the experiences of a number of people who have died and managed to transmit their experiences in the beyond. 128pp. S&S 72

WORDEN, J. WILLIAM and WILLIAM PROCTOR. *PERSONAL DEATH AWARENESS,* c7.95. Dr. Worden spent eight years as Research Director for Harvard University's Omega Project, a study of terminal illness and suicide. During this time he came to the conclusion that many of life's problems, both emotional and practical, stem from an inability to confront the inevitability of one's own death. *The book contains a number of awareness exercises, many of which I use in teaching death awareness to medical students, psychiatric residents, and university students.*—from the preface. Many case studies are included and the book is designed to encourage personal reflection. Bibliography, index, 196pp. PrH 76

WYSCHOGROD, EDITH, ed. *THE PHENOMENON OF DEATH,*
3.45. This is another collection of essays about death. It goes beyond the problem of individuals to explore also the question of
the dying of a civilization. 235pp. H&R 69

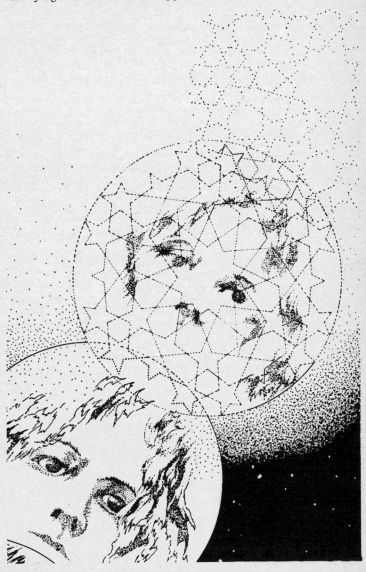

Healing

Your body is a three million year old healer. Over three million years of evolution on this planet it has developed many ways to protect and heal itself. When you get a cut you do not have to think about healing that cut. Your body knows how to handle it. If you were asked to take a peanut butter sandwich and a glass of milk, and heal the cut with these things, there would be no way you could do that, but your body can easily heal a cut "without you," using the ingredients of these foods. In a similar way your body cures its infections, mends its broken bones, and heals its diseases.

You have all the knowledge, tools, materials, and energy necessary to keep yourself healthy. The way to allow your three million year old healer to heal you is to get out of its way. It is not a matter of teaching your body to heal and mend; it is a matter of first learning how you *prevent* your three million year old healer from working, then learning conscious skills to provide your three million year old healer with the space and energy it needs to keep itself well.

The things your body does to heal a simple cut are so complex that only the most advanced medical scientists are even beginning to understand them. Yet compared to the other healing processes that your body knows how to do, a cut is a simple job. It also knows how to analyze thousands of substances from the external environment that can cause disease, and how to protect itself from them by creating incredibly complex protein molecules, called *antibodies,* which neutralize these otherwise harmful substances.

In your blood are many different kinds of cells, each a unit of life in itself, and each with a specific job to do: some bring nutriment to other cells; some break down bacteria and carry it away; some carry away the waste produced by cells; some produce antibodies, etc. Each cell knows exactly what to do—without any conscious directions from you. *But you can stand in the way of these processes.* For one thing, if you tense your muscles, you prevent blood from freely circulating in the tense area. This means that that part of your body may not get the full benefits of these specialized cells.

How do you choose between harmony and health on the one hand, and disease on the other? Let's take the example of a cut hand. *A choice for disease* might go something like this: You cut yourself while working in the garden. Immediately you become angry. You tense up in the area that's cut. You wipe the blood off on your work pants, and then you're back working again with your hands in the dirt. For a day or two, you're mildly angry at your hand for hurting. Maybe you're also becoming a little worried about it. Then, two days hence, you're surprised when you discover that you're "struck down" by an infection where you cut yourself. You may feel, at that point, that you have been dealt a cruel blow. Now your body needs outside help to heal itself. That's when you go to a doctor.

A choice for harmony and health might go like this: You cut yourself while working in the garden. You realize the cut is a message telling you to pay attention to your work. You rest for a moment, you relax the area of the cut, knowing that your body knows exactly how to heal the cut. You help it a little by washing it off with clean water, and you protect it from the dirt as you work for the rest of the day. You might stop work a little earlier than you planned, to take a warm bath and relax in order to bring greater circulation to the area of the cut, further helping your three million year old healer to heal you. All of these things are what we call working for harmony and health. Put another way, it is *working in harmony with Nature.*

Your mind has a great deal to do with helping your three million year old healer. Medical scientists are now proving what Indian yogins and other healers from the eastern world have known and practiced for thousands of years: that by conscious control you can influence blood flow, heart beat, blood pressure, glandular secretions, and muscular tensions in all areas of your body. These are skills which can be learned in the same way that you learn to drive a car, play tennis, ride a bicycle, or anything else.

When the mind holds ideas such as worry, fear, anger, jealousy, hate, etc., your body manifests thse feelings as muscle tension, decreased blood flow, and abnormal hormonal secretions. Eventually these states of consciousness result in disease. In this way people literally create their own diseases.

When your mind entertains ideas and feelings of love, joy, peace, harmony, and openness (knowing and understanding fcar, anger, jealousy, hate, etc., but also understanding that you need not *hold onto* these feelings) your body manifests these feelings as relaxation, acceptance, radiance, alertness, and a natural flow of blood, energy and hormones. This is a healthy state. Through your thoughts and feelings you create your own well body.

When you let your body receive the energies of the universe, when you are open to them and not closed, when you are relaxed and not tense, when you have positive ideas and not negative ideas, the energies of the universe will flow into your body to keep you well or heal you. Your body's use of these energies is more powerful than any drug or herb, more powerful than any surgeon, than any healer known to man. All effective healing makes use of these energies. You can make use of these energies yourself.

–from **The Well Body Book** by Mike Samuels, M.D. and Hal Bennett

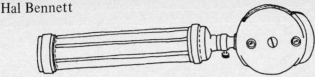

ACADEMY OF PARAPSYCHOLOGY AND MEDICINE. *THE DIMENSIONS OF HEALING*, 10.00. Transcript of the Fall 1972 program, including individual research as well as theoretical constructs for viewing the "whole man." It contains addresses of Drs. Puryear, Worrall, Grad, Chaudhuri, Green, Puharich, Tiller, McGarey, Moss, Bradley, Simonton, Sister Justa Smith, Mr. Dean and Mr. Johnson, and Edgar Mitchell. Includes questions and discussion as well as two lectures from the professional medical seminar on acupuncture by Drs. McGarey and Puharich. 8½"x11", 172pp. APM 72

ACADEMY OF PARAPSYCHOLOGY & MEDICINE. *THE VARIETIES OF HEALING EXPERIENCE*, 5.00. The complete transcript of the Academy's October 1971 interdisciplinary symposium. Includes addresses of Drs. Holland, Lilly, Green, Puharich, Tiller, McGarey, and Bradley on a variety of healing phenomena related to the parapsychological capabilities of man. 8½"x11", 112pp. APM 72

AIROLA, PAAVO. *HEALTH SECRETS FROM EUROPE*, 1.65. An excellent report by a Swedish naturopath revealing the nutrition and vitamin-mineral therapies now in use in some of Europe's leading natural health centers and progressive medical clinics. This book is composed of easy-to-follow, do-it-yourself instructions based on European studies and experiences. Notes, index, 224pp. Arc 70

AIROLA, PAAVO. *HOW TO GET WELL*, c8.95. This is Dr. Airola's magnum opus, a complete handbook of natural healing, written for professionals and informed laymen. This is the comprehensive reference work on therapeutic uses of foods, vitamins, food supplements, juices, herbs, fasting, baths, heat, and other nutritional and biological modalities in the treatment of most common diseases. The first 160 pages provide this information in relation to a wide variety of diseases and conditions ranging from acne and alcoholism to warts and worms. This is followed by sections on protection against common poisons in our environment, directions for recommended therapies, recipes and charts and tables. This is our favorite home medical encyclopedia. Extensive notes and index, 301pp. HPP 74

AMBER, R. *PULSE IN THE OCCIDENT AND ORIENT,* c15.00. A detailed, scholarly study of the pulse and pulse diagnosis in the East and West. The material is arranged in almost outline form and the text includes an abundance of notes. Index, 218pp. NYA 66

Arthritis

It is estimated that over thirteen million Americans are afflicted with arthritis in its various forms. Arthritis is, perhaps, the most crippling and agonizing of all degenerative diseases. Although not as great a direct killer as, for example, cancer and heart diseases, arthritis causes more pain, despair, and suffering to more people than any other single disease. The most distressing fact about arthritis is that thirteen million or more arthritis sufferers are given no hope for cure or even relief from their discomfort and misery.—Paavo Airola, **There Is A Cure For Arthritis.**

The Arthritis Foundation, which is the leading authority in the United States, has flatly stated: *The relationship between diet and arthritis has been thoroughly and scientifically studied. The simple proven fact is: no food has anything to do with causing arthritis and no food is effective in treating or curing it.* Along with this view, conventional medicine has little to offer the arthritic except aspirin and sympathy.

Fortunately, there are a number of doctors who didn't accept the Foundation's simple proven fact and who have explored the relationship between arthritis—which is not one but many different diseases—and metabolic, nutritional and biochemical factors. They have frequently had remarkable success in treating arthritis by treating the whole person. If you are one of the twenty million in this country who suffer from arthritis and want more than aspirin and sympathy, you would do well to start reading among these books and decide if you wish to make the changes in eating and living habits that might bring the relief so desperately sought.

AIROLA, PAAVO. *THERE IS A CURE FOR ARTHRITIS,* 2.95. Airola reports on biological methods of treating arthritis which are widely used in European clinics. He has studied the therapies first hand and has used them in his own practice. A complete program is outlined and many case studies are included. This is a very useful book which we highly recommend. Index, 219pp. PrH 68

BECKETT, SARAH. *HERBS FOR RHEUMATISM AND ARTHRITIS,* 1.35. See the Herbs section.

BIRCHER-BENNER. *BIRCHER-BENNER NUTRITION PLAN FOR ARTHRITIS AND RHEUMATISM,* 1.50. Recipes and treatment suggestions by the staff of the Bircher-Benner Clinic. 127pp. Pyr 72

CAMPBELL, GIRAUD. *A DOCTOR'S PROVEN NEW HOME CURE FOR ARTHRITIS,* 2.95. Written by an osteopath, this book recommends avoidance of all processed and adulterated foods, use of raw and natural foods, good elimination, and a certain amount of osteopathic manipulation and exercise as needed. Although written with a little too much hype for our taste, the concepts appear sound and certainly worth trying by anyone suffering from arthritis. Bibliography, index, 224pp. PrH 72

CLEMENTS, HARRY. *ARTHRITIS,* 1.35. A discussion of causes, symptoms, and treatment. 64pp. TPL 73

DONG, COLLIN H. and JANE BANKS. *NEW HOPE FOR THE ARTHRITIC,* 1.95. Dr. Dong, who has treated thousands of arthritics over forty years, hypothesizes that the inciting factors are food allergens. The Dong diet avoids milk products, most meats, and fruits and fruit juices, as well as the usual chemical additives, etc. It's not too different from the recommendations of many nutritionists for good health and a long life. This book contains a review of standard treatments of arthritis, many case histories, discussion of the Dong diet, menus and several dozen recipes. There is also a chapter on use of acupuncture in arthritis. Extensive bibliography, index, 269pp. RaH 75

JARVIS, D.C. *ARTHRITIS AND FOLK MEDICINE,* 1.50. Dr. Jarvis is the M.D. who made an extensive study of Vermont folk medicine, observed the care of plants and animals, and reached many important conclusions for his medical practice that differed from what he had been taught in medical school. This book is fascinating reading because it goes back to basics and lets us see why things work the way they do. In particular, he advocates the use of vinegar and honey to keep blood calcium in solution so that it doesn't precipitate in the cells. How and why this works is explained in the text. In addition to any other book you read about arthritis, we think you'll find a great deal of interest in this one to help you understand how the body works. Index, 144pp. Faw 60

JENSEN, BERNARD. *OVERCOMING ARTHRITIS AND RHEU-MATISM,* 3.95. A collection of diet suggestions, and healing hints based on Dr. Jensen's experience with patients and on traditional naturopathic methods. 55pp. Jen nd

SCIENCE OF LIFE BOOKS. *RHEUMATISM AND ARTHRITIS,* 1.35. An outline of common causes and corrective measures including dietary treatments, vitamin therapy, and hydrotherapy. 62pp. SLB 75

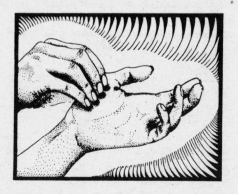

SPEIGHT, PHYLLIS. *OVERCOMING RHEUMATISM AND AR-THRITIS*, 1.10. A discussion of homoeopathic, herbal, and dietary remedies for rheumatism and arthritis. Each of the possible remedies is surveyed individually and there's also a homoeopathic index of symptoms. There's material in this small book which cannot be readily found elsewhere. 64pp. HSP 74

TOBE, JOHN. *HOW TO CONQUER ARTHRITIS*, c10.50. A scattered, badly written collection of possible arthritis cures and including Tobe's usual abundance of digressions. A tremendous amount of information is presented, though virtually none of the material is documented. Bibliography, index, 217+pp. Prv 76

WADE, CARLSON. *ARTHRITIS, NUTRITION AND NATURAL THERAPY*, 1.95. Wade discusses the causes of arthritis, and explores remedies, preventative measures, and palliatives. He also gives a number of warning signals and offers practical advice and recipe suggestions. The latest research is cited. 118pp. Kea 76

WARMBRAND, MAX. *HOW THOUSANDS OF MY ARTHRITIS PATIENTS REGAINED THEIR HEALTH*, 1.65. Similar to the following book, but written in a somewhat more popular vein. Includes diet suggestions, how to use water for relief of pain, exercises and helpful manipulative techniques. Dr. Warmbrand also surveys the role of vitamins and food supplements, and provides recipes and a guide to meals and beverages. Index, 225pp. Arc 70

WARMBRAND, MAX. *NEW HOPE FOR ARTHRITIS SUFFERERS*, c4.95. Dr. Warmbrand points out that the use of cortisone demonstrates that arthritis is a metabolic disorder; however, cortisone, like other drugs, has undesirable side effects. His method of therapy relies primarily on proper diet as part of a new way of life that will bring to play the natural healing power inherent in the organism. This book covers dietary and exercise requirements, tells what to expect during the transition period (problems that may be encountered), and also discusses related afflictions such as gout, rheumatic fever, bursitis and slipped discs. 153pp. TPL 68

WARMBRAND, MAX. *OVERCOMING ARTHRITIS AND OTHER RHEUMATIC DISEASES*, c8.95. This book presents an extremely positive, practical approach to treatment. Detoxification and raw foods form the basis of Dr. Warmbrand's approach. The elimination of stress and a life in harmony with nature are equally important, as is appropriate exercise. This is a simply written account, replete with case studies which should inspire and aid all arthritis sufferers. Dr. Warmbrand is one of America's best known naturopathic physicians. 220pp. DAC 76

WELSH, PHILLIP. *HOW TO BE FREE FROM ARTHRITIS,* 7.95. Dr. Welsh is a dentist and naturopath, with more than fifty years of experience treating people nutritionally. He considers white sugar, white flour, and salt to be the three leading offenders in arthritis. All additives must also be avoided. He prescribes a cleansing course and then a basic diet primarily of fresh fruit and vegetables. This book is written in a simple style, easy to follow. It also includes quotations from many other writers who have treated arthritis nutritionally, plus a large number of recipes. Spiral bound, bibliography, 8½"x11", 107pp. WoP 74

Bach Flower Remedies

Edward Bach was an English physician who felt that sickness and disease were primarily due not to physical causes, but to some deeper disharmony within the sufferer himself. These conclusions were strengthened and confirmed by his observations during sixteen years of practice. In 1930 he determined to devote all of his time to the search for a simple method of treatment and harmless remedies among the wild flowers of the countryside. He worked with them until his death in 1936 and found thirty-eight remedies; all, with one exception, the flowers of plants, trees, and bushes. The remedies are prescribed not directly for the physical complaint, but rather according to the sufferer's state of mind, according to his moods of fear, worry, anger or depression. The patient himself decides which remedies s/he should take and how long to continue taking them. The remedies are absolutely benign in their action. Therefore they can be safely prescribed and used by anyone.

BACH, EDWARD. *HEAL THYSELF,* .85. Dr. Bach's first book on his philosophy of healing, subtitled *An Explanation of the Real Cause and Cure of Disease.* This small book is one of the most inspiring works we have ever read and we highly recommend it to all who are interested in the philosophy of natural healing. 56pp. Dan 31

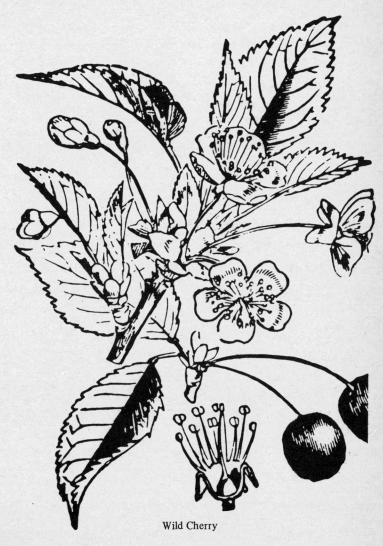

Wild Cherry

BACH, EDWARD. *TWELVE HEALERS,* .60. Dr. Bach's basic book, in which he describes the thirty-eight remedies, one for each of the most common negative states of mind, or moods that afflict mankind. He divides these negative states of mind into seven groups under the following headings: fear, uncertainty, insufficient interest in present circumstances, loneliness, oversensitivity to influences and ideas, despondency or despair, and overconcern for the welfare of others. In addition, he gives directions for preparation of the remedies and dosage. 30pp. Dan 33

CHANCELLOR, PHILIP, ed. *HANDBOOK OF THE BACH FLOWER REMEDIES,* c7.20. This is the newest and most comprehensive of the books on the remedies. Much of the material is taken from *The Bach Remedy News Letter,* edited by Nora Weeks. Includes an excellent section "Prescribing and the Interview: for Oneself, for Pregnancy and Childbirth, for Children, for Mental Distress, for Animals, for Plants." There's also a separate chapter on each of the remedies and notes on prescribing, together with many case histories to illustrate the use of the remedies in the home as well as by the practitioner. Bibliography, index, 251pp. Dan 71

EVANS, JANE. *INTRODUCTION TO THE BENEFITS OF THE BACH FLOWER REMEDIES,* .70. 19pp. Dan 74

WEEKS, NORA. *THE MEDICAL DISCOVERIES OF EDWARD BACH, PHYSICIAN,* c4.80. Ms. Weeks runs the Bach Healing Centre in England. This is the only critical account of Dr. Bach's work available. 144pp. Dan 40

WEEKS, NORA and VICTOR BULLEN. *BACH FLOWER REMEDIES,* c7.25. Contains botanical descriptions and colored illustrations of the remedy flowers and the exact method of preparing each one. 98pp. Dan 64

WHEELER, F.J. *THE BACH FLOWER REMEDIES REPERTORY,* .60. A supplementary guide to the use of the herbal remedies discovered by Dr. Bach, designed as an aid to those seeking to develop their own ability to choose and administer the right remedy. In outline form. 28pp. Dan 52

BAILEY, ALICE. *ESOTERIC HEALING,* 6.75. *In this book the seven ray techniques of healing are described, the laws and rules of healing are enumerated and discussed, the requirements for healing are given in detail, and basic causes of diseases are shown. We learn, for example, that much disease can be karmic in origin, that certain diseases are inherent in the soil and the substance of the planet, and that many others are psychological arising in the mental and emotional bodies.* 771pp. LPC 53

BAILEY, HERBERT. *GH3: WILL IT KEEP YOU YOUNG LONG-ER?* 1.95. GH3 (Gerovital H3) has been widely used in Europe. It slows down the aging process and helps to regenerate cells. It is also used as an antidepressant and to reduce hypertension and arthritis. Bailey devoted many years to the preparation of this detailed survey of GH3. The bulk of the book is twenty-five technical appendices written by members of the medical profession which evaluate GH3 in specific instances. As yet, GH3 is not able to be prescribed in the U.S. Bibliography, notes, index, 350pp. Ban 77

BAKER, DOUGLAS. *ESOTERIC HEALING,* 14.00. This is the most comprehensive treatise we have seen on the title subject. Baker is an English surgeon, among other things. This 11¾"x8" tome is profusely illustrated, including many full color plates, and is divided into four parts: *The Origin and Nature of Esoteric Healing, Some Common Disorders, Some Esoteric Healing Methods* and *Nutrition and Preventive Medicine.* The techniques and background material emphasize the energy centers and rays and the use of healing energy in general. The material is practical and many illustrations illuminate the text. 266pp. Bak 75

BAKER, DOUGLAS. *ESOTERIC HEALING: STRESS DISORDERS,* 14.00. A fully illustrated discussion of four topics: stress disorders, the Bach flower remedies, alcoholism, and the completion of cycles. Dr. Baker is at his best when he is writing about the esoteric aspects of health and healing. In this book he covers a great deal of interesting information, albeit in his usual scattered way. Many color plates, very fully indexed, 8"x11¼", 260+pp. Bak 76

BENJAMIN, HARRY. *EVERYBODY'S GUIDE TO NATURE CURE,* c11.70. A comprehensive and illuminating treatise on the nature of disease and its treatment by natural methods written by an English naturopath. Includes in depth discussions of diseases of all parts of the human organism, with specific as well as general treatments. Index, 487pp. TPL 61

BLAINE, TOM. *GOODBYE ALLERGIES,* 2.95. Judge Blaine suffered severely from allergies, tried many treatments with scant results, and finally learned of what was for him and many others most successful—a combination of an anti-hypoglycemic diet with treatment of hypoadrenocorticism. Blaine has researched the literature and checked his findings with many M.D.'s. Recommended to all allergy sufferers. 159pp. CiP 65

BLYTHE, PETER. *DRUGLESS MEDICINE,* c6.70. This is a sympathetic, well researched journalistic survey of herbalism, homoeopathy, naturopathy, osteopathy, and chiropracty. The author is a British psychotherapist, best known for his work in hypnotism. Many case studies of practitioners and patients are cited. The account is fragmented and incomplete, nonetheless the reader can learn a fair amount about each of these alternative methods of healing from Blythe's presentation. Notes, index, 175pp. Wdf 74

BOYD, DOUG. *ROLLING THUNDER,* 3.45. Rolling Thunder is an American Indian medicine man. As a medicine man, or shaman, he is guardian of a wealth of knowledge that has been passed down through countless Indian generations. This knowledge includes the power to cure disease and heal wounds, to find and use medicinal herbs, to make rain, to transport objects through the air, and to communicate telepathically. These powers come out of his special relationship with nature, with what can only be called a *spirit of the earth.* This remarkable book is a record of an attempt to learn something about the sources of the medicine man's powers. With Rolling Thunder's full cooperation, Doug Boyd, on a research field trip for the Menninger Foundation, spent a long time observing him and he reports in detail on his observations here. A fascinating account. 283pp. Del 74

BRENA, STEVEN. *YOGA AND MEDICINE,* 2.45. See the Yoga subsection of Body Work.

BRICKLIN, MARK. *NATURAL HEALING,* 12.95. This is an extremely complete presentation of both the theories and practical applications of natural healing. The author is the Executive Editor of **Prevention Magazine.** The material is topically arranged and the book itself is fully indexed. Annotated bibliographies are included

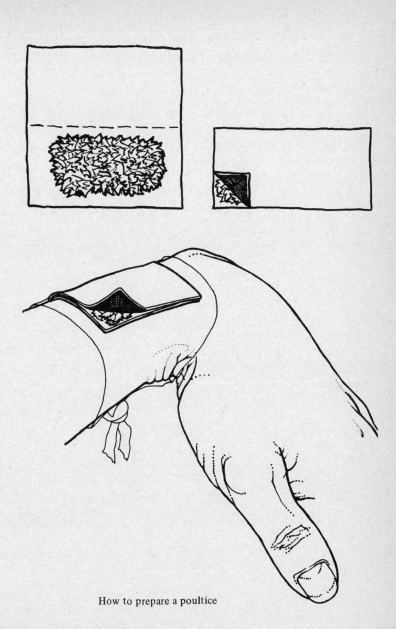

How to prepare a poultice

for some of the major sections along with descriptions of related schools. 602pp. Rod 76

BROWN, BARBARA. *STRESS AND THE ART OF BIOFEED-BACK,* c12.50. Dr. Brown here presents the first comprehensive formulation of how to use biofeedback to treat a variety of illnesses and, especially, to relieve conditions related to stress. She also outlines a number of related concepts and psychotherapeutic measures. This is a technical work which outlines clinical procedure. Nonetheless, the interested layman should be able to understand the material. Bibliography, index, 309pp. H&R 77

BURANG, THEODORE. *TIBETAN ART OF HEALING,* 5.00. *The medicine indigenous to Tibet is highly respected throughout Central Asia and has a remarkable record of success in healing. Its philosophy and curative methods transport us into a strange web of macrocosmic and microcosmic interrelations. In contrast to the standpoint of Western research, it acquaints us with unusual spiritual foundations. . .and often displays a masterful observation of nature.* The material is divided into the following parts: *The Cosmic Humours, The Second Body, Tibetan Medical Writings, Materia Medica, Tibetan Methods of Healing, About Cancer, Mental Illness and Possession,* and *Co-operation Between Western and Tibetan Doctors.* The style is not overly technical and the general reader can gain much from the book. 117pp. Wat 74

Cancer

Cancer is insidious, generally pain-free in the initial stages, and frequently deadly by the time it is detectable. It has been described as savage cells which somehow evade the laws of the body, corrupt the forces which normally protect the body, invade the well-ordered society of cells that surround it, colonise distant areas, and as a finale to this cannibalistic orgy of flesh consuming flesh, commit suicide by destroying the host. A more prosaic definition is that cancer is a disorder in which cells in the body multi-

ply in a seemingly unchecked way, a proliferation in which they tend to lose or change their normal biochemical characteristics.

Every second of every day, a man, woman, or child dies of cancer. The malignant, crab-like cellular malfunction, which begins to multiply at bewildering speed in their body tissue, will for those countless millions, tragically bring the realisation that their cancer could not be cured, controlled, or even contained, by the usual methods of surgery, radiotherapy and chemotherapy. Four out of every five persons who receive one, or all, of these treatments die within five years. That is not only an indication of the destructive power of the disease, but also a sobering reflection on the limits of standard techniques, and the concepts of cancer on which they are based.

These methods have one common factor. They treat cancer "in loco." The failure of these methods usually means the patient is left to die—unaware that there is another proven and positive treatment still available, one that totally discounts the popular concept that cancer is a "local" disease. Because it involves the entire bodily defense systems, it is called whole-body treatment. It is my contention, based on twenty-five years of clinical experience with over eight thousand cancer patients, that only by recognising that the disease is, and always has been, one affecting the whole body from the outset, can it be more effectively arrested. —condensed from **Cancer** by Josef Issels.

In the United States the only legal treatments for cancer are surgery, radiation or chemicals. Each of these is destructive to the body. Any other treatments, even though completely non-toxic, require approval by the FDA—a process that takes years and can be additionally hampered by the prejudices of the establishment. As the American Cancer Society has stated: *Research is to be strongly encouraged— but only in the framework of the accepted ideology.* The Government has gone to great lengths to prosecute non-orthodox researchers: witness the imprisonment of Wilhelm Reich and the burning of his books.

The unorthodox approach to cancer treatment swings away from the attempt to destroy cancer cells themselves (dealing with the symptoms) to a concerted effort to restore the sick host to a state of health by mustering up the inherent natural defense mechanisms of the body (dealing with the cause). Cancer is thus regarded as a degenerative disease of the entire system and much of the treatment (detoxification and nutritional improvement) is essentially the same as for any other degenerative disease. There is considerable evidence that these unorthodox methods work if the individual is willing to make the necessary changes in his/her living habits and the cancer is not too far advanced. For example, the author of **A Program for Prevention, Detection and Reversal of Pre-Cancerous Conditions** reports following some 400 cancer victims over a ten year period. Of 268 who followed their (unorthodox) doctor's instructions and did not change their living habits, 7% survived. Of 57 early and precancer involvements who followed the recommended approach without professional help, 100% survived. Of 41 advanced cases who followed the recommendations (and in some cases got therapy outside the U.S.), 90% survived. And of 39 *terminal cases* who followed the recommendations, 46% were still alive at the time of writing.

There are three organizations championing non-toxic cancer therapies and promoting public awareness of alternatives: International Association of Cancer Victims and Friends, Inc. (PO Box 707, Solana Beach, CA 92075), Cancer Control Society (2043 N. Berendo, Los Angeles, CA 90027), and Committee for Freedom of Choice in Cancer Therapy, Inc. (146 Main Street, Suite 408, Los Altos, CA 94022).

AGRAN, LARRY. *THE CANCER CONNECTION AND WHAT WE CAN DO ABOUT IT,* c8.95. Agran is an attorney who was director of UCLA's History of Cancer Control Project, a federally funded investigation of the U.S.'s national cancer policy. He contends that ninety percent of human cancer originates in the artificial environment that pollutes our air, land, and water—thus our food and lungs. Cancer therefore is largely a man made disease, and it is up to us to do something about it. Agran's message is that we, as voters, consumers, politicians, teachers, must work toward the limitation of carcinogens in the environment. Notes, index, 256pp. HMC 77

AIROLA, PAAVO. *CANCER: CAUSES, PREVENTION AND TREATMENT,* 2.00. An excellent overview of twenty-two causes of cancer, possible cures, and a discussion of the biological anticancer program. Includes many addresses of clinics and references to the literature. 40pp. HPP 72

BORDERLAND SCIENCES. *THE KOCH REMEDY FOR CANCER,* 4.45. Includes three separate essays: *The Koch Treatment* (involving blood purification), *The Occult and Karmic Causes of Cancer,* and *The Electro-Magnetic Approach to Health*—restoring the balanced polarity of body cells with soft radio waves and/or homoeopathic remedies. This is a detailed, graphically illustrated account, designed for practical use and inspiration. Includes newspaper clippings, quotations, and comments by N. Meader Layne and Riley Crabb. Bibliography, oversize, 70pp. BSR 71

CULBERT, MICHAEL. *FREEDOM FROM CANCER,* 2.95. This is a comprehensive review of the laetrile story by a man who started out as a skeptical newspaper reporter and went on to become a laetrile activist. Despite the obstruction and obfuscation of the authorities laetrile proponents are slowly winning the war: it has been made legal in Alaska, several state judges have issued orders permitting cancer victims to bring it into the country for their own use, the Sloan-Kettering studies were bottled up by the Institute but leaked by insiders who wanted to see them made public. This book will not only raise your ire but will also give you a good overview of what laetrile is and is not good for. Includes recipes and advice on getting laetrile from natural sources. Bibliography, index, 238pp. SSP 76

EAST WEST FOUNDATION. *A DIETARY APPROACH TO CANCER ACCORDING TO THE PRINCIPLES OF MACROBIOTICS,* 2.95. Transcription of a lecture by Michio Kushi and reproductions of a series of case studies and two technical papers. 38pp. EWF nd

FERE, MAUD. *DOES DIET CURE CANCER,* 4.70. Dr. Fere cured herself of cancer of the bowel. Her hypothesis is that cancer is a constitutional disease, like rheumatism or the common cold. She believes that it is almost always caused by excessive sodium, plus a constitution that has been debilitated through breaking the "Laws of Good Health"—which are listed and explained in detail. Dr. Fere is a medical doctor and she details her cure in terms other doctors as well as laymen can understand. In the process she provides a succinct biochemic explanation of what causes cancer and how it starts forming in the body. 112pp. TPL 71

FYFE, AGNES. *MOON AND PLANT: CAPILLARY DYNAMIC STUDIES,* 6.75. An analysis of the capillary-dynamolysis studies of the formative or etheric forces in plants suggested by Rudolf Steiner and researched by some of his followers. The theoretical basis of the technique is discussed, experiments are cited, and practical instruction is offered. Many photographs illustrate the results of some studies. 30pp. SCR 75

GERSON, MAX. *A CANCER THERAPY—RESULTS OF FIFTY CASES,* 7.95. A detailed, technical book by one of the great pioneers of nutritional therapy of cancer. Directed primarily to physicians with a theoretical discussion, complete dietary directions, and fifty case histories. 402pp. Can 58

GLASSER, RONALD. *THE GREATEST BATTLE,* c6.95. *The cancers we are seeing today did not begin yesterday or the day before, but twenty, thirty and even forty years ago. Scientists now agree that most adult malignancies have their beginning in childhood, adolescence and early life, some indeed even before birth. Not everything, by any means, is known about the causes of cancer, but enough is known for physicians to say unequivocally that 75 to 85 percent of all cancers have nothing to do with viruses or even genetics, that they do not develop from trauma or because of infections, but result solely from exposure to environmental causes and industrial pollutants. . . .For many of us, exposed for most of our lives, it may already be too late. But there is no reason why our children too should be doomed. There is still time to save them. That is what this book is all about.*—from the preface. 188pp. RaH 76

GRIFFIN, EDWARD. *WORLD WITHOUT CANCER,* 4.00/set. A two volume set: **The Science of Cancer Therapy** and **The Politics of Cancer Therapy.** Griffith is a member of the John Birch Society and much of the books are devoted to polemics against international cartels and governmental monopolies. The subject that Griffith devotes the most energy to is an energetic defense of laetrile and he cites data and cases. A journalistic report. Index, 558pp. AmM 74

HAUGHT, S.J. *HAS DR. MAX GERSON A TRUE CANCER CURE?* 1.50. The late Dr. Max Gerson developed a method of cancer treatment that relied heavily on diet and body cleansing. He became controversial due to the apparent success of his method and the simultaneous obstruction and vituperation by the AMA and the American Cancer Society. This is a fascinating account by a journalist who planned an expose and the more he dug into the story the more he was convinced of the value of what Dr. Gerson was doing. 160pp. Par 62

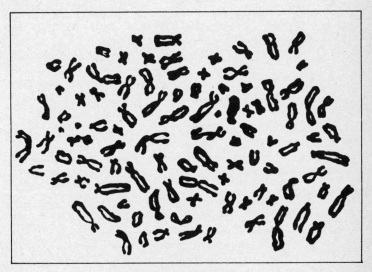

Cancerous Cell Chromosomes

INTERNATIONAL HEALTH COUNCIL. *A PROGRAM FOR THE PREVENTION, DETECTION AND REVERSAL OF PRE-CAN-CEROUS CONDITIONS,* 1.75. This booklet is written by a layman who devoted himself to a thorough study of cancer after his son died from it. In addition to reviewing the literature, he interviewed several hundred cancer victims, following them to success or death. The booklet contains a good summary of the nutritional, detoxification, enzyme, and laetrile approaches. It also provides addresses and full details on obtaining urine and blood tests to diagnose cancer earlier than is possible by orthodox approaches. We recommend this as the best brief treatment of the subject we've seen. 44pp. IHC 74

ISSELS, JOSEF. *CANCER: A SECOND OPINION*, c11.98. Dr. Issels is a noted German cancer specialist who has treated over 8000 patients with considerably better than average results. He is known for his *ganzheitstherapie*—whole body treatment—which views cancer as a systemic disease and supplements surgery or other conventional therapies with a whole array of methods to help the body build up its own resistance and immunities. This is an excellent, comprehensive book, which surveys much of the history of medicine, provides a pointed short course in relevant physiology, and covers broadly the state of knowledge about cancer and its origins. It is written primarily for physicians but can be read with great profit by anyone else who can handle the technical terminology. Dr. Issels writes from a basis of extensive European research which is not hung up by our unfortunate American legalities. Extensive bibliography, but mostly in German. 216pp. Hod 75

KELLEY, WILLIAM. *NEW HOPE FOR CANCER VICTIMS*, 1.55. An excellent simple discussion. Kelley, a dentist by background, cured himself of cancer and now studies and treats cancer. He considers cancer a symptom of protein metabolism malfunction—a deficiency disease, which can be treated by detoxification, proper nutrition, and ingestion of pancreatic enzymes. 42pp. NuB 69

KELLEY, WILLIAM. *ONE ANSWER TO CANCER*, 1.50. This is Kelley's latest book with the regimen he favors described in some detail. While he gives general recommendations regarding nutritional supplements and enzymes in the book, he is unable, for legal reasons, to recommend specific brands. For that, one can go to a series of three interviews with him printed in the **Cancer News Journal** of the International Association of Cancer Victims and Friends. Can

KITTLER, GLENN. *LAETRILE, CONTROL FOR CANCER*, 1.50. A journalist's account of the development of what has been called the most effective drug against cancer which is also harmless to other tissues, and the struggle with medical orthodoxy to have it tested and used. Includes case histories and evaluations from many research scientists. 255pp. War 63

KREBS, ERNEST, et al. *THE LAETRILES-NITRILOSIDES IN PREVENTION AND CONTROL OF CANCER,* 3.00. Technical papers on laetrile treatment by the leaders in its development. Directed to physicians. 88pp. McN nd

LAYNE, N. MEADE and RILEY CRABB. *THE KOCH REMEDY FOR CANCER AND OTHER DISEASES,* 4.40. A collection of three non-technical polemical style papers: *The Koch Treatment for Cancer and Allied Allergies, The Occult and Karmic Causes of Cancer,* and *The Electro-Magnetic Approach to Health.* Many far out ideas and theories are suggested and practical applications are offered along with case studies. Bibliography, 8½"x11", 71pp. BSR 71

LEROI, A. *THE CELL, THE HUMAN ORGANISM AND CANCER,* .95. Leroi is a doctor at the Society for Cancer Research in Arlesheim, Switzerland. Here he points out that the causes of cancer should be sought in the entire organism, not just in the cells. The problem is not eradicating the diseased cells, but rather healing the diseased human being. Includes references, mainly from European sources. 24pp. NKB 61

LIVINGSTON, VIRGINIA. *CANCER: A NEW BREAKTHROUGH,* 5.80. Dr. Livingston is an outstanding, long time cancer researcher who believes cancer is infectious. Her treatment involves use of autogenous vaccines (i.e., prepared from one's own blood) plus good diet, blood transfusions, vitamins and antibiotic and other medicines. All are intended to build up the body's self-healing powers instead of using surgery, radiation and chemotherapy. Much of the book is highly technical. It also provides many vivid details of the efforts of the FDA and American Cancer Society to prevent research on non-toxic approaches which differ from the established ideology. Laetrile is discussed sympathetically. Illustrations, index, 269pp. Dut 72

MCNAUGHTON FOUNDATION. *PHYSICIANS HANDBOOK OF VITAMIN B-17 THERAPY,* 2.00. A collection of a number of technical suggestions. Notes, 32pp. McN 75

MAE, EYDIE. *HOW I CONQUERED CANCER NATURALLY,* 3.95. This is a personal story of one woman's search for a better way to deal with cancer. She followed the method of Ann Wigmore which emphasizes thorough cleansing, eating only organic raw foods, and, in particular, use of wheat grass juice. As in other nutritional approaches, it cannot be said that the cancer is cured; only that it is held in remission as long as the strict diet is continued. The book is a little too folksy in tone for our taste, but its essence can be invaluable to cancer sufferers. Includes instructions on how to do everything and many recipes. Bibliography, index, 211pp. HvH 75

MEDEXPORT, V.O. *VITAMIN B-15 (PANGAMIC ACID),* 1.40. Indications for use and efficacy in internal disease. 33pp. McN 60

REICH, WILHELM. *THE CANCER BIOPATHY,* 5.95. In his controversial theories, reprinted here for the first time, Reich defines cancer not as a tumor—the tumor is merely a late manifestation of the disease—but as a systemic disease due to chronic thwarting of natural sexual functioning. The material here was originally published as Volume II of **The Discovery of the Orgone**, Volume I being **The Function of the Orgasm.** See the Reich subsection in Life Energies for more on his work. Illustrations, photographs, index, 458pp. FSG 73

SCIENCE PUBLISHING HOUSE. *VITAMIN B-15 (PANGAMIC ACID): PROPERTIES, FUNCTIONS AND USE,* 7.00. A translation of various studies carried out by the U.S.S.R. Academy of Sciences on Pangamic Acid and on one of its analogs, Dipan. Very technical material. Ernst Krebs has contributed a foreword. 205pp. Can 65

SCOTT, CYRIL. *VICTORY OVER CANCER,* 3.00. Scott is a naturopath who believes that there are several prime causes of cancer, including oxygen starvation and the consumption of over-salted foods. In this volume he explains these causes and seeks to establish the concept that cancer is a blood disease. He advances reasons for the increase of cancer and reveals the failure of orthodox research and treatment. Drugs, food, and chronic constipation are also discussed in relation to cancer. The second half of the book is devoted to a review of unorthodox cancer treatments. Notes, 168pp. HSP 39

SUN, WONG HON. *HOW I OVERCAME INOPERABLE CANCER,* c6.00. A self-published book, subtitled *The true account of a man who conquered the dread disease by using the principles of natural healing.* Wong Hon Sun is now a naturopath. 125pp. ExP 75

TOBE, JOHN H. *HOW TO PREVENT AND GAIN REMISSION FROM CANCER,* c12.85. Tobe is an outspoken iconoclast who has written a great many books on different nutritional and naturopathic subjects. Here he takes on the whole cancer establishment, which he accuses of having a vested interest in cancer rather than its cure. Much of the book discusses the various foods and drugs to avoid, some well recognized and some not fully established as carcinogenic, but probably worth avoiding anyway. He reviews a number of the non-toxic cancer treatments such as laetrile, but comes out most strongly in favor of an all raw food diet. Tobe has obviously done a great deal of research but the book is marred by a lack of footnotes or complete citations and a tendency to quote from newspaper accounts or refer to unknown (to us) persons as the famous Dr. So and So. For all our criticisms, there is a lot of value for anyone doing serious reading on cancer. Bibliography, index, 402pp. Prv 75

WAERLAND, EBBA. *CANCER—A DISEASE OF CIVILISATION,* 1.50. Brief discussion of the biological basis of cancer, in particular disturbed cellular respiration. Advocates the Waerland diet—primarily raw food. 54pp. Prv 70

CARLSON, RICK, ed. *THE FRONTIERS OF SCIENCE AND MEDICINE,* 3.95. Transcription of a collection of papers delivered at a conference on the title theme. The following selections give a good idea of the coverage: *Consciousness and Commitment* by Werner Erhard, *Is Primitive Medicine Really Primitive* by Lyall Watson, *Biofeedback and Voluntary Control of Internal States* by Elmer Green, *The Role of Psychics in Mental Diagnosis* by Norman Shealy, *The Role of the Mind in Cancer Therapy* by Carl Simonton, *In-depth Studies of Uri Geller* by Andrija Puharich. Notes, 224pp. Reg 75

CARMEN, RICHARD. *OUR ENDANGERED HEARING,* c7.95. Almost thirty-two million Americans suffer some degree of hearing loss, and the number is on the increase. Carmen, a clinical audiologist, examines the psychological and social effects of hearing loss. He discusses various sources of noise in our environment, and how we can and must protect our hearing. A long section of the book is devoted to the various hearing disorders, their causes and treatments. Another chapter surveys hearing aids. Questions and answers and case histories are also included. Illustrations, index, 224pp. Rod 77

CARTER, MARY ELLEN and WILLIAM MCGAREY. *EDGAR CAYCE ON HEALING,* 1.50. *This book is about a psychic and his work in suggesting methods by which healing might come to the human body.* These suggestions centered on the field of medicine and spread out over osteopathy, chiropractic, physical therapy, herbal therapy, nutrition, spiritual therapy, hypnotherapy, dentistry, and what is best described as *"other methods."* The major part of the book consists of Ms. Carter's narrative of the lives of several people (some critically ill) who, through Cayce's suggestions, regained their health as well as a different perspective on life. Each of Ms. Carter's accounts is followed by Dr. McGarey's discussion of the physiological concepts and the various therapies which Cayce suggested. Dr. McGarey is Director of the A.R.E. Clinic. 205pp. War 72

CASSELL, ERIC. *THE HEALER'S ART,* c8.95. *An important and timely book that emphasizes the difference between curing the disease and healing the patient—or rather helping the patient heal himself.*—Rene Dubos. Dr. Cassell fully explores the role of doctor as healer and discusses the complex interaction between doctor and patient that makes sick people get well. He also explains why the doctor's ability to connect with his patient is as important as his scientific skills. Dr. Cassell provides dramatic case histories which illustrate how the sick person can become an active partner in treatment. The book ends with a powerful chapter, *Overcoming the Fear of Dying* which details Dr. Cassell's remarkable success in helping terminally ill patients. Bibliography, index, 240pp. Lip 76

CAYCE, EDGAR. *MEDICINES FOR THE NEW AGE,* 1.50. This is the most detailed account of the remedies suggested in the Cayce readings. The material is alphabetically arranged by remedies and is paraphrased from the original readings with some background information on the remedy. The appropriate circulating files are cited by number (these files are available only to A.R.E. members) and manufacturers' product names for Cayce formulas are also given. Appendices contain an alphabetical listing of publications and files on related subjects, a cross-reference guide to selected conditions and recommendations, a partial listing of medical circulating files available from the A.R.E., and a list of products recommended in the readings that are not currently available. 47+pp. Her 74

CAYCE, J. GAIL. *OSTEOPATHY,* 3.00. A comparison of various parallel concepts expressed by A.T. Still, the founder of Osteopathy, and Edgar Cayce. Excerpts from both sources are examined with brief comments between the extracts. The material is topically arranged and an appendix explores several topics in further detail. *It is hoped that this survey will serve as a tool and as a foundation for expansion of the various points presented in the outline. . . .* Bibliography, oversize, 64pp. ARE 73

CERNEY, J.V. *HANDBOOK OF UNUSUAL AND UNORTHODOX HEALING METHODS,* c8.95. In the introduction Cerney summarizes his book as follows: *Section I tells the story of those amazing "Z" zones that not only treat you, but can be used to diagnose your own problems. Section II is composed of healing agents called herbs, cell salts, raw juice and fasting. Section III has to do with physical therapy procedures you can use in your home, procedures such as somatherapy, the body cure, spinal concussion, percussion, vibration, and aquatonics.* The orientation is toward the general reader and the emphasis is on practical advice and case studies. Index, 217pp. PrH 76

CERNEY, J.V. *MODERN MAGIC OF NATURAL HEALING WITH WATER THERAPY,* c8.95. Dr. Cerney has had over thirty years of experience with water therapy, mainly in the line of physical fitness for athletes. He devotes a separate section to water treatments for each of the following parts of the body: the head, the neck, the shoulder, the upper extremities, the chest, the back, the abdomen, the lower extremities, and the skin. The treatments are clearly presented and can be followed with ease. Index, 216pp. PrH 75

CHAITOW, LEON. *OSTEOPATHY,* 4.50. A practicing osteopath explains the origin of osteopathy and its development. The ailments which respond well to osteopathic treatment—including lumbago, sciatica, brachial neuritis, neuralgia, slipped disc, migraine, insomnia, asthma, cardiac conditions, and bronchial and catarrhal disorders—are discussed and a selection of case histories drawn from the author's own experience is presented. Dr. Chaitow also reviews the latest trends in osteopathic research and training. The text is very well illustrated and many exercises and techniques are presented. Glossary, 92pp. TPL 74

CHALLONER, H.K. *THE PATH OF HEALING,* 3.25. An inspiring book on the true nature and function of spiritual healing. 175pp. TPH 72

CHERASKIN, E. and W.M. RINGSDORF. *NEW HOPE FOR IN-*

CURABLE DISEASES, 1.65. An easily understood, concise work which shows scientifically that nutrition and diet play a large role in the determination of a disease. The book presents medical findings which show that glaucoma, multiple sclerosis, schizophrenia, alcoholism and other problems, including aging, can be controlled or prevented with proper diet and nutrition. Notes, 187pp. Arc 71

CHERASKIN, E., W.M. RINGSDORF and J.W. CLARK. *DIET AND DISEASE,* 5.95. Dr. Cheraskin, trained both in medicine and dentistry, is one of the leading academic nutritional researchers today. Together with his colleagues at the University of Alabama Medical Center, he here presents a thorough review of findings about the relationship of diet and disease. Originally written as a college text, with voluminous footnotes, it has recently been given wider circulation because of its value to concerned general readers. Index, 369pp. Rod 68

CHRISTOPHER, JOHN. *THE COLD SHEET TREATMENT AND AIDS FOR THE COMMON COLD,* 1.25. A number of detailed suggestions on dealing with the flu and with the common cold based on herbalogy and on the principles of naturopathy. Dr. Christopher is a naturopath. 10pp. Crs 76

CHRISTOPHER, JOHN. *THE INCURABLES,* 1.50. A collection of graduated healing recommendations for those with cancer and other degenerative diseases. Specific suggestions are offered. 10pp. Crs 76

CLARK, LINDA. *GET WELL NATURALLY,* 1.95. Ms. Clark is a reporter who has a deep interest in nutrition and alternative healing techniques. In this compendium she begins by presenting a good review of many healing techniques including homoeopathy, Bach flower remedies, herbs, acupuncture and pressure therapy, radiesthesia, and material from the Edgar Cayce readings. From there she goes on to summarize the various nutritional therapies. The main body of the book is a section entitled "Treating Diseases Naturally" in which the author devotes a separate section to many ailments and reviews the applicable remedies and the literature on the subject, and also cites sources (with addresses) for many of the items and individuals mentioned in her survey. There's also a good, albeit outdated, bibliography. A well written, informative survey. Index, 406pp. Arc 65

CLARK, LINDA. *HANDBOOK OF NATURAL REMEDIES FOR COMMON AILMENTS,* c9.95. This is Ms. Clark's newest and most organized compendium of healing hints. The book is arranged by ailments and a variety of types of treatments are suggested. The discussion is quite complete and well written and incorporates the latest research. Bibliography, notes, index, 291pp. DAC 76

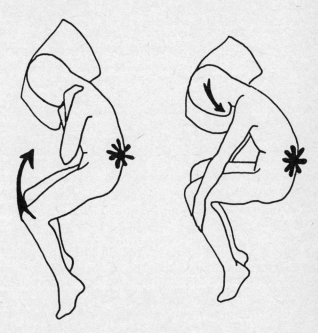

CLARK, LINDA. *HELP YOURSELF TO HEALTH,* 1.75. An inspirational approach to healing through prayer and positive thinking. Topically arranged and basically composed of case histories of countless individuals. Bibliography, index, 267pp. Pyr 72

CLEMENTS, HARRY. *BANISHING BACKACHES AND DISC TROUBLES,* 1.35. An osteopath investigates backaches and related disorders. Details of treatment are provided, based on a sensible diet, corrective exercise, and relaxation. 64pp. TPL 74

CLEMENTS, HARRY. *THE CAUSES AND TREATMENT OF HEADACHES AND MIGRAINE,* 1.35. Clements emphasizes that a headache is a symptom, not a disease. 64pp. TPL 73

CLEMENTS, HARRY. *PAINFUL JOINTS,* 1.35. A selection of natural measures for eliminating the pain and discomfort resulting from strains and minor injuries to joints. Also includes simple tests for determining the amount of free-play movement within joints. 64pp. TPL 73

CLEMENTS, HARRY. *SELF-TREATMENT FOR HERNIA,* 1.35. A selection of useful exercises for hernia problems, including details on the "sloping board" method of influencing the muscles of the lower abdominal wall. Specific diets are also offered. 64pp. TPL 73

COCA, ARTHUR. *THE PULSE TEST,* 1.95. Based on the fact that allergens speed up the pulse, this book provides a simple method by which the reader can conduct his own allergy tests simply and effectively. Dr. Coca was President of the American Association of Immunologists and founder of the **Journal of Immunology**, the foremost medical publication in this field. 189pp. Arc 56

CRABB, RILEY and JUDY. *THE HEART TO HEART TRANS-PLANT,* 1.75. A scattered tract on the conscious use of the subconscious to promote health through positive thinking from a metaphysical point of view, with relation to the energy centers and the etheric body. Oversize, 44pp. BSR nd

DAVIS, ADELLE. *LET'S GET WELL,* **1.95. This is our favorite Davis: we keep it on our shelf along with Airola's** *How to Get Well* **as our two home medical encyclopedias. When anything ails us we look it up in the excellent index. It's all here, including fifty-five pages of medical references in small print! Her final chapter, "A Fortress Against Disease" summarizes the unfortunate state of our national health as well as anything we've seen. 476pp. NAL 65**

DAVIS, ROY EUGENE. *HEALTH, HEALING AND TOTAL LIVING,* 2.95. A practical collection of guidelines on our innate potential to fully express health and creativity. The following chapter headings give a good idea of the approach: *How to Live as a Life-Giving Spirit, How to Prepare for Health and Fulfillment, How to Breathe for Health, How Yoga Poses Can Enhance Awareness, How to Eat for Sound Nutrition, How Gems and Metals May Influence the Human Body.* Davis has written many spiritual self-help books. Illustrations, 126pp. CSA 76

DECKER, NELSON and RILEY CRABB. *PSYCHIC SURGERY,* 2.35. A collection of scattered material entitled fully **Psychic Surgery in the Philippines (and in Brazil), Bible Kahuna Healers in Hawaii, New Age Therapy in California.** Some interesting material is presented, none of it in any way verified. Illustrations, stapled, 8½"x11", 51pp. BSR 74

DEXTREIT, RAYMOND. *OUR EARTH, OUR CURE,* 4.95. This book is compiled, edited, and translated by Michael Abehsera from the forty-three books written by Dextreit. *Mr. Dextreit brings something new to medical practice. . .for in addition to his authoritative use of food, herbs, and baths, and his extensive knowledge of the human organism, Mr. Dextreit has mastered the use of clay for curative purposes. . . .A basic principle in Mr. Dextreit's medicine is that when undertaking to heal ourselves, treating the general condition is more primary than relieving a specific manifestation, for a "local disease is usually the consequence of a general disorder."* The clay remedies suggested here have been the "rage" in France and they have created quite a stir among natural healers in the U.S. This edition is oversized and beautifully illustrated. Includes many specific remedies and preparations. Index, 203pp. SwH 74

The Digestive System

To understand digestive disorders—their problems and their solutions—it is helpful to take a worm's-eye view of what happens to food after you've chewed and swallowed it. Its initial destination is the stomach. There, your food is churned with acid and with digestive enzymes that begin the process of breaking it down into its constituents. The body (with good reason not trusting your choices) will later assemble these into the compounds that meet its nutritional needs.

Contrary to the popular concept, absorption of food and its constituents isn't a prime function of the stomach. Absorption takes place all the way from the mouth to the rectal exit. If that astonishes you, remember that there are medications given sublingually (under the tongue) that are promptly absorbed, and that the drugs in rectal suppositories readily enter the body from the lower bowel.

Exiting from the stomach (and on occasion probably leaving it in a state of disbelief), your churned and predigested food enters the small intestine, so called because of its small diameter, not its length, which is over twenty feet. Here food is treated with other digestive substances needed to break it down; these originate principally in the liver and the pancreas.

The small intestine is a miracle of anatomical engineering, for the absorption surfaces there would, if rolled out flat, cover more than half a basketball court. The majority of the nutritional elements in your foods reach the body through the walls of the small intestine. Then, by the rippling conga dance the medical man calls *peristalsis,* the residue is extruded, like ointment from a large tube, into the colon—the large intestine. Here the body manages somehow to separate liquid and solid. The intestinal wall absorbs excess fluid after the solid portion of the stool has journeyed toward the rectum.

If the food we eat is so highly overprocessed that it doesn't yield enough natural residue to stimulate elimination, not only will constipation result, but the transit time for the stool in its progress through the bowel will be prolonged. That lingering process gives added opportunity for the gut bacteria to attack certain chemicals normally produced by the body as part of the digestive process and normally excreted with the stool. The compounds that result when those chemicals are broken down are known to be powerful and effective triggers of cancer.

The disease is not produced by a mistake of nature, for what happens is the product of unnatural reactions to unnatural foods. Nature doesn't make starches and sugars devoid of fiber, nor does she strip them of vitamins, minerals, and fats. We must take the responsibility for the mischief

146

perpetrated by white flour, white sugar, white rice, degerminated corn, overmilled rye, and overprocessed barley. Not only are these foods that "keep," but when we eat them, we tend to keep the unnatural residues within us long enough for trouble to begin.

The studies of primitive Africans show that these people stay healthy because their diets stimulate elimination, which is to say that their starches and sugars are unmilled, unfractionated, high in bran and fiber, rich in vitamins and minerals. The primitive African obeys the laws of nature, and remains healthy unless we change his internal environment with our westernized foods.

—from **Carlton Fredericks' High-Fiber Way to Total Health** by Carlton Fredericks

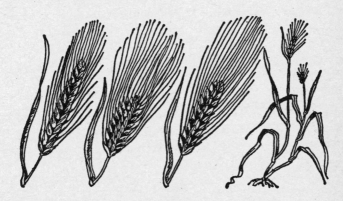

BIRCHER-BENNER. *NUTRITION PLAN FOR DIGESTIVE PROBLEMS,* 2.75. Written by the staff of the Bircher-Benner Clinic, this is one of fifteen guides to diet for particular purposes. It includes both menus and recipes for a variety of digestive disorders. 142pp. Nas 71

CHRISTOPHER, JOHN. *DR. CHRISTOPHER TALKS ON REJUVENATION THROUGH ELIMINATION,* 1.75. A survey of what and how we digest, absorb, and assimilate combined with a number of specific elimination and cleansing hints and herbal aids. 24pp. Crs 76

FLATH, CARL. *THE MIRACLE NUTRIENT,* 1.95. One out of every two Americans is now, or is on the way to becoming, a laxative addict, and collectively they are shelling out about one quarter of a billion dollars to support the habit. Flath, a health-care administrator, begins this book with a review of laxatives and the problems they create, goes on to survey the gastrointestinal tract, and then discusses the values of bran. He covers all the usual ground. Despite the title, this book is a good brief general book on good bowel health, not just a rehash on the case for bran. Recipes, glossary, index, 169pp. Ban 75

FREDERICKS, CARLTON. *HIGH-FIBER WAY TO TOTAL HEALTH,* 1.95. Fredericks has been advocating a high-fiber diet for years. One can expect then, that this book will be more about Carlton Fredericks' views on health than just a resume of the high-fiber hypothesis. There's more background information, and a discussion of the dangers of sugar and the delights of yogurt and wheat germ. If you just want to learn about fiber, we'd recommend the Galton book. If you want to use the growing awareness of the importance of fiber as a handle to turn some of your friends on to better diet and better health habits in general, this book should do an effective job. In addition to an extensive medical bibliography, Dr. Fredericks lists eight all-time great books on nutrition. Three of them turn out to be his own! Index, 208pp. S&S 76

GALTON, LAWRENCE. *THE TRUTH ABOUT FIBER IN YOUR FOOD,* c8.95. This, we think, is the best of the fiber books. Galton, an experienced writer on medical topics, has gone to the source—the various British doctors who did most of the basic research on the fiber hypothesis. Chief among them is Dr. Denis Burkitt, whose epidemiological data are derived from his communications with a network of 110 mission hospitals throughout Africa. Dr. Burkitt has contributed an introduction to this volume. Galton tells the full story of Burkitt's research and that of many others, so that the reader can follow the evidence as it unfolds and judge it for himself. One singular contribution of this book is a discussion of the importance of eating foods with their natural fiber, rather than merely adding bran to a refined diet. Appendices provide tables of fiber and caloric contents of over 1000 foods and some 130 high fiber recipes. Bibliography, index, 246pp. Crn 76

HILL, RAY. *BRAN,* 1.50. An introductory discussion, reviewing the benefits of bran, its value in treating constipation and all colonic diseases, and an explaining of how bran can replace the fiber missing from processed food. A selection of recipes is included. 64pp. TPL 76

MOYER, ANNE, ed. *THE FIBER FACTOR,* 3.95. This is a straightforward presentation of the arguments for fiber. The information is derived from articles in **Prevention Magazine,** the leading magazine in the field of nutrition in the U.S. today. The book includes an explanation of how dietary fiber works in the intestinal tract and presents a selection of recipes and charts. Index, 146pp. Rod 76

MOYLE, ALAN. *CONQUERING CONSTIPATION,* 4.55. Most of the basic causes of constipation, and the complaints associated with that condition, can be traced to modern methods of food production and consumption. Recently a rash of books has appeared suggesting that a major factor in constipation is the lack of suitable roughage in our food. In this book an experienced naturopath explains the nutritional deficiencies which precipitate constipation, and how to remedy them. All the related ailments are also discussed in some depth. Index, 126pp. TPL 76

MOYLE, ALAN. *DIGESTIVE TROUBLES,* 1.35. Moyle begins his discussion with an explanation of how the digestive organs work and the nature of food. He follows with a course of self-treatment designed to eliminate digestive upsets. 64pp. TPL 73

REUBEN, DAVID. *THE SAVE YOUR LIFE DIET,* 1.95. This is a pioneering book on the subject and it remains the most popular book about the role of fiber in health. Based on a study of over 500 medical authorities in 600 articles (the book is extensively footnoted with special notes to other M.D.'s), Reuben points out the high correlation between our Western low-fiber diets and our high rates of cancer of the colon and rectum, heart attacks, diverticulosis, appendicitis, hemorrhoids and obesity. He recommends a natural food diet which avoids white sugar and white flour but holds out hope for those who insist on eating junk food if they take three teaspoons to three tablespoons of bran per day. Bibliography, 173pp. RaH 75

SCIENCE OF LIFE BOOKS. *CONSTIPATION, HAEMORRHOIDS AND COLITIS,* 1.35. A discussion of treatment, with notes on the twelve causes of constipation, the case against laxatives, and the value of enemas. 60pp. SLB 75

SNEDDON, J. RUSSELL. *GASTRIC AND DUODENAL ULCERA-TIONS,* 1.35. A collection of diet suggestions, exercises, and a course of drugless self-treatment for the gastric sufferer. 64pp. TPL 75

SUBAK-SHARPE, GENELL. *THE NATURAL HIGH FIBER LIFE SAVING DIET,* 1.95. This book begins with a review of the medical researches that led to our understanding of fiber, treated somewhat like a detective story. It covers the various diseases related to fiber and gives considerable attention to the problem of weight reduction, in general, and in relation to a high fiber diet. Ms. Subak-Sharpe is editor of **Medical Opinion**; she is also a cook and some of her favorite recipes are included. This is the fiber book for the overweight reader. Bibliography, 190pp. G&D 76

SCIENCE OF LIFE BOOKS. *STOMACH ULCERS AND ACIDITY,* 1.35. An examination of symptoms, causes, and treatment based on natural principles along with a variety of dietary suggestions. 63pp. SLB 73

SMITH, WILLIAM. *HERBS FOR CONSTIPATION,* 1.35. See the Herbs section.

DINTENFASS, JULIUS. *CHIROPRACTIC: A MODERN WAY TO HEALTH,* 1.50. Presents a good overview of the subject. 189pp. Pyr 66

DOOLEY, ANNE. *EVERY WALL A DOOR,* 2.95. An engrossing study of spirit healing and psychic surgery. Ms. Dooley traces the awakening of her interest in psychic phenomena and her study of various mediums. She was invited to a healing session given by Lourival de Freitas, a Brazilian psychic surgeon, and following it she went to Brazil to study his work more thoroughly. The bulk of the book is devoted to her recreation of De Freitas' remarkable healings and surgical operations. She herself underwent an operation. She also gives us a comprehensive picture of the Brazilian spiritist scene and reports on the work of other healers. Photographs, bibliography, 206pp. Dut 74

DRESSER, HORATIO, ed. *THE QUIMBY MANUSCRIPTS,* 5.95. Heretofore unpublished documents dealing with techniques and theories of mental and spiritual healing. Dr. Quimby was the physician who treated Mary Baker Eddy, the founder of the Christian Science Church, and he was instrumental in the development of her theories. The selections explain how Quimby developed his silent method of healing and his "science and health" theory. Index, 461+pp. CiP 61

DUZ, M. *A PRACTICAL TREATISE OF ASTRAL MEDICINE AND THERAPEUTICS,* 5.00. An in depth study of the relationship between medicine and astrology. Many diagrams, 252pp. HeR 12

EDMUNDS, H. TUDOR, et al., eds. *SOME UNRECOGNIZED FACTORS IN MEDICINE,* 3.25. A group of scientists, physicians, and clairvoyants presents a philosophy of medicine and healing based upon the concept of man as a complex being consisting of a spirit, soul, and physical body. The authors suggest that health, in its fullest sense, means the alignment of the whole of man's being to his spiritual nature. They also feel that diagnosis can only be accurate if consideration is given not only to the effect of a disease, but also to the cause of the disease. Here they discuss special diagnostic techniques and include a complete section on the principles of the treatment of diseases. Index, 209pp. TPH 76

EDWARDS, HARRY. *A GUIDE TO THE UNDERSTANDING AND PRACTICE OF SPIRITUAL HEALING,* c8.40. Harry Edwards is England's most noted spiritual healer. In this book he has drawn upon his vast healing experience and his unparalleled knowledge of spiritual science to explain how spiritual healing is accomplished and how we can develop our own healing potential. Edwards prepared a series of Healing Study Courses for members of the National Federation of Spiritual Healers, and these courses are now embraced in this volume, which in itself is an extended and revised edition of his earlier book *A Guide to Spirit Healing,* which was considered to be the leading textbook for healers. Major sections include "Absent Healing and the Seeking of Attunement with Spirit," "The Theory of Spirit Healing," "Healing Practice," "The Science of Spirit Healing," "Psychosomatic Conditions and Mental Healing," and "An Enquiry into the Cause, Prevention, and Cure of Cancer." Photographs, index, 360pp. SHS 74

EDWARDS, HARRY. *THE HEALING INTELLIGENCE,* 2.50. In clear and precise language the author explains the laws at work behind spiritual healing. Drawing material and insight from numerous

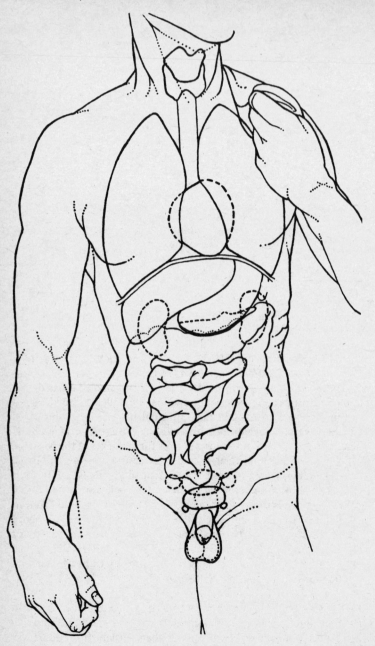

experiences in his own career in the healing art he explains the inner spiritual factor in man that may be released in order to vanquish disease and illness of both psychological and physical varieties. 189pp. Haw 65

EDWARDS, HARRY. *THE POWER OF SPIRITUAL HEALING,* c3.35. *This book is not so much a scientific appreciation of spiritual healing as an effort to present the healing story in a simple way to enable everyone to have a measure of understanding of its powers, processes and purpose and how all who are in need can benefit from it.* 173pp. SHS 63

EDWARDS, HARRY. *SPIRIT HEALING,* c3.95. Outlines some fundamental principles of spirit healing, its relationship to the Church and the medical profession and its actual application in cases of disease. 170pp. SHS 60

EDWARDS, HARRY. *THIRTY YEARS A SPIRITUAL HEALER,* c3.95. Edwards' autobiography, in which he discusses how he first realized his healing faculty and relates many of his healing experiences. Photographs, index, 167pp. SHS 68

EHRENREICH, BARBARA and DEIRDRE ENGLISH. *WITCHES, MIDWIVES AND NURSES: A HISTORY OF WOMEN HEALERS,* 1.70. Women have always been healers. They were the unlicensed doctors of western history. They were pharmacists, cultivating healing herbs and exchanging the secrets of their uses. They were also midwives. They learned from each other, passing their experience from neighbor to neighbor and mother to daughter. This book traces the history of women as healers and analyzes the takeover of medicine by male professionals. Bibliography, 64pp. WRP 73

EICHENLAUB, JOHN. *HOME TONICS AND REFRESHERS FOR DAILY HEALTH AND VIGOR,* 1.25. A selection of natural tonics and remedies for various common ailments—with instructions on how to prepare them, and some background material. Index, 221pp. ASC 63

EICHENLAUB, JOHN. *A MINNESOTA DOCTOR'S HOME REMEDIES FOR COMMON AND UNCOMMON AILMENTS,* 2.95. This is an excellent collection of useful tips which is well organized and covers every conceivable area. All the remedies are simple to prepare. Dr. Eichenlaub writes in a simple down-home style and includes many anecdotes. We have found this book very useful and we think you will too. Fully indexed, 262pp. PrH 72

Fasting

Fasting is the oldest therapeutic method known to man. Even before the advent of the "medicine man" and the healing arts, man instinctively stopped eating when feeling ill and abstained from food until his health was restored. Or perhaps he learned this, the most efficient means of correcting any disease, from animals, which always fast when not feeling well. Certainly, nature provided man with a definite protective and health-restoring alarm signal, which suggests to him to abstain from eating by taking away his appetite for food.

Throughout the long medical history fasting has been regarded as one of the most dependable curative and rejuvenative measures. Hippocrates, "the Father of Medicine," prescribed it. So did Galen, Paracelsus, and all the other great physicians of old. Fasting was practiced by many great thinkers and philosophers, such as Plato and Socrates, to *attain mental and physical efficiency*. Most Eastern philosophers and super-yogis, known for their long life, mental efficiency and spiritual awareness, fast regularly, along with meditation, to attain long life and a high level of spirituality.

With the advent of modern, drug-oriented medicine, fasting has fallen into disregard in the eyes of the orthodox practitioners. We are living in the age of "diets," when almost half of the population is constantly trying to "reduce" by way of countless restricted diets of every imaginable description. But the classic, and the best form of reducing—the total abstinence from food, or fasting—is seldom tried. Those who employ fasting, either for healing or reducing, are still looked upon as crackpots, quacks, and health-nuts, to say the least.

Fasting has been used throughout history, and is used quite extensively now, not only for the therapeutic purpose of healing disease, but also for its obvious rejuvenating and revitalizing effect. Thousands of people throughout the world fast regularly not to cure any particular disease, but because they consider fasting to be an effective way to cleanse the body from accumulated wastes, build up the physical stamina and resistance against disease, and revitalize and rejuvenate the functions of all their vital organs.—from **How to Keep Slim and Healthy with Juice Fasting** by Paavo O. Airola

AIROLA, PAAVO. *HOW TO KEEP SLIM AND HEALTHY AND YOUNG WITH JUICE FASTING,* **3.25. Dr. Airola considers juice fasting to be the number one healer and rejuvenator. He gives theory, case histories, information on fasting to reduce, how to fast, why juice fasting is better than water fasting; he advocates enemas and gives complete advice on what to do while fasting. Bibliography, 79pp. HPP 71**

BRAGG, PAUL. *THE MIRACLE OF FASTING,* **3.00. Bragg, who is now in his nineties, is the best example of health through good diet principles that we know of, and this is one of the most popular books on fasting. Contrary to most authors, he believes we should fast on distilled water only (possibly with a little honey and lemon added) and should not take enemas during fasts. He urges the reader to start with easy twenty-four to thirty-six hour fasts and gradually work up to longer ones. Bragg himself fasts a day a week and for seven to ten days four times a year. This book, in addition to giving much practical advice on fasting, contains a lot of other advice about healthful eating and living. 197pp. HeS nd**

BRANDT, JOHANNA. *THE GRAPE CURE,* 1.95. Johanna Brandt was a South African who, in 1925, cured herself of cancer by fasting on nothing but grapes. She recommends eating one to four pounds of grapes a day, chewing the skins and seeds, and continuing for a week to a month. The grapes apparently act to break up diseased tissue and purify the blood. Later other fruits, buttermilk, etc. can be added. The grape cure for various diseases has a long history. Needless to say, it is controversial. However, it can't hurt you and if you like grapes as well as we do, you might want to give this idea a try next grape season for whatever good it might do you. 191pp. Lus 67

CARRINGTON, HEREWARD. *SAVE YOUR LIFE BY FASTING,* 2.95. This is a reprint of an old (pre-World War II) book by one of the best known early hygienists. He makes an interesting case for not eating any more than the minimum amount of food needed to sustain life. (This has been corroborated by more recent studies with rats showing that those who ate twice as much lived half as long!). *We are not nourished by the amount of food we eat, but by the amount we can properly use and assimilate.* The last half of the book deals with fasting, per se, although it is more concerned with arguing the merits of the case than it is with giving practical advice. 226pp. Prv 69

EHRET, ARNOLD. *MUCUSLESS DIET HEALING SYSTEM,* 1.50. Near the beginning of this century, Arnold Ehret came into prominence as an exponent of the mucusless diet. He argued that meat, dairy products, and starchy foods tend to produce large quantities of mucus which provides an ideal medium for germs. He favored fasting and a fruit diet. This book is his major statement and it continues to be extremely popular. His writing style (or perhaps it is the translation) is terrible and he tends to make outlandish claims which he does not back up with facts. Nonetheless, his work is important and almost everyone that we know has at least sampled Ehret. Diets and menus are included. 194pp. Ehr 22

EHRET, ARNOLD. *RATIONAL FASTING,* 1.25. This book gives useful information about fasting in addition to extolling the benefits to be derived. Professor Ehret favored use of lemon juice and enemas during fasts. 175pp. Lus 71

GHAZZALI, AL-. *THE MYSTERIES OF FASTING,* 1.50. The practice of fasting as a spiritual discipline is both ancient and widespread, found in virtually all religious traditions. Al-Ghazzali, a fourteenth century poet and mystic, wrote this piece to discuss fasting from the Islamic point of view, rather than strictly from a health standpoint. Fasting *stands alone as the only act of worship which is not seen by anyone except God. It is an inward act of worship performed through sheer endurance and fortitude. . .it is a means of vanquishing the enemy of God, Satan, who works through the appe-*

tites and carnal lusts. Translated by Nabih Amin Faris. 52pp. Asf 68

CHRISTOPHER, JOHN. *DR. CHRISTOPHER'S THREE DAY CLEANSING PROGRAM AND MUCOUSLESS DIET,* 2.00. A detailed collection of dietary and healing instructions which aid the eliminative and regenerative process. A number of specific preparations are suggested. 20pp. Crs 76

COTT, ALLAN. *FASTING: THE ULTIMATE DIET,* 1.75. This is a book by a medical doctor for people from a more conventional background who may feel that fasting is a very strange activity. It attempts to set their minds at rest and make the case for fasting. It recommends that no one fast for more than a day without consultation with a doctor. Dr. Cott is a psychiatrist who specializes in megavitamin therapy. Extensive bibliography, 148pp. Ban 75

COTT, ALLAN. *FASTING AS A WAY OF LIFE,* 1.75. This discussion of fasting is intended as a complement to Cott's earlier book. He includes information on how to get started on a fast, how long you can fast, how fasting acts on the body and spirit, and much else. He also provides suggestions on after the fast menus and reviews places where you can have a fasting vacation. The book ends with a series of questions and answers. It is geared toward the general reader who knows little about fasting and does not want to be overwhelmed by a lot of technical jargon and is a more than adequate presentation of the case for fasting. Bibliography, 136pp. Ban 77

KIRBAN, SALEM. *HOW TO KEEP HEALTHY AND HAPPY BY FASTING,* 3.35. A simplified discussion of the benefits of fasting, filled with cartoons, photographs, and many biblical quotations. It's a scattered book, nonetheless it covers material not found elsewhere. 183pp. HrH 76

KIRSCHNER, H.E. *LIVE FOOD JUICES,* 3.00. Kirschner, an M.D., cites many case histories of near miraculous cures through the use of juices, including one woman who drank only carrot juice for eighteen months. There is a table of the nutritional content of various juices, a discussion of the values of individual juices, and a listing of conditions which shows the juices considered helpful. Also includes a brief chapter on the virtues of a low protein diet. 120pp. WoP 74

LUST, JOHN. *DRINK YOUR TROUBLES AWAY,* 1.95. An excellent presentation of the argument for raw juice therapy. Lust covers the general benefits and presents recipes for both general health and for specific ailments. This is an excellent book which both updates and complements **Raw Juice Therapy.** Appendices offer a number of technical tables and there's also a glossary and a lengthy index. 189pp. Lus 67

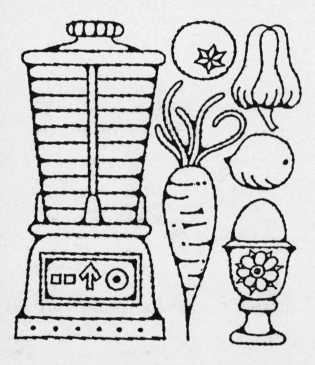

LUST, JOHN. *RAW JUICE THERAPY,* c3.90. This is our favorite of the raw juice books. Dr. Lust provides the theory of raw juice therapy without oversell, and then he goes on to give a great deal of useful information including an extensive listing of vitamin and mineral deficiency symptoms and the juices to take to overcome them, a table of the vitamin content of foods which can be juiced, extensive juice recipes with discussion of the health values thereof, lists of ailments with juice formulas to treat them, menus, and many other assorted tables of useful information. Excellent index, 173pp. **TPL 74**

NEWMAN, L. *MAKE YOUR JUICER YOUR DRUG STORE,* 1.95. Dr. Newman is a naturopath who spent some thirteen years compiling the information in this book. After general treatment of raw juices and cleansing, he considers a wide variety of diseases in separate chapters, relating each to his dietary suggestions. These include hardening of the arteries, digestion, elimination, glands, circulatory troubles, respiratory troubles, female troubles, nerves, eyes, teeth, weight, and children's ailments. He concludes with a discussion of various juices, including alfalfa, clover and dandelion. 191pp. Lus 72

ROSS, SHIRLEY. *FASTING: THE SUPER DIET,* 1.75. This is a well researched general survey of fasting which brings together scientific and biological data with case studies of spiritual fasts and health fasts. It's an easy book to read and has useful information which is not covered in other books on fasting. Practical suggestions on how to fast are also included, although these do not form the bulk of the book. Glossary, bibliography, 131pp. RaH 76

ROSS, SHIRLEY. *NATURE'S DRINKS,* 1.75. After a discussion of nutrients in many fruits and vegetables and how to process them (e.g., never put garlic in your juicer—you can't get the smell out), Ms. Ross gives us some 200 mouth-watering recipes for preparing delicious, energizing, nutritious drinks, free of preservatives and sugar. If you have a juicer and want ideas on new combinations to try, this is the book for you. The latter part of the book deals in great detail with coffee and tea, how to buy, brew and use them. 154pp. RaH 74

SCIENCE OF LIFE BOOKS. *RAW JUICES FOR HEALTH,* 1.35. An overview, including sections on the uses of juices, properties of juices, and raw juice therapy. 64pp. SLB 72

SHACKLETON, BASIL. *THE GRAPE CURE,* 3.90. This book begins with an account of Shackleton's miraculous kidney cure. The author follows with a discussion of the grape cure along with a hodge-podge of other healing hints. 128pp. TPL 69

SHELTON, HERBERT. *FASTING CAN SAVE YOUR LIFE,* 1.75. This is the book that introduced us to the benefits of fasting. Dr. Shelton is top man in the American Natural Hygiene Society and this book includes a good deal about natural hygiene. It reviews the whole area of fasting, what it can accomplish and what problems to watch out for. Shelton favors plain water fasting, without enemas.

The latter half of the book discusses therapeutic values of fasting in relation to many conditions, among them weight loss and gain, asthma and hay fever, arthritis, high blood pressure, psoriasis, multiple sclerosis and gonorrhea. Index, 200pp. NHP 64

SHELTON, HERBERT. *FASTING FOR RENEWAL OF LIFE*, 2.45. Shelton's latest book is the most comprehensive and scholarly treatment of the subject we've seen. He gives a great deal of historical background, analogies with animals, and information about fasting in other cultures. He also gives all the necessary advice about conducting a fast, though it is not as immediately accessible as in some of the briefer books. The last part of the book discusses the use of fasts in many different kinds of diseases. Index, 314pp. NHP 74

SMITH, FREDERICK. *JOURNAL OF A FAST,* c7.95. This is the inner journal of the thirty days that the author fasted. It records an extraordinary record of his odyssey to the innermost recesses of his being. While fasting he approaches a pure state of spiritual awareness and as he ponders the meaning of what he is sensing he relates his insights to those of some of the great mystics. Bibliography, 216pp. ScB 76

SZEKELY, EDMUND BORDEAUX, tr. *THE ESSENE GOSPEL OF PEACE*, 1.00. This is a translation of a third century Aramaic manuscript, preserved in the Vatican archives, which gives Christ's views on healing and health. *For I tell you truly, except you fast, you shall never be freed from the power of Satan and from all diseases that come from Satan. . . .Seek the fresh air of the forest and of the fields, and there in the midst of them shall you find the angel of air to embrace all your body. . . .After the angel of air, seek the angel of water. . . .Think not that it is sufficient that the angel of water embrace you outwards only. . . .Seek, therefore, a large trailing gourd, having a stalk the length of a man; take out its innards and fill it with water from the river which the sun has warmed. Hang it upon the branch of a tree, and kneel upon the ground before the angel of water, and suffer the end of the stalk of the trailing gourd to enter your hinder parts, that the water may flow through all your bowels. . . .Then let the water run out from your bowels that it may carry away from within it all the unclean and evil-smelling things of Satan. . . .Renew your baptising with water on every day of your fast, till the day when you see that the water which flows out of you is as pure as the river's foam. Then betake your body to the* *coursing river, and there in the arms of the angel of water render thanks to the living God that he has freed you from your sins.* 72pp. Aca 75

SZEKELY,EDMUND. *THE ESSENE SCIENCE OF FASTING,* 2.80. A detailed guide to fasting and sobriety based both on the principles advocated by the ancient Essenes and on Mr. Szekely's own experience in his health spas. The instructions are based on classical naturopathic ideas. The tone is more spiritual than most of the fasting books. 48pp. Aca 75

WALKER, N.W. *RAW VEGETABLE JUICES,* 3.10/1.25. This book was first published in 1936 and ever since has been the bible of the juicer contingent. In fact, Dr. Walker is the inventor of the Norwalk juicer—the most effective one on the market. The book begins with a discussion of the importance of juices and the reasons for drinking them in quantity, then follows with information on the values of many different kinds of juice from alfalfa to watercress. Finally, Walker discusses the therapeutic use of juices in different ailments ranging from acidosis to varicose veins. These are keyed to eighty-seven different juice mixture formulas. The $3.10 edition is larger and has bigger type. 171pp. Pyr 70

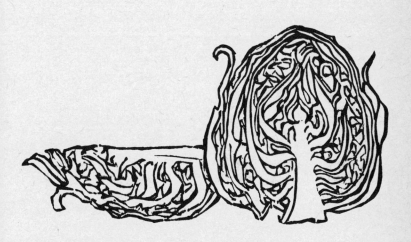

FEINGOLD, BEN. *WHY YOUR CHILD IS HYPERACTIVE,* c7.95. Dr. Feingold, a noted pediatrician, received considerable newspaper publicity when he found that the problem of hyperkinesis—learning disability which affects more than five million children in the U.S. could in many cases be traced to the additives in their food. By eliminating all synthetic food colorings and flavorings from their diet, he found his patients became much calmer, more responsive, less distractable, more able to cope, and their school work improves markedly. What a contrast to the recent scandal in Iowa in which the school system was systematically drugging many of the children to try to get the same results. In this book, Dr. Feingold relates how his discovery came about and its scientific basis, and provides details about the diet and how parents should apply it. Recipes are included. 211pp. RaH 74

FISHER, RICHARD. *DICTIONARY OF DRUGS,* 2.75. Describes the uses, effects, chemical make-up, and side effects of the fifty-six drugs most commonly used by physicians. The book cannot be used for self medication (dosages are not given) but will enable the serious reader to better understand and question what his doctor is up to. Indexed by trade names, chemical names, and diseases. 252pp. ScB 71

FLAMMONDE, PARIS. *THE MYSTIC HEALERS,* c8.95. This survey of spiritual healers through the ages is mainly a series of anecdotes and biographical material. The emphasis is on modern day healers beginning with Mary Baker Eddy and on Christian-oriented healers such as Oral Roberts and Katherine Kuhlman. Most of the individuals discussed were totally unfamiliar to us. The book lacks depth and serves merely as an introductory overview from which the reader can pick out those healers that interest her and get a more in depth study elsewhere. Glossary, bibliography, index, 252pp. S&D 74

FRIEDMANN, LAWRENCE and LAWRENCE GALTON. *FREEDOM FROM BACKACHES,* 1.95. This is the best book we've seen on back troubles. Dr. Friedmann, Medical Director of the Institute for the Crippled and Disabled, Research and Rehabilitation Center in New York City, points out that most persons can themselves relieve an acute attack quickly, determine the basic cause of their trouble, and reduce or eliminate recurrences. Surgery is rarely necessary. So if you think you have a slipped disc and might need surgery, read this book first. Replete with exercises, manipulations, home remedies and excellent line drawings wherever needed to explain the text. Index, 240pp. S&S 73

FULLER, JOHN. *ARIGO: SURGEON OF THE RUSTY KNIFE,* 1.50. Arigo had only a third grade education and no medical training, yet thousands flocked to the small village where he lived to be cured by him. He performed hundreds of operations daily usually with an ordinary kitchen knife or jackknife, without anaesthetics, without major bleeding, and without the benefits of modern science. He made thousands of correct diagnoses without even examining the patient. And, one after another, patients left his primitive "clinic" cured. He saved many from cancer and other fatal diseases who had been given up as hopeless by the leading medical authorities. He never charged for his services nor would he accept any remuneration. Arigo's healings were witnessed by both Brazilian and American doctors. Explicit motion pictures of his operations were taken, and stills from these illustrate the book. This is a spellbinding book in which John Fuller has reconstructed the story of Arigo, and has carefully researched and documented his presentation. Afterword by Andrija Puharich. Bibliography, index, 282pp. S&S 74

GARTEN, M.O. *THE HEALTH SECRETS OF A NATUROPATHIC DOCTOR,* 2.95. This is a good, clear layman's guide to naturopathy, covering many therapies and giving detailed diet suggestions. 238pp. PrH 67

GARTEN, M.O. *THE NATURAL AND DRUGLESS WAY FOR BETTER HEALTH,* 1.65. Garten's books are very good practical guides to living a more healthy life—this one specifically details exercises and remedies for every part of the body. 240pp. Arc 69

GLASSER, RONALD. *THE BODY IS THE HERO,* c8.95. A vividly written account of how our body defends itself against disease. Dr. Glasser tells how the immune system works, describes the discoveries of its explorers, and explores what happens when the system goes haywire. He recreates a daily drama as the defense systems surround, coat, and detonate the invading bacteria; as they block off and destroy the advancing viruses and intra-cellular parasites. *It has to be a total war; not one single enemy can be left alive. Just one survivor, by continuing to grow, would eventually mean death.* This is an illuminating book which helps us to understand just how amazing the human machine is and how complex is our biological functioning. Many case studies are included, and a final chapter surveys the

HEALING/*General*

role of immunology in curing cancer. 248pp. RaH 76

GLICK, JOEL and JULIA LORUSSO. *HEALING STONED: THE THERAPEUTIC USE OF GEMS AND MINERALS,* 5.50. This is an excellent modern discussion of the healing properties of countless gems and minerals. The authors are spiritual teachers and this vibration is evident in their presentation. Every conceivable aspect, both negative and positive, of each gem is considered. 92pp. MiP 76

GUIRDHAM, ARTHUR. *OBSESSION,* c5.60. Subtitled *Psychic Forces and Evil in the Causation of Disease,* this is a study based on the author's years of psychiatric and medical experience Dr. Guirdham believes that obsessional symptoms are often due to the repression of psychic gifts and here he explores this thesis through many case studies. He writes very clearly and his work is useful both for the layman and the professional. 181pp. Spe 72

GUIRDHAM, ARTHUR. *A THEORY OF DISEASE,* c5.45. *The aim of this book is to produce a comprehensive theory of disease. Proneness to disease is related to the degree of development of the personality and to the individual's awareness of it. The pattern of disease depends to a large extent on the religious and philosophical outlook of the community in which he finds himself.* 204pp. Spe 57

HALL, GEORGE. *HEALTHY FEET,* 1.35. A collection of treatments for a variety of foot ailments in both adults and children along with a series of preventive suggestions. 62pp. TPL 73

HALL, GEORGE. *HOW TO BANISH COLDS AND INFLUENZA,* 1.35. Suggestions for natural treatments for the underlying causes of colds and influenza. 64pp. TPL 73

HALL, GEORGE. *OVERCOMING ANAEMIA,* 1.35. Explains what anaemia is, its symptoms and causes, and points out its relationship to faulty diet. Hall also gives a variety of natural treatments. 64pp. TPL 74

HALL, MANLY P. *HEALING,* c7.75. A fascinating account tracing the history of healing from the earliest times and discusses the major figures in the field. Hall analyzes various types of healing and relates them to esoteric psychology and to physiology and anatomy. He includes material on the etheric bodies of man and nature, the

164

human will, the factor of conscience, and the energies underlying the physical processes of the body. There is a special section on the pineal gland and on the effects of mental attitudes on health. The book concludes with a group of case histories, showing how the individual causes many of his health problems, and discussing techniques for self help. 341pp. PRS 71

HAMMOND, SALLY. *WE ARE ALL HEALERS,* 1.95. Ms. Hammond is a reporter with an intense personal and professional interest in healing. She feels that the ability to heal psychically is innate in all humans—although dormant in most of us—and that it can be developed to greater or lesser degree. The only requirements for that development are a sense of compassion and a willingness to acquire the necessary training. In researching this book Ms. Hammond visited the most noted healers and healing centers in the U.S. and the U.K. including The National Federation of Spiritual Healers, Harry Edwards, Gordon Turner, Mary Rogers, Ronald Beesley, The Academy of Parapsychology and Medicine, and Rolling Thunder. This is a very personal, well written account and includes edited transcripts of her dialogues with healers. Index, 296pp. RaH 74

HAND, WAYLAND. *AMERICAN FOLK MEDICINE,* c12.95. This book comes out of the proceedings of the UCLA Conference on American Folk Medicine. It makes available for the first time a general collection of studies on folk medicine in North America. The book includes essays on a wide variety of subjects by twenty-five scholars in folklore and related fields. Most of the essays are of a technical nature. Notes, index, 347pp. UCa 76

HARTMANN, FRANZ. *OCCULT SCIENCE IN MEDICINE,* c6.50. A reprint of a philosophical treatise first published in 1893. Hartmann wrote a number of things on Paracelsus, the pioneering alchemist physician, and he incorporates many alchemical concepts into the material presented here. He includes information on the esoteric constitution of man, on the development of medicine through the ages (it is here that he delves most deeply into alchemy), on the causes of disease from the spiritual point of view, and on the five types of diseases and the five related types of physicians and treatments. Hartmann does not write terribly clearly and this is definitely a work for those interested in esoteric science only. 100pp. Wei 75

HEINDEL, MAX. *ASTRO DIAGNOSIS: A GUIDE TO HEALING,*

4.50. An introductory text explaining certain fundamental principles of the methods of medical diagnosis based on an understanding of the astrological factors influencing a patient. Index, 482pp. Ros 29

HEINDEL, MAX. *OCCULT PRINCIPLES OF HEALTH AND HEALING,* 4.00. A treasury of material concerning the health and healing of the human organism as considered from the occult point of view. Discusses specific ailments as well as the origin, functions and proper care of the physical vehicle. 248pp. Ros 38

HEWLETT-PARSONS, J. *ABC'S OF NATURE CURES,* 1.45. This is the best overall introduction to naturopathy that we know of. It is written for the layperson and includes sections on dietetics, hydrotherapy, fasting, vitamin therapy, and various specialty treatments such as mono diets and eliminative diets. It also contains a great deal of information on basic nutrition and on the role of the various micro-nutrients and minerals. Dr. Hewlett-Parsons is a practicing naturopath. He bases his work on the classic teachings of naturopathy and stresses a balanced lifestyle. Glossary, index, 192pp. Arc 68

HILGARD, ERNEST and JOSEPHINE. *HYPNOSIS IN THE RELIEF OF PAIN,* c12.95. Two distinguished researchers, a psychologist and a psychiatrist, present an assessment of the role of hypnosis in relation to pain—based both on studies in the experimental laboratory and on clinical practice. A detailed study, geared toward the general reader. Bibliography, notes, index, 271pp. Kau 75

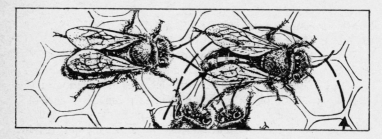

HILL, RAY. *PROPOLIS: THE NATURAL ANTIBIOTIC,* 1.50. Propolis is used by bees in making and repairing their hives. It has also been found to be a powerful, non-toxic antibiotic. Some believe that the bees protect themselves against infection by using propolis so extensively in their hive. The medicinal properties of propolis, although known for about 2,000 years, have only recently been rediscovered. Hill reports on current research, traces the history of this remedy, tells of the forms in which propolis is now available, and gives treatment and dosage suggestions for specific ailments. 64pp. TPL 77

HOLZER, HANS. *BEYOND MEDICINE,* 1.50. Presents the latest research about unorthodox healing, including documented case studies, a discussion of various healing theories, and a long section devoted to noted healers, including some in the medical profession. A fascinating study. 209pp. RaH 73

HOMOLA, SAMUEL. *A CHIROPRACTOR'S TREASURY OF HEALTH SECRETS,* c7.95. Each chapter of this book outlines a complete self help program for a specific ailment, along with general nutritional information. Includes many practical exercises, with illustrations. 224pp. PrH 70

HOMOLA, SAMUEL. *DR. HOMOLA'S LIFE-EXTENDER HEALTH GUIDE,* c7.95. Dr. Homola has been a practicing chiropractor, using natural methods, for nearly two decades, and he is a prolific writer. This book contains a wealth of good nutritional information and simple, practical home remedies for a wide variety of ills. It covers in detail ways to get rid of body poisons, restore good digestion, control weight and build energy. Index, 223pp. PrH 75

HOMOLA, SAMUEL. *DR. HOMOLA'S NATURAL HEALTH REMEDIES,* c6.95. Dr. Homola details here practical home remedies for numerous ailments—combining naturopathy and chiropracty into what he calls naturomatic healing methods. This is an interesting study, fully indexed. 250pp. PrH 73

HUMAN DIMENSIONS INSTITUTE. *APPROACHES TO HEALING: LAYING ON OF HANDS,* 3.50. A collection of fairly technical articles on the title theme. 55pp. HDI 76

HURDLE, J. FRANK. *A COUNTRY DOCTOR'S COMMON SENSE MANUAL,* 2.95. This is a topically organized collection of health and healing tips written by an experienced physician. The suggestions are varied and unusual and all are of a self help nature. Index, 266pp. PrH 75

ILLICH, IVAN. *MEDICAL NEMESIS,* c8.95. This is an extremely important book. Illich argues that modern medicine has reached the stage where it itself is a major threat to our health. With incredibly comprehensive documentation, he shows that during the past century doctors have affected epidemics no more profoundly than did priests during earlier times, and that, indeed, much of modern illness is doctor-caused. ". . .one out of every five patients admitted to a typical research hospital acquires an iatrogenic disease (i.e., caused by the treatment there), sometimes trivial, usually requiring special treatment, and in one case in thirty leading to death. Half of these episodes result from complications of drug therapy; amazingly, one in ten comes from diagnostic procedures. Despite good intentions and claims to public service, a military officer with a similar record of performance would be relieved of his command, and a restaurant or amusement center would be closed by the police." No wonder malpractice insurance rates are skyrocketing. But Illich's major attack on the medical establishment is even more basic. The doctors have mystified healing to such an extent that they have taken away from us the faith and ability to heal ourselves. Illich's concern is a profound humanism which would return to people control over the most basic elements of their own lives. This book has received wide acclaim and attention in the media. It may turn out to be one of the most important influences in hastening the revolution in attitudes and approaches to healing that we now see taking place. It's difficult reading often, but highly recommended nonetheless. Subject and author indices, 294pp. RaH 76

Irisdiagnosis

Irisdiagnosis, also known as iridology and iridiagnosis, is the science of diagnosing physical illness and imbalance from the marks and color changes in the iris of the human eye. Irisdiagnosis in its present form was discovered by a Hungarian physician, Ignatz von Peczely (1822-1911). On the basis of several decades of comparative study, von Peczely realized that certain indications in the iris were related to organic diseases. He developed an iris topography in which every organ had its corresponding point in the eye. Many others built on his work and today irisdiagnosis is accepted as an excellent diagnostic tool.

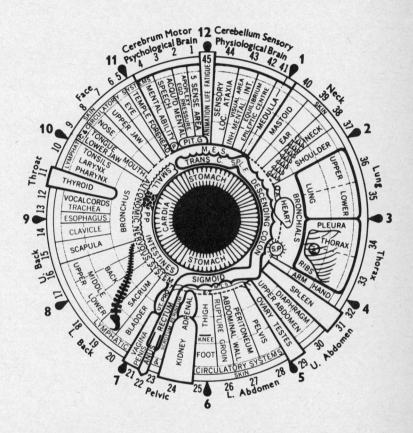

JENSEN, BERNARD. *CHART FOR IRIDOLOGY,* 8.40. An 8½"x 14" chart, laminated in heavy plastic. Both eyes are reproduced and the various points on the eyes can be clearly seen. Jen

JENSEN, BERNARD. *THE SCIENCE AND PRACTICE OF IRIDOLOGY,* c18.50. Dr. Bernard Jensen, D.C., N.D., is the foremost exponent of irisdiagnosis in the U.S. today. He believes it is more accurate than any other single method of diagnosis. The iridologist can determine the inherent structure and working capacity of an

169

organ, can detect environmental strain, can tell if a person is anemic, can determine the nerve force, the responsive healing power of tissue and the inherent ability to circulate the blood. This is a technical book, for professionals, profusely illustrated and including many color plates Index, 372pp. Jen 74

KRIEGE, THEODOR. *FUNDAMENTAL BASIS OF IRISDIAGNOSIS,* c9.35. This is a very complete technical presentation. The early chapters explain how to develop a diagnostic approach and the later ones review the appropriate signs for typical conditions in each physiological system. Excellent diagrams support the textual descriptions and an appendix contains twelve monochrome iris photographs with diagnostic comments. 120pp. Fow 75

LINDLAHR, HENRY. *IRIDIAGNOSIS, AND OTHER DIAGNOSTIC METHODS,* 12.50. This is an offset reprint of an important early study. Iris diagnosis is explored as fully here as in any modern study and many of Dr. Lindlahr's insights and diagnostic suggestions are not available elsewhere. Index, 327pp. HeR 22

TRIAD RESEARCH COMPANY. *IRIS ANALYSIS WALL CHART,* 10.95. This is the best iris chart available. Each iris diagram is 8½" in diameter. In the center is a large, detailed drawing of the human body. The various organs shown are connected by red lines to iris-diagnosis points. There's also a spinal nerve relationship chart and ten photographs of common iris indications. 20"x30", two-color, plastic-coated. Asl

TRIAD RESEARCH COMPANY. *IRIS INDEX KEY,* 10.95. This 8½"x14¾" chart is plasticized on heavy cardboard. One side has 5½" in diameter iris drawings and a zone indicator. The other side has eight photographs of textures and lesions and fifteen photographs of common iris indications. Asl

TRIAD RESEARCH COMPANY. *VEST POCKET KEY FOR IRIS ANALYSIS,* 5.50. Contains a 3½" in diameter set of iris charts and a set of blank charts of the same size which can be filled in by the practitioner. Plastic laminated, 8½"x4" folded size. Asl

WILBORN, ROBERT and JAMES and MARCIA TERRELL. *HANDBOOK OF IRIDIAGNOSIS AND RATIONAL THERAPY,* 16.50. This a comprehensive volume which is essential reading for all interested in irisdiagnosis. The information is arranged by both diseases and parts of the body and many charts and line drawings accompany the text. Two important early works, **Iridology: The Diagnosis from the Eye** by Henry Lahn (detailing the pioneering work of Dr. von Peczely) and **Irisdiagnosis Notes** by Ralph Weiss are also bound into this book. Spiral bound, index, 8½"x11", 355pp. HeR 61

ISMAEL, CRISTINA. *THE HEALING ENVIRONMENT,* 4.95. An exploration of a variety of paths to wholeness and healthiness. There's nothing unique about the book and the reader can expect no more than a superficial introduction to a wide number of subjects. Nonetheless, it has a nice feeling to it and the orientation is spiritual in the best sense of this word. *If our external conditions are unpleasant, then hope lies in our belief in ourselves—in our capacity to change, affect and enhance our environment. If you are among those who feel trapped, who feels alone and unimportant, I urge you to try introducing into your own life the environmental changes, inner and outer, discussed in this book. If you feel strong and solid, secure in yourself, I urge you to find ways in which you can help make the healing environment a reality for all.* Bibliography, index, 206pp. CeA 76

JACKSON, MILDRED and TERRI TEAGUE. *THE HANDBOOK OF ALTERNATIVES TO CHEMICAL MEDICINE,* 4.95. This is one of the nicest healing guides we have seen. The authors write clearly and well and they offer many unusual and sound suggestions. The book begins with some basic information, followed by a comprehensive discussion of ailments and problems common to different parts of the body. The authors' recommendations are taken from a variety of healing disciplines and they cover every area we can think of. Ms. Jackson is an experienced naturopath and Ms. Teague is involved in alternative healing in the San Francisco Bay area. Fully indexed, 176pp. LTP 75

JARVIS, D.C. *FOLK MEDICINE,* 1.50. This book has sold over three million copies. Dr. Jarvis is a respected physician who went beyond what he learned in medical school to observe the animal laws of health and the way native Vermonters used simple natural remedies: honeycomb, cider vinegar, kelp, etc. There is a lot of

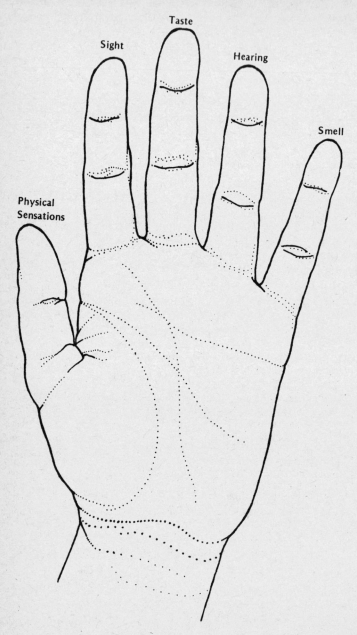

Taste

Sight

Hearing

Smell

Physical
Sensations

useful information in here for those who are trying to wean themselves away from the AMA and drugs. 192pp. Faw 58

JENSEN, BERNARD. *SEEDS AND SPROUTS FOR LIFE,* 1.75. Jensen is a well known West Coast chiropractor who practices preventive therapy. Here he gives a detailed survey of the medicinal value of seeds and grains. There's also a recipe section. 50pp. Jen nd

JENSEN, BERNARD. *WORLD KEYS TO HEALTH AND LONG LIFE,* 6.65. This is a collection of forty observations about health that Jensen has made in his world-wide travels. The writing style is informal and case studies and photographs illustrate a variety of healing techniques. 305pp. Jen 75

JENSEN, BERNARD. *YOU CAN MASTER DISEASE,* 5.50. This book is subtitled *Lessons Dealing with the Causes of Disease and How they can be Prevented.* It includes chapters on Starvation in the Midst of Plenty, What Determines Ideal Health, Intestinal Disorders, Fasting and Eliminative Diets, Surgery, Diabetes, Cancer, Colds, The Mental and Spiritual Aspects of Healing, and much else. Dr. Jensen's approach emphasizes purification of the body through good food (usually uncooked) and good thoughts. He includes many case studies illustrating his experiences. 229pp. Jen nd

JOHARI, HARISH. *DHANWANTARI,* 4.95. *This is a book for anyone who is seeking a logical, scientific and practically tested set of principles for daily life. It is a book about waking up, cleansing, eating, drinking, massage, sex and home remedies. It is a book about right living, about synchronizing the individual organism with the cycles of the Cosmos which has given him birth. It is a book about becoming normal. There are chapters on meditation, exercises and the cycle of breath—these are ways of tuning the system in shorter spans of time. . . .This is a book about techniques of centering, about stabilizing one's energy, about creating a place within one's being to which he can return at will. . . .This book is based upon my own cultural experience* [Johari is a Hindu] *and the ageless traditions of India. On the pages which follow are practices from Yoga, from Ayurvedic medicine, from the ancient Yunani system of the Greeks and Moslems, and from the timeless tribal cultures which people the plains, deserts and mountains of the Indian subcontinent. But the validity of these practices is not limited to Indians. There is nothing on these pages which has not been tried successfully on and by those born and raised in America. Truth, to be worthy of its* *name, must be universal.*—from the preface. Illustrations, 225pp. RHI 74

KELSO, ISA. *THE CAUSES AND TREATMENT OF WOMEN'S AILMENTS,* 1.35. 64pp. TPL 73

KERVRAN, LOUIS. *BIOLOGICAL TRANSMUTATIONS,* 3.50. The only English edition of Kervran's controversial book in which he shows that the mechanisms for the transmutation of biochemic elements exist within man. For example, if you need iron you can take organic manganese and your body will convert this element into iron. The field of transmutations has been widely applied in France by both physicians and agronomists. This is a detailed account of Kervran's research and discoveries, suitable for the layman who has some knowledge of the biological sciences. Bibliography, 183pp. SwH 72

KHAN, HAZRAT INAYAT. *THE BOOK OF HEALTH,* 3.95. **The Book of Health** is a collection of teachings on the spiritual aspects of healing, originally intended only for Inayat Khan's pupils. In a long introductory section he discusses the basic laws governing the mind's influence over the body, which he considers greater than the physical body's influence on mental existence. In Part Two Khan presents an excellent review of healing; Part Three is devoted to the psychological nature of disease; Part Four reviews the development of healing power; Part Five, the application of healing power; and Part Six, methods of healing. The material is not discussed in depth—however, the spiritual philosophy behind the teaching is evident and the material is very clearly presented. 106pp. SPC 62

KHAN, HAZRAT INAYAT. *SUFI HEALING,* 1.95. Inayat Khan was a great Sufi healer, and this newly discovered transcription of his 1925 healing seminar, is his most lucid and succinct presentation of Sufi healing, from cause to cure, from dis-ease to health. 40pp. Rai 75

KIEV, ARI, ed. *MAGIC, FAITH AND HEALING.* 2.95. A collection of anthropological papers on the beliefs, rituals, and symbols of the aborigines of Western Australia, the Sea Dayaks of Borneo, the Mescalero Apache of North America, and the Yoruba of Nigeria. Most of the essays are dry and academic but there are occasional insights into the healing practices of the groups discussed. Notes, index, 475pp. McM 64

KIRBAN, SALEM. *DR. CAREY REAMS' HEALTH GUIDE FOR SURVIVAL,* 4.50 Dr. Reams is a biophysicist who has discovered an ingenious "urine/saliva test" which yields information to mathematically analyze the entire body chemistry and also makes it possible to detect the location and severity of most physical maladies. This book is a journalistic report of Dr. Reams' discovery and its practical applications. Dr. Reams runs a health clinic and many case histories are included. He is also a minister and his views on the biblical health message are interspersed throughout. 180pp. HvH 76

KORTH, LESLIE. *THE PYONEX TREATMENT,* 1.40. The pyonex treatment was developed by a German physician in the nineteenth century. It involves inserting an instrument made up of thirty-three needles into an area of the body which has been infested by toxic substances. A special combination of three oils is then rubbed into the pores made by the instrument. This has the effect of not only alleviating pain, but of eliminating the toxic matter. This book includes case studies and practical treatment guidelines. 64pp. HSP 68

KORTH, LESLIE. *SOME UNUSUAL HEALING METHODS,* 5.45. Dr. Korth was trained in traditional medical practices. However, he has devoted his career to the search for alternative practices. This book is a review of the therapies he himself encountered. The material is presented in terms of practical usage and background information is also given. Topics include respiratory therapy, osteopathy, foot reflexology, acupuncture and pulse diagnosis, iris diagnosis, colds and coughs, color therapy, magnetism, and much else. A chapter is devoted to each topic. 148pp. HSP 67

KORTH, LESLIE. *TENSIONS,* 2.40. A collection of short chapters giving a number of self-help techniques for relieving tension including the use of color, word pictures, and relaxation techniques. 78pp. HSP 71

KRIPPNER, STANLEY and ALBERTO VILLOLDO. *REALMS OF HEALING,* 6.95. This volume discusses many of the most notable healers practicing today. The following chapter headings give a good idea of the contents: *The Case Against "Psychic Sur-*

gery," Paranormal Healing in the Laboratory, Three North American Healers: Rolling Thunder, Dona Pachita, and Olga Worrall, Hernani Andrade and the Spiritist "Healers" of Brazil, The Esoteric and the Intuitive Paths: Peru's Fausto Valle and Czechoslovakia's Josef Zezulka, Josephina Sison and the Filipino Spiritists, and *How Healing Happens.* Each of the individual healers is discussed at length and much of the material comes from the authors' first hand research and observation. Photographs accompany the text. Bibliography, index, 336pp. CeA 76

KROEGER, HANNA. *OLD TIME REMEDIES FOR MODERN AILMENTS,* 2.85. This little book is a remarkable collection of natural remedies, modern nutritional knowledge, spiritual healing, fasting, magnetism, etc. 105pp. NAF 71

KRUGER, HELEN. *OTHER HEALERS, OTHER CURES,* c.8.95. This is a scattered survey of alternative forms of healing and other aspects of the new consciousness. The material is not well arranged and does not seem to be well researched. Most every technique is mentioned somewhere in the volume and the format makes a general scanning possible, but those seeking any depth or good general information on a topic should look elsewhere for their information. Fully indexed, 403pp. BoM 74

KULVINSKAS, VIKTORAS. *SURVIVAL INTO THE 21ST CENTURY,* 8.00. This is a very popular book covering all aspects of alternative healing—albeit in a scattered fashion. The reader can dip into this volume and learn a bit about an incredible variety of things and go from there into more detailed discussions of the topics that interest her the most. The layout and general tone of the book is not very pleasing to us, nonetheless it is a welcome effort which should help to turn many people on to natural healing methods. Illustrated throughout and including many practical suggestions. 8½"x11," 318pp. Oma 76

KURLAND, HOWARD. *QUICK HEADACHE RELIEF WITHOUT DRUGS,* c7.95. Dr. Kurland is a Professor of Psychiatry at Northwestern University Medical School and he also has a large private practice. This book is a presentation of the technique he has developed which he calls autoacupressure. It is based on extensive studies he has made in the U.S. and China and it integrates many aspects of Chinese medicine with traditional Western medicine. Dr. Kurland explains how you can locate the pressure points that directly relate to headache pain and how you can use the pressure of your thumbnail to obtain quick relief. Very clear instructions are given and each point is fully illustrated. The book contains many testimonials from both physicians and patients about the efficacy of autoacupressure. Index, 224pp. Mor 77

KUTUMBIAH, P. *ANCIENT INDIAN MEDICINE,* 9.20. This is a comprehensive picture of ancient Indian medicine written by an Indian physician who is well versed in the ancient Indian medical classics. A fifty-two page introduction traces the origin and development of ancient Indian medicine. The rest of the book is devoted to a presentation of the treatment techniques of the ancient Indians and much practical information is included. The book is more detailed than most individuals would want, and it is also not very clearly written. Glossary, notes, index, 285pp. OLL 62

LANSON, LUCIENNE. *FROM WOMAN TO WOMAN,* 4.95. This is a sympathetically written, useful collection of information written by a gynecologist in a question and answer format. Topics include the gynecological examination, irregular periods, menstrual cramps, fertility, menopause, and much else—all considered from a psychological as well as a physical point of view. The author's goal is to help women understand the workings of their bodies. Illustrations, glossary, index, 389pp. RaH 75

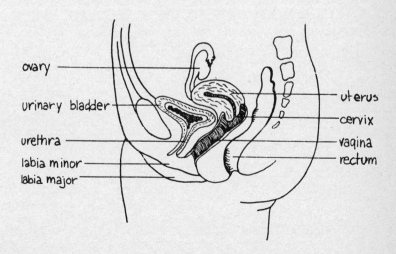

LAW, DONALD. *A GUIDE TO ALTERNATIVE MEDICINE,* 2.50. This is the best encyclopedic work we have seen. We have referred to it often in writing background for the reviews. The material is alphabetically arranged and each entry is brief and informative. The more important topics are discussed at length. There is also a good topically arranged bibliography and a listing of where to go for further information (usually the addresses of related societies), also topically arranged. Every conceivable (to us anyway!) area is surveyed. 212pp. Dou 74

LAW, DONALD. *HOW TO KEEP YOUR HAIR ON,* 2.40. This book begins with a discussion of hair—how it grows, why it sometimes stops growing, and what causes such stoppages. This is followed by a discussion of the nutrients needed by hair and a selection of diet suggestions for specific problems. Next, herbal and naturopathic remedies are given. Bibliography, 70pp. HSP 68

LAWS, PRICILLA. *X-RAYS: MORE HARM THAN GOOD,* c8.95. Diagnostic x-rays expose Americans to more man made radiation than nuclear power plants, color television sets, and microwave ovens. In today's health care system, x-rays are standard medical practice, even when there is no sign of trouble. This is an in depth analysis, based on extensive research. Dr. Laws stresses ways in which we can protect ourselves from unnecessary radiation by understanding the uses and misuses of diagnostic x-rays. Illustrations, glossary, notes, index, 271pp. Rod 77

LAWSON-WOOD, D. and J. *GLOWING HEALTH THROUGH DIET AND POSTURE,* 1.40. A collection of suggestions for ways of improving one's general health based largely on the principles of oriental medicine and macrobiotics. Basic concepts such as yin-yang and the laws of the universe are discussed in the first chapters. The Lawson-Woods follow with some specific suggestions including a regime of self-massage. The information on yin-yang is the clearest we have read anywhere. Illustrations, 62pp. HSP 73

LESLIE, CHARLES, ed. *ASIAN MEDICAL SYSTEMS,* c16.50. Three great traditions of medical science evolved during antiquity in the Chinese, Indian, and Mediterranean civilizations—all based on humoral conceptions of health and illness. This is a scholarly collection of essays by individuals trained in history, sociology, anthropology, public health, pharmacology, epidemiology, cosmopolitan medicine, and philosophy. All aspects of the traditional medical systems and their cosmopolitan counterparts are discussed at length. Notes, index, 419pp. UCa 76

LETTVIN, MAGGIE. *MAGGIE'S BACK BOOK,* c10.95. Maggie Lettvin has taught a number of exercise classes on public television. In this book she offers a series of exercises for those with back pain. Over 300 line drawings accompany the step-by-step instructions. The exercises can accompany and become part of your daily life routine. There are also specific exercises for particular kinds of pain, for rebuilding flexibility, and for keeping your back pain free. Bibliography, 8½"x9½", 173pp. HMC 76

LONG, JAMES W. *THE ESSENTIAL GUIDE TO PRESCRIPTION DRUGS: WHAT YOU NEED TO KNOW FOR SAFE DRUG USE,* 5.95. An extensive analysis of the 200 most commonly prescribed generic drugs in the U.S. and Canada and of a selection of over-the-counter medications. Each of the profiles includes the following information: brand names, available dosage forms, how this drug works, cautions, possible adverse effects, and much else. Every possible subject has been covered in depth. The book is also fully cross-referenced and there are a number of tables. This is an extremely well researched work which should be available to all people who use drugs. 131pp. H&R 76

LOOMIS, EVARTS and J. SIG PAULSON. *HEALING FOR EVERYONE,* c8.95. A physician and a minister blend their experience to explore the physical, mental, and spiritual elements that make up a complete human being. Both men have had extensive healing experience. The book begins with a conversation between the two and from there Dr. Loomis goes on to analyze man's being from a spiritual point of view. He devotes the next chapter to nutrition and gears his discussion toward the need for maintaining physical harmony. Other chapters review the diabetic and hypoglycemic states and provide advice on muscle use and breathing. Various alternative healing systems are also discussed and evaluated. Sig Paulson then follows up with the minister's view, emphasizing the importance of proper mental and emotional attitudes. Notes, index, 234pp. Haw 75

LOWENKOPF, ANNE. *OSTEOPUNCTURE,* 5.95. Osteopuncture is a technique discovered by a California neurologist, Dr. Ronald Lawrence. Osteopuncture was developed as a technique to deal with chronic pain. In osteopuncture, the surface of the bone is stimulated by a needle prick. It is most effective in treating problems that are located in the joints in any area of the body and least effective in eliminating pain caused by internal medical problems. Dr. Lawrence has been treating patients with osteopuncture at his clinic for over three years and has had an amazing success rate. He is currently teaching many others his techniques and in this book one of his patients outlines the technique, presents many actual case studies and presents both a theoretical and practical discussion of the subject. Bibliography, notes, index, 187pp. MAr 76

MCGAREY, WILLIAM. *EDGAR CAYCE AND THE PALMA CHRISTA,* 4.95. A detailed study of the use of castor oil packs as suggested in the Edgar Cayce readings and as observed in case histories from the readings and in Dr. McGarey's own practice. Cayce suggested the packs as remedies for over fifty different ailments and the results have often been remarkable. Notes, oversize, 133pp. ARE 70

MCGINNIS, TERRI. *THE WELL CAT BOOK,* c10.00. If you are a cat owner, this book will tell you just about everything you can handle about your pet's body, preventive medicine, diagnostic medicine, home medical care, and breeding and reproduction. It will save on vet bills and provide information halfway between that of the trained vet and that of the average cat owner. Many line drawings, index, 279pp. RaH 75

MCGINNIS, TERRI. *THE WELL DOG BOOK,* c10.00. Just the same as the above, but for dogs. 237pp. RaH 74

MCGUIRE, THOMAS. *THE TOOTH TRIP,* 4.95. Our dentist doesn't like this book. He says it makes his patients too suspicious. If you think maybe you ought to be a little more suspicious, this is for you. Written by a dentist, it tells you all you'll need to know about your teeth and how to care for them (including good advice on nutrition), plus such chapters as: *A Manual for Survival in the Dental Office, Portrait of the Bad Dentist as Con Artist.* and *How to O.D. Your Teeth.* Written in hip style with many amusing illustrations. 233pp. RaH 72

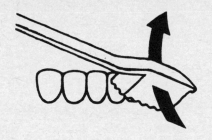

MACKARNESS, RICHARD. *EATING DANGEROUSLY: THE HAZARDS OF HIDDEN ALLERGIES,* 6.95. Dr. Mackarness is a British physician, specializing in the treatment of obesity and the ecological and allergic aspects of mental illness. In this book he contends that the ailments which millions suffer from can often be traced to food allergies. He urges us to examine our diets when we feel awful and warns us not to be surprised when our favorite foods turn out to be the culprits. For many food allergies are masked—something that gives us a lift can trap us in a pernicious cycle where highs are followed by increasingly severe and dangerous letdowns. Dr. Mackarness has devised a number of tests to prove and isolate allergies and their effects. In this book he discusses his testing procedures and offers a number of case histories. Bibliography, notes, index, 179pp. HBJ 76

MAJNO, GUIDO. *THE HEALING HAND,* c25.00. Illustrated with hundreds of photographs, many in full color, this is a well researched account of man's attempts over the centuries to promote good health and conquer pain and disease. Dr. Majno, Chairman of the Department of Pathology at the University of Massachusetts, spent over ten years researching the material. He reviews the techniques and documented experiences of physicians in Egypt, Greece, Rome, India, and China. A mammoth, oversized volume—well documented, but still suitable for the general reader. Extensive notes, fully indexed, 594pp. HUP 75

MAPLE, ERIC. *THE ANCIENT ART OF OCCULT HEALING,* 1.00. A brief treatise incorporating material from many areas. 64pp. Wei 74

MEARES, AINSLIE. *A SYSTEM OF MEDICAL HYPNOSIS,* c15.00. Meares is a respected Australian psychiatrist. This is considered the definite text on the subject. It gives a good explanation of the principles and uses of hypnosis in medicine, explicit details of the five fundamental techniques of induction, and many case histories that vividly portray the problems and the successes that attend the use of hypnotism. A very detailed account, recommended for the serious student. 484pp. Jul 60

MELLOR, CONSTANCE. *NATURAL REMEDIES FOR COMMON AILMENTS,* c10.50. This is a modern, up-to-date encyclopedia of common ailments and their remedy by purely natural methods, including homoeopathy, herbalism, and biochemistry. The author is a physiotherapist and nutritionist. She discusses not only the general nature of disease but the treatment of its many signs and symptoms. Preventive suggestions and diets for specific ailments are given in great detail, as are other therapies. The book is alphabetically arranged by the diseases, and fully indexed. Recommended. 240pp. Dan 73

Mental Health

In recent years research has brought about a much greater awareness of the relationship between the chemical balance in our cells and our emotional and mental states. Most dramatic is the growth of orthomolecular medicine and megavitamin therapy in treating schizophrenia. While still vigorously opposed by many psychotherapists, this metabolic approach is finding new converts within the medical profession as further evidence of its effectiveness becomes known. The Canadian Schizophrenia Foundation found an 85% recovery rate and the Princeton Brain Bio Center found a 90% recovery rate using the biochemical approach, compared to a 35% spontaneous recovery rate and a 50% rate using traditional therapies. The leading organization promoting research and understanding in this field is the Huxley Institute for Biosocial Research (parent of the American Schizophrenia Assn.) at 56 West 45th Street, New York City 10036. In addition to the books below, also see the subsection on Sugar, because hypoglycemia is involved in most cases of schizophrenia, alcoholism, etc., and is central to the whole problem of disturbed metabolism that underlies much mental and emotional disturbance.

ADAMS, RUTH and FRANK MURRAY. *BODY, MIND AND THE B VITAMINS,* 1.95. If you get as confused about all the different B vitamins as we do, you will welcome this book. Clearly written, with a wealth of research findings, it details the effects of the various B vitamins on physical ills, mental illness, depression, and the stresses of modern life. Lengthy foreword by Abram Hoffer. Bibliography, index, 258pp. War 75

ADAMS, RUTH and FRANK MURRAY. *MEGAVITAMIN THERAPY,* 1.95. This book is largely devoted to various forms of drug abuse and addiction—particularly alcohol and sugar—and their relationship to nutritional deficiencies. The cure includes but is not limited to megavitamin therapy. A good, occasionally rambling, account. Includes a list of addresses where further information on megavitamin therapy may be found. Index, 277pp. War 75

BLAINE, TOM. *MENTAL HEALTH THROUGH NUTRITION,* 3.45. Judge Blaine's concern with allergies led him to hypoglycemia and adrenal cortex insufficiency; these in turn led him to schizophrenia and alcoholism—all the various diseases that respond to diet and megavitamin therapy. Citing a wealth of medical evidence (but lacking footnotes, alas) he alleges that most mental disorders, major and minor, have their genesis in improper or inadequate nutrition. 203pp. CiP 69

CHERASKIN, E. and W. RINGSDORF, JR. *PSYCHO-DIETETICS,* 1.95. With the obvious help of Arlene Brecher, a popular writer on medical subjects, the authors present their most up to date survey of the relationship of diet and psychological states. Covers alcoholism, schizophrenia, hypoglycemia, depression, etc. Written in popular style with lots of quizzes by which you can see how you rate on mental states or diet. Useful appendices with further sources of information and an excellent bibliography. Index, 228pp. S&D 74

FREDERICKS, CARLETON. *PSYCHO-NUTRITION,* c7.95. Another book on megavitamin, orthomolecular therapy. Fredericks is not only one of the best known and most knowledgeable nutritionists, but is also the President of the International Academy of Preventive Medicine. He discusses hypoglycemia, schizophrenia, autism, allergies—the whole range of problems reflecting biochemical abnormalities which can frequently be cured nutritionally. Many case histories and research findings are cited. Because Dr. Fredericks is an authority, not just a popular writer, this is a good book to give to someone with a personal need to be turned on to this new therapy which is still damned by much of the medical and psychiatric orthodoxy. An appendix, *Where to Seek Help,* is also included. Index, 224pp. G&D 76

HOFFER, ABRAM and HUMPHRY OSMOND. *HOW TO LIVE WITH SCHIZOPHRENIA,* c8.95. This is a new edition of the classic book on schizophrenia by the two doctors who pioneered niacin therapy. Briefly, they view schizophrenia as basically a physical illness due to disturbances in the biochemical balance of the body. It appears to involve a defective adrenal metabolism which results in production of a subtle poison in the blood of the victims—a poison which is counteracted by megavitamin therapy. Written for lay persons, it should be the first book read by persons facing this problem. Index, 224pp. UnB 74

LILLISTON, LYNN. *MEGAVITAMINS,* 1.50. An excellent, up to date summary of the whole field: the development of megavitamin therapy for schizophrenia, alcoholism, hypoglycemia, heart attacks, senility, drugs. An interesting chapter details the use of fasting for treatment of schizophrenia and allergies. The final chapter discusses organizations in the forefront of research and publicity regarding this new therapy. Clear and readable, notes, index, 224pp. Faw 75

NEWBOLD, H.L. *MEGA-NUTRIENTS,* c11.95. This is a worthy addition to the do-it-yourself medical books. Dr. Newbold is a psychiatrist with excellent medical credentials who, like most of his profession, ridiculed or ignored nutritional medicine until he, himself, came down with hypoglycemia which the best doctors he could find did not diagnose. He tells his own story in the book and that is one of its delights—the reader gets a good feeling about who the author really is. After hitting on an accurate self diagnosis he began to read up on nutritional medicine and since then has been able to help his patients much more than he ever did before. In this book Dr. Newbold assumes you don't have access to a physician who is knowledgeable about preventive medicine so he tells you what you need to know (and your doctor ought to know), advising you what tests you can give yourself, and what ones you should ask your doctor to give or authorize. In particular, he gives details on how to establish your own vitamin and mineral regimen, what are the minimum tests you need, and how you can gradually step up dosages of each vitamin and tell when you've hit the right level. Other chapters deal with hormone deficiencies, alcoholism, beauty and weight control, the importance of the right kind of light, aging, and how to save money on your nutritional needs. A final chapter suggests some ways to go about finding a nutritionally-oriented doctor. Recommended. Index, 360pp. Wyd 75

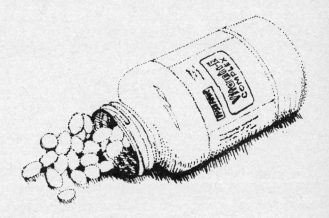

PFEIFFER, CARL. *MENTAL AND ELEMENTAL NUTRIENTS,* c9.95. See the Nutrition section.

STEINER, LEE. *PSYCHIC SELF-HEALING FOR PSYCHO-LOGICAL PROBLEMS,* c7.95. Dr. Steiner, a psychologist, shows how Kirlian photography can serve as an important diagnostic tool. She found that the health and fullness of Kirlian photographs correlate precisely with clinical diagnoses of nervous breakdown, schizophrenia, psychosomatic illness, and brain damage. Kirlian photographs can also show the effectiveness of new techniques such as megavitamin therapy. Dr. Steiner documents the implications of this discovery through case histories of her own patients and over forty Kirlian photographs. Index, 6"x9", 224pp. PrH 77

WADE, CARLSON. *EMOTIONAL HEALTH AND NUTRITION,* 1.50. Carlson Wade is one of the most prolific of all the popular health writers. His writing is generally sound, although at times a bit overenthusiastic for our taste. This book covers hypoglycemia, schizophrenia, megavitamin therapy, effects of caffeine, tension, fatigue and many related topics. 155pp. ASC 71

WATSON, GEORGE. *NUTRITION AND YOUR MIND,* c1.95. This has been quite a popular book. Dr. Watson was Professor of Philosophy of Science at USC before devoting full time to psychochemical research and treatment. He contends that mental and emotional disorders are caused almost exclusively by physical malfunctioning of the body's metabolism. His unique contribution is the concept of fast oxidizers and slow oxidizers and he provides a simple test by which the reader can determine which metabolic type he is. This, in turn, greatly affects the kind of food each of us needs to be in best physical and mental shape. The book gives practical diet and vitamin suggestions for both types. 204pp. Ban 72

MESSEGUE, MAURICE. *OF MEN AND PLANTS,* c6.95. An autobiography of the world's greatest plant healer, with anecdotes about the thousands he has healed, and a full account of his actual methods of treatment. Even more engrossing than the anecdotes is the plant lore throughout the book. It has been a bestseller in Europe. 327pp. McM 70

MEYER, CLARENCE. *AMERICAN FOLK MEDICINE,* 3.95. A collection of early American remedies, arranged topically by ailment, from a wide variety of people, utilizing ingredients usually found at hand (at least back in the good old days!). Includes a listing of common and Latin names. 296pp. NAL 73

MICHELE, ARTHUR. *ORTHOTHERAPY,* c6.95. One out of every three Americans is born with a musculoskeletal imbalance which ultimately puts stress on every muscle of the body—a stress that results in pain. Every painful muscle is a tightened and shortened muscle that can only be relaxed through exercise. The core of this book is a series of corrective exercises, each keyed to a particular muscular problem. There are exercises to help hip pain, exercises for sciatica, exercises for cricks in the neck, headaches, and leg cramps. To help ascertain which of them you need, Dr. Michele also includes a series of tests based on the diagnostic procedures he uses in his own private practice. Dr. Michele himself is an orthopedic surgeon and in this book he summarizes the results of over thirty-five years of medical study. Illustrations, index, 223pp. EvC 71

MILLER, DON. *BODY MIND,* 1.50. Calling itself the *Whole Person Health Book,* this one, written by a martial arts instructor, deals with movement, breathing, flexibility and relaxation, centeredness, sex and love, and food. It's very general, so only suggested for people just beginning to take an interest in these things. 217pp. Pin 74

MONTGOMERY, RUTH. *BORN TO HEAL,* 1.75. Here Ms. Montgomery gives us the life story and experiences of Mr. A—whom she says is one of the greatest healers of our time. Mr. A heals by laying on of hands and some of his most interesting cases are cited here along with interpretation of his healing abilities. 224pp. Pop 73

MOORE, MARCIA and MARK DOUGLAS. *DIET, SEX, AND YOGA,* c6.95. See the Yoga subsection of Body Work.

MOYLE, ALAN. *ASTHMA AND HAY FEVER,* 1.35. This discussion focuses on removal of the root causes of asthma and hay fever, and on a variety of unorthodox treatments. 63pp. TPL 75

MOYLE, ALAN. *INSOMNIA,* 1.35. A discussion of the basic causes of insomnia and a variety of treatments. 64pp. TPL 74

MOYLE, ALAN. *NATURAL HEALTH FOR THE ELDERLY,* 4.55. Moyle, a British naturopath, begins this book with an explanation of the aging process and how it is complicated by such degenerative diseases as rheumatism, arthritis, bronchitis, emphysema, and asthma. He gives details of simple therapies and diets designed to overcome these and other disorders in the aged. Index, 128pp. TPL 75

MURAMOTO, NABORU. *HEALING OURSELVES,* 4.95. Traditional Oriental medicine does not conceive of the body in parts; it considers each organ a part of the whole, and disease a deterioration of the entire body system. This book presents a number of simple principles which we can use to heal ourselves. Muramoto explains how to diagnose diseases and determine the foods, herbs, or external treatments necessary to cure them. The material in this book came from a series of lectures and classes which Muramoto gave, and the material is uniquely adapted to an American audience. A great deal of philosophy is included and many sensitive drawings. 8½"x11", 150pp. Avo 73

MURPHY, JOSEPH. *HOW TO USE YOUR HEALING POWER,* 3.00. A discussion of Jesus' healing power and techniques, and an explanation of how the same principles can be applied to every individual. 158pp. DeV 57

NITTLER, ALAN. *HEALTH QUESTIONS AND ANSWERS,* 1.75. The questions and answers in this book first appeared in Dr. Nittler's monthly *Let's Live* magazine column. They are topically organized by ailments. Index, 383pp. Pyr 76

NOLEN, WILLIAM. *HEALING,* 1.75. Nolen, a surgeon, conducted an investigation into faith healing and psychic surgery. The book is organized into five parts, the first of which sets the stage and relates how Dr. Nolen got interested in these things. Then he devotes three long chapters to analyses of Norbu Chen, Katherine Kuhlman, and Filipino psychic surgeons. A final section sums up his thoughts on healing and the healers previously discussed. Nolen presents interviews with each of the individual healers and does follow up research on many of the healed patients. He attempts to be objective, but we get the feeling that he just does not believe that the type of healing he is investigating *is* possible—therefore he finds that most of the healing miracles are hoaxes. In the process he provides a fascinating narrative. 308pp. Faw 74

NULL, GARY. *THE COMPLETE QUESTION AND ANSWER BOOK OF NATURAL THERAPY,* 1.25. Arranged alphabetically by ailment, disease, and organ. Index, 287pp. Del 72

OKI, MASAHIRO. *YOGA THERAPY,* 5.95. In this volume Master Oki presents a series of techniques which are a combination of controlled breathing, mental concentration, and physical movement and which produce concentrated effects on specific organs, muscles, and bodily functions. Master Oki is Japan's foremost yoga teacher and is also adept at Oriental and North African healing arts. 150 illustrations, index, oversize, 128pp. Jap 76

OYLE, IRVING. *THE HEALING MIND,* 4.95/1.95. Dr. Oyle organized New York City's first free clinic. More recently he founded a clinic in Bolinas, California which incorporates herbal medicine, osteopathy, traditional medicine, psychic healing, acupuncture massage, sonopuncture (his own technique utilizing high frequency sound rather than needles), and many other ancient and modern techniques. This narrative relates his experiences in an informal style and emphasizes specific cases and practical self-healing instructions. A well written, informative account. Illustrations, bibliography, notes, 125pp. CeA 75

PARAMANANDA, SWAMI. *SPIRITUAL HEALING,* 2.75. A short, religious treatise, with chapters on spiritual healing, control of breath and healing, the source of healing power, healing of body and mind, and healing in meditation. 86pp. VdC 75

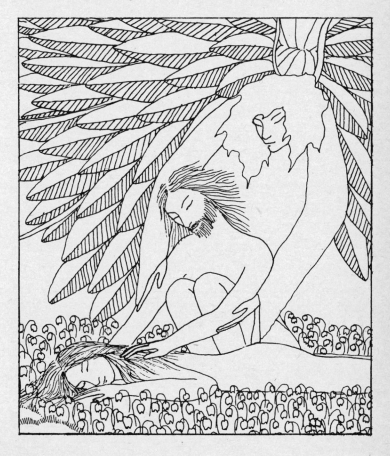

PELLETIER, KENNETH. *MIND AS HEALER, MIND AS SLAYER,* 4.95. Dr. Pelletier is a research psychologist at the Langley Porter Neuropsychiatric Institute of the University of California. In this book he defines the role of stress in four major types of illnesses: cardiovascular disease, cancer, arthritis, and respiratory disease. The book's three major sections cover a survey of the sources of stress, guidelines for the evaluation of one's own stress levels, profiles of various disease prone personalities, practical suggestions for the prevention of stress related diseases using such techniques as meditation and biofeedback. Gay Luce says that *This book is not only going to call for a significant new look at our practice of medicine, it is going to allow people to finally realize there is something definite and positive they can do about their own health by preventing sickness and creating a more satisfying life.* Bibliography, index, 381pp. Del 77

POWELL, ERIC. *HEALTH FROM EARTH, AIR, AND WATER,* 1.10. Health from the earth covers clay and mud treatments, from the air covers breathing exercises, and health from water deals with the skin and a variety of baths and water packs. The final chapter outlines the Kneipp water cure, modified and abbreviated. A simple naturopathic presentation. 64pp. HSP 70

POWELL, ERIC. *THE NATURAL HOME PHYSICIAN,* c11.90. This is an encyclopedic handbook which contains remedies for a host of ailments. The treatments are taken from a variety of natural healing areas including herbalism, biochemistry, homoeopathy, spiritual healing, and zone therapy. Powell himself is a naturopath and he brings years of experience to this compendium. The arrangement is alphabetical, with ailments and remedies mixed together and unfortunately there is no index. Nonetheless, this is one of the most useful handbooks that we know of. 284pp. HSP 75

POWELL, MILTON. *HOW TO STRENGTHEN WEAK NERVES,* 1.35. Clear instructions on building sound, healthy nerves. Special attention is given to the mental and emotional causes of weak nerves and to effective ways of building a sound psycho-physical system. 64pp. TPL 74

PRENSKY, JOYCE, ed. *HEALING YOURSELF,* 1.50. This small, multilithed booklet contains a great deal of useful information about home remedies for a wide variety of ailments. It also covers babies and children, birth control, vitamins and minerals, and suggests a complete home remedy self help kit. Written in hip style with a do-it-yourself layout (not always too readable), it is oriented toward good nutrition and natural remedies, but also contains up-to-date medical knowledge. It started with a printing of 500 copies and kept growing as people passed it on and word about it spread. Illustrated with line drawings and some photographs. Index, 65pp. HeY 75

PREVENTION MAGAZINE STAFF. *THE ENCYCLOPEDIA OF COMMON DISEASES,* c19.95. A voluminous handbook which explains the causes and symptoms of hundreds of familiar health problems, and provides the latest authoritative information on treatment and cure. The emphasis is on methods for the prevention of disease, not just the cure of ailments. The discussion is non technical and is easy to read. The book is fully indexed and the 227 chapters cover virtually every topic we can think of. 1296pp. Rod 76

QUICK, CLIFFORD. *NATURE CURE FOR CYSTITIS,* 1.30. A simply written explanation of cystitis—including information on how and why it occurs, its effects on the urinary and other vital body systems, and how to cure it and allied ailments by a combination of diet, exercise, and fasting. 64pp. TPL 75

QUICK, CLIFFORD. *SINUSITIS, BRONCHITIS AND EMPHYSEMA,* 1.95. Describes the nature of these diseases, why they happen, and how they can be treated with drugless, natural methods. A variety of diet suggestions, helpful breathing exercises, and other programs are included. 128pp. Kea 75

RAMACHARAKA, YOGI. *THE PRACTICAL WATER CURE,* 1.00. A comprehensive survey of various water cures practiced in India and the Orient. 123pp. YPS 37

RAMACHARAKA, YOGI. *THE SCIENCE OF PSYCHIC HEALING,* c6.00. A simple introductory explanation of healing through the understanding of natural laws and cooperation with them. Many theories are introduced to acquaint the reader with various aspects of healing. 190pp. YPS 09

RECHUNG, RINPOCHE. *TIBETAN MEDICINE,* 6.95. English translations of the most important Tibetan medical texts, and a history of Tibetan medicine. A very extensive, illustrated treatment. Bibliography, 327pp. UCa 76

REGARDIE, ISRAEL. *THE ART OF TRUE HEALING,* 2.00. Subtitled *A Treatise on the Mechanism of Prayer, and the Operation of the Law of Attraction in Nature,* this pamphlet suggests a number of techniques for generating healing energy based on the Western esoteric tradition. 42pp. Hel 64

REILLY, HAROLD J. and RUTH HAGY BROD. *THE EDGAR CAYCE HANDBOOK FOR HEALTH THROUGH DRUGLESS THERAPY,* c10.95. Dr. Reilly is a physiotherapist who was referred many cases by Edgar Cayce and has worked with Cayce methods for some forty-five years. In this book he presents a fusion of his own knowledge and experience and Cayce's recommendations. Subjects covered include diet and nutrition, exercise, hydrotherapy, massage, internal cleansing, weight reduction, complexion and skin care, and how to age without growing old. The chapter on massage is particularly good, with extensive instructions and line drawings on how to give a massage. For followers of Cayce's health ideas, this is the most comprehensive, useful book to come along yet. Index, 348pp. McM 75

REYNER, J.H. *PSIONIC MEDICINE,* c5.95. A new approach to orthodox medicine, involving the assessment and treatment of the underlying causes of clinical symptoms, is described here. Dr. George Laurence discovered that from the scientific application of medical dowsing, precisely determined homoeopathic or allied remedies can be prescribed to restore vital harmony to the body. Reyner, in collaboration with Dr. Laurence, describes the basis and practice of psionic medicine—including case histories and explanations of techniques. Bibliography, index, 139pp. Wei 74

ROSSITER, FREDERICK. *WATER FOR HEALTH AND HEALING,* 2.00. The virtues of hydrotherapy or water treatment have been known since ancient times. *It is the purpose of this book to present a practical guide to the use of water for the promotion of health by simple methods which may be used in the home, and to present vital information about the marvels of water and its relation to human well-being. The book stresses the connection between water and the circulation of the blood and other fluids of the body, and its relations to functions of the mind.*—from the introduction. 112pp. Wte 72

ROWSELL, HENRY and HELEN MACFARLANE. *HENRY'S BEE HERBAL,* 1.80. Subtitled *Modern Applications of Honey Therapy,* this book presents a beekeeper's researches into the therapeutic benefits of bee venom, honey, and pollen extract, and emphasizes the efficacy of these in breast cancer, rheumatism, and other degenerative diseases. Index, 128pp. TPL 74

SAMUELS, MIKE and HAL BENNETT. *BE WELL,* 3.95. The authors believe that each person contains inborn healing abilities which s/he can use to make herself well. This impulse toward healthiness represents a guiding force which is available to us every moment of our lives and which is manifest in many forms throughout the world in which we live. In this volume Samuels and Bennett suggest a variety of ways to recognize your inborn healing abilities and to learn what you can do to free them to work at their best. The techniques are simple and can be incorporated into your daily life. It is a very positive message and it is well stated. Illustrations, glossary, bibliography, index, 164pp. RaH 74

SAMUELS, MIKE and HAL BENNETT. *THE WELL BODY BOOK,* c12.95/7.50. This is the most comprehensive home medical handbook we've seen. Samuels, a physician, describes in excellent detail how to do a complete physical exam, how to diagnose common diseases, how to practice preventive medicine and how to get the most from your doctor if you do need to go to one. Includes wonderful step-by-step illustrations and an annotated bibliography. Highly recommended. 8½"x11", 350pp. RaH 73

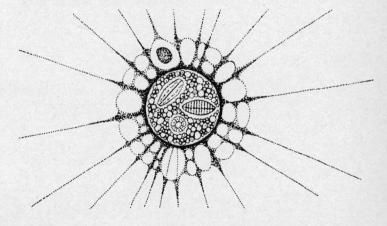

SCIENCE OF LIFE BOOKS. *CARING FOR PETS,* 1.35. Suggestions for natural treatments of cats, dogs, and cage birds. 46pp. SLB 71

SCHNEIDER, L.L. *OLD FASHIONED HEALTH REMEDIES THAT WORK BEST,* c8.95. An experienced self help writer and a naturopath have teamed up to present another compilation of *dozens of tried-and-true home remedies that can help you get quick, long-lasting relief from just about anything that ails you.* The following selections from the table of contents give a feeling of the authors' approach: *Special Foods That Exert Amazing Curative Power Over Supposedly Incurable Conditions, Common Ailments You Can Get Rid of Uncommonly Fast Nature's Way, Little Things That You Do That Pay Off In Health Dividends.* Index, 227pp. PrH 77

SCIENCE OF LIFE BOOKS. *THE COMMON COLD,* 1.35. A discussion of causes and remedies based on natural treatments. Includes specific suggestions for influenza, bronchitis, catarrh, sinus trouble, hay fever, and asthma. 61pp. SLB 64

SCIENCE OF LIFE BOOKS. *LIVER AILMENTS AND COMMON DISORDERS,* 1.35. Topically arranged natural treatments of migraine headeaches, kidney and bladder troubles, glandular disturbances, enlarged tonsils and adenoids, goiter, anaemia, underweight, unhealthy hair, varicose veins, and ulcers. And all in 62 pages! SLB 69

SCIENCE OF LIFE BOOKS. *SKIN TROUBLES,* 1.35. A discussion of how the causes of skin problems and their remedies. Includes specific treatments for acne, boils, carbuncles, hives, eczema, dermatitis, erysipelas, shingles, psoriasis, dandruff, and much else. 64pp. SLB 73

SCIENCE OF LIFE BOOKS. *WOMAN'S CHANGE OF LIFE,* 1.35. A general survey which includes information on all aspects of menopause and a variety of suggestions for making this period flow more smoothly. 62pp. SLB 69

SCOFIELD, ARTHUR G. *CHIROPRACTIC: THE SCIENCE OF SPECIFIC SPINAL ADJUSTMENT,* c7.80. A comprehensive, scholarly presentation of the principles and history for laymen and doctors. Chiropractic consists of an analysis by x-ray of interference with normal nerve transmission followed by manual adjustment of the vertebral column. This is the best overall book available. Glossary, 222pp. TPL 68

SEHNERT, KEITH and HOWARD EISENBERG. *HOW TO BE YOUR OWN DOCTOR (SOMETIMES),* c9.95. This is an extremely useful handbook▪which is designed to help people handle minor illnesses and emergencies without medical help and major ones without panic. Dr. Sehnert calls his patients (and readers) *Activated Patients* and he bases his presentation on his own medical practice and his experience as Director of the Center for Continuing Health Education, Georgetown University, Washington, D.C. Basic chapters —designed to help you recognize and understand your own medical problems and learn to correct them—present information on basic drugs, the language that physicians use when discussing symptoms, how to keep a medical history, and much else. *The Self-Help Medical Guide,* a section within the book, outlines clearly and in layman's terms, the symptoms, treatment, and call the doctor signals for fourteen illnesses, thirteen injuries, and nine emergencies. Dr. Sehnert's orientation is allopathic, but he is sympathetic to alternate techniques. 364pp. G&D 75

SELYE, HANS. *THE STRESS OF LIFE,* c8.95. This book is a classic. Dr. Selye has received eight honorary degrees, and his pioneer work on stress has been compared with the contributions of Pasteur, Ehrlich and Freud. It is in five parts: I, the discovery of stress; II, the dissection of stress, analyzing the mechanism through which our body is attacked by, and can defend itself against, stress-producing situations; III, the diseases of adaptation: maladies such as cardiovascular diseases, digestive disorders and mental derangements considered to result largely from failures in the stress-fighting mechanism; IV, a sketch for a unified theory; and V, the implications and applications, not only in medicine but also as regards man's ability to devise a natural, healthy philosophy of life. Difficult reading for laymen but it has a good glossary and various aids by the author to make his findings accessible. This new revised edition is somewhat more readable than the original. It incorporates the findings of the last twenty years and eliminates some of the original lengthy arguments for matters which are now commonly accepted. Glossary, bibliography, index, 515pp. MGH 76

SELYE, HANS. *STRESS WITHOUT DISTRESS,* 1.75. Dr. Selye again takes us through a discussion of the mechanism of stress as a nonspecific response of the body to any demand made upon it. He goes on to develop a philosophy of life which is in harmony with the demands of nature and which uses stress as a positive force for personal achievement and happiness. He calls for an altruistic egotism which is both biologically sound and consonant with the teachings of most religions. For those of us who talk about living in harmony with nature, this book presenting the scientific views of a physician can reveal many valuable new perspectives. Glossary, excellent annotated bibliography, index, 171pp. NAL 74

SHEALY, C. NORMAN. *OCCULT MEDICINE CAN SAVE YOUR LIFE,* c7.95. When we first heard of this book we were put off by the title. Despite the title, this is a fine overview of contemporary healing movements. Dr. Shealy has held professorships in neurosurgery at three American medical schools and he has devoted himself to learning about these techniques and incorporating them into his practice. This book traces what Dr. Shealy has learned about alternative medicine and discusses his experiences with it. It is a personal account which often makes fascinating reading. Dr. Shealy begins with an account of faith healing and then he relates how he got interested in all this. The next section is devoted to an historical study of occult medicine. This is followed by surveys of the medical benefits of psi phenomena, astrology, palmistry, graphology, and much else. The final sections discuss when conventional medicine should be used and when alternative techniques should be applied. Bibliography, index, 214pp. Dia 75

SHEALY, C. NORMAN. *90 DAYS TO SELF-HEALTH,* c7.95. Dr. Shealy believes that just as emotional and physical problems can cause ill health, you can also achieve good health by maintaining conscious control over your autonomic nervous system. He has developed a series of biogenic exercises which, practiced daily for three months, help to create good health, increase energy, promote relaxation, control pain, and minimize the effects of daily stress. In this book he presents a daily health and exercise plan developed in his work with over 1300 patients and in a number of clinical research projects. Both mental and physical exercises on a number of levels are included. This is an excellent program which we recommend. Bibliography, index, 190pp. Dia 77

SHEALY, C. NORMAN. *THE PAIN GAME,* 4.95. Dr. Shealy believes that drugs and surgery should be used as little as possible in treating pain. In this book he discusses in transactional analysis terms the games patients and doctors play, and shows how much the condition and the treatment is a game. He has developed a clinic in which drugs are withdrawn and operant conditioning (learning to live normally despite the pain) and biofeedback and autogenics are used. The object is to help the patient understand where the pain is really coming from and what s/he can do to take responsibility for dealing with it. The book includes both a discussion of the theoretical aspects of pain, and practical exercises that the reader can do at home. Bibliography, index, 145pp. CeA 76

SHERMAN, HAROLD. *"WONDER" HEALERS OF THE PHILIPPINES*, 5.25. Sherman investigated claims that psychic surgery was being done by persons in the Philippines without drugs or instruments, and causing no pain to patients even though they remained in full consciousness. The operations were reported to have been accomplished only with the use of the surgeon's hands. The facts and results of these highly successful, unorthodox surgeries are presented allowing the reader to decide for himself upon the evidence gathered. Included are a series of pictures of a successful surgery being performed on a woman with an internal stomach growth. 328pp. DeV 66

SHERMAN, HAROLD. *YOUR POWER TO HEAL*, 1.50. An excellent overview of healing techniques and important healers, including practical suggestions and case studies. 223pp. Faw 72

SIMEONS, A.T.W. *MAN'S PRESUMPTUOUS BRAIN*, 2.95. This is the best book we have ever seen on psychosomatic disorders. Dr. Simeons contends that man's brain battles with and submerges his animal instincts and that this battle grows more serious with every advance of our civilization. The book begins with a review of the evolution of the body, psyche, and culture, and provides a medical and historical background for the thesis. Dr. Simeons next discusses the many physical complaints caused by the unceasing struggle between the cortex and the source of our instincts (the diencephalon). Included are disorders of the upper and lower digestive tract, of the heart and blood vessels, the thyroid and metabolism (obesity), some forms of diabetes, arthritis, and sexual deviations. A fascinating, important contribution. Index, 290pp. Dut 60

SMEDT, EVELYN DE, et al. *LIFEARTS: A PRACTICAL GUIDE TO TOTAL BEING–NEW MEDICINE AND ANCIENT WISDOM*, 5.95. As the title suggests this book covers many topics in an introductory way. The book is divided into four sections: *knowing yourself, nourishing yourself, healing yourself* and *being in the*

197

world. As you might imagine spirituality is integrated into the discussion, even when the authors are covering apparently mundane subjects such as basic nutrition. Each of the subjects is covered in a fair amount of depth. Unfortunately the reader is not guided to sources of additional information. Nonetheless, the book is well written and is a good general primer. 8¼"x11", 197pp. SMP 77

SNEDDON, J. RUSSELL. *HAIR DISORDERS,* 1.35. Suggestions on ways to eliminate hair troubles such as alopecia, dandruff, and baldness by first cleansing the bloodstream and then revitalizing scalp and hair by special natural methods. 64pp. TPL 74

SNEDDON, J. RUSSELL. *HEALING YOURSELF WITH WATER,* 1.50. Hydrotherapy, or the use of water to gain and maintain good health, originated centuries ago and was praised by Hippocrates. But it was not until the beginning of the nineteenth century that pioneers like Priessnitz, Schroth, and Kneipp developed what we think of today as the water cure. This book outlines water treatments for many specific ailments including arthritis, bronchitis, fever, hernia, and prolapse of the abdominal organs. Hydrotherapy treatments are also useful for maintaining health and many preventive suggestions are also offered in the book. Index, 64pp. TPL 77

SNEDDON, J. RUSSELL. *HIGH BLOOD PRESSURE,* 1.35. A collection of methods for the diagnosis and treatment of hypertension. 64pp. TPL 73

SNEDDON, J. RUSSELL. *LIVER TROUBLES,* 1.35. A naturopath explains how liver troubles are caused and provides detailed advice for overcoming them without harmful drugs through an intense elimination diet. 63pp. TPL 73

SPAULDING, C.E. *A VETERINARY GUIDE FOR ANIMAL OWNERS,* c9.95. A practical reference guide to the care and treatment of cattle, goats, sheep, horses, pigs, poultry, rabbits, dogs, and cats. Each chapter includes information on general care and management, and on specific health problems to which that particular animal is susceptible. A final chapter explains such basics as drug administration, antibiotics, viruses, and bacteria, handling animals in shock, and first aid. There's also an extensive glossary. The author is an experienced veterinarian. Many line drawings accompany the text. 431pp. Rod 76

STEARN, JESS. *DR. THOMPSON'S NEW WAY FOR* YOU *TO CURE YOUR ACHING BACK,* c7.95. Plagued by lower back problems, Stearn finally discovered Dr. Alec Thompson, a well known Southern California osteopath who developed a simple exercise that anyone can do to relieve the many forms of mis-alignment which cause a variety of pains in the back and limbs. It seems unnecessary to write a whole book to explain this; a short article or even a couple of pictures would do. Nevertheless, anyone with lower back problems would probably consider $8.00 cheap enough for relief and possibly a cure. Much of the book is case histories; the rest gives details that will help you to understand what it is all about and maybe convince you that you can indeed do something about your aching back. Illustrations, glossary, 203pp. Dou 73

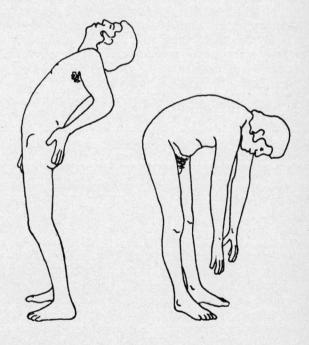

STEBBING, LIONEL, ed. *MUSIC: ITS OCCULT BASIS AND HEALING VALUE,* 9.10. An excellent, comprehensive selection of writings on music in the light of Rudolf Steiner's Spiritual Science by people in diverse disciplines. 212pp. NKB 58

STEINER, RUDOLF. *SPIRITUAL SCIENCE AND MEDICINE,* 5.25. The twenty lectures in this volume were given by Steiner in response to requests by a number of physicians. Their form and content were also determined by specific questions asked by those attending the course. Basically the lectures led to a deepened understanding of man's being, without which, in Steiner's words, *it has actually become impossible to investigate the true nature of health and disease.* Many case studies included in the lectures show the importance of spiritual insights in true healing. The language is often technical. Illustrations, index, 277pp. RSP 48

STODDARD, ALAN. *MANUAL OF OSTEOPATHIC PRACTICE,* c20.00. This book is a companion to the author's **Manual of Osteopathic Technique.** It describes many facets of manipulation and is written for students and practitioners. The main emphasis is clinical and practical, although the first chapter is devoted to a summary of the principles and theory of osteopathy. The second chapter deals with mechanical diagnosis, the third classifies the various spinal syndromes—twenty-four of which are described and the most effective treatments are suggested. The final chapter discusses the art of osteopathy. Appendices list contraindications to manipulation and review the osteopathic research literature. Many photographs accompany the text. Notes, index, 321pp. HPG 69

STODDARD, ALAN. *MANUAL OF OSTEOPATHIC TECHNIQUE,* c15.90. *This is one of the best texts on osteopathic techniques that has ever been published. Well organized and written and beautifully illustrated.*—**Journal of the American Osteopathic Association.** The methods and the procedure of the techniques described are easy to follow and are illustrated by an excellent series of photographs. Index, 275pp. HPG 62

STONE, RANDOLPH. *HEALTH BUILDING (THE CONSCIOUS ART OF LIVING WELL),* 3.00. A concise expression of Dr. Stone's Polarity Therapy. *When we are ill and have pains, we think that it is the body which hurts and is sick, when in reality it is the life-breaths or Prana Currents in the body which operate it and sustain it, which are all out of balance or coordination in their polarity function of attraction and repulsion. . . . The body itself has no sensation, as it is matter. But these energy currents which permeate and run it are living messengers to the life within at its core, and to the consciousness which is the Soul. All pain is but an obstruction* *to this energy flow.* Many specific diet suggestions are offered here. 75pp. CRC 62

Sugar

John Yudkin writes in **Sweet and Dangerous** that *Sugar is common enough in all our lives, and almost everyone believes that it is simply an attractive sweet—one of many carbohydrates in the diet of civilized countries. But sugar is really quite an extraordinary substance. It is unique in the plant that makes it, in the materials that chemists can produce from it, and in its use in foods at home and in industry. And research is only now beginning to show that it also has unique effects in the body, different from those of other carbohydrates. Since it now amounts to about one-fifth of the total calories consumed in the wealthier countries, it is essential that everyone know more about what it does to people when it enters the body in food and drink.*

The fact that so much about the effects of sugar is still being discovered is in itself an illustration of how different these effects are from those of other common foods. You might have imagined that the realization that there were differences would have stimulated the sugar producers and refiners themselves to initiate studies into the properties of their product. Other industries that produce foods like meat or dairy products or fruits have spent a great deal of money over the years to carry out or support nutritional studies on their products, even though these foods form a much smaller proportion of the Western diet than sugar now does. But the sugar people seem quite content to spend their money on advertising and public relations, making claims about quick energy, and simply rejecting suggestions that sugar is really harmful to the heart or the teeth or the figure or to health in general.

I can make two key statements that no one can refute:

First, there is no physiological requirement for sugar; all human nutritional needs can be met in full without having to take a single spoon of white or brown or raw sugar, on its own or in any food or drink.

Secondly, if only a small fraction of what is already known about the effects of sugar were to be revealed in relation to any other material used as a food additive, that material would promptly be banned.

A hundred years ago the average annual consumption of sugar in the United States was several pounds a year. Now it is over a hundred pounds—more than a teaspoon per hour, every hour of the day or night for every man, woman and child in this country. Virtually every food you buy in the supermarket has some sugar in it. White sugar is not a natural product, but is a highly concentrated form which our bodies were never designed to be able to handle. It goes right to the bloodstream, where it calls forth the production of insulin to balance it. Then it is quickly metabolized (quick energy!) and the insulin is left floating in the bloodstream, causing a low blood sugar condition. Overconsumption of sugar leads to hypoglycemia (low blood sugar) and often then to diabetes, which is increasing in incidence every year in this country. Hypoglycemia is possibly the most widespread and generally undiagnosed disease in America today. Estimates of those affected range from ten to fifty million persons. Hypoglycemia is implicated not only in alcoholism and schizophrenia—the two diseases that lead to more long-term institutionalization than any others—but also in allergies, heart disease, and probably most forms of degenerative disease. Thus we sometimes refer to sugar as America's number one drug addiction problem. And we are delighted to see so many books on the subject now being published. We hope that the general public will begin to wake up to the problem, despite the efforts of the sugar and processed foods industries to convince us that sugar is good for us.

ABRAHAMSON, E.M. and REZET, A.W. *BODY, MIND AND SUGAR,* 2.95. This was the first book to alert the public to the problem of low blood sugar, here called hyperinsulinism, and often called hypoglycemia. Written by a medical doctor, it relates it to chronic fatigue and allergies, alcoholism and insanity. A thorough presentation of symptoms and effects, enlivened by many case histories and dietary advice. 240pp. Avo 51

ADAMS, RUTH and FRANK MURRAY. *IS LOW BLOOD SUGAR MAKING YOU A NUTRITIONAL CRIPPLE,* 1.75. Adams and Murray are two of the most prolific medical and health writers around and their books are balanced and well informed. This is an excellent review of the literature, not only concerning the diseases most often implicated in hypoglycemia, but also including toothache, neurasthenia, psoriasis, hyperactivity, epilepsy, peptic ulcers, gout, and multiple sclerosis. If you have a problem with any of these, you'll be interested in the research reported herein. Food value tables, bibliography, index, 174pp. Lar 75

AIROLA, PAAVO. *HYPOGLYCEMIA: A BETTER APPROACH,* 4.95. Dr. Airola explains what hypoglycemia is, how to know whether you have it, and how his common sense approach and diet suggestions can eliminate the symptoms and begin to cure the disease. The book includes menus, recipes, doctors' reports, case histories, food charts, glucose tolerance test charts, exercises, information on special vitamins and herbs, and much else. HPP 77

BRENNAN, R.O. *NUTRIGENETICS,* c8.95. Dr. Brennan is past President of the American College of General Practitioners in Osteopathic Medicine and founder of the International Academy of Preventive Medicine. This book argues the case for better nutrition in preventive medicine. Hypoglycemia keeps coming into the picture because it is so central to virtually all of the problems our cells and organs face from inadequate nutrition. The title comes from Dr. Brennan's view that hypoglycemia results from the combination of genetic and nutritional factors. Appendices include food value tables, menus, recipes, and some suggestions for converting your favorite recipes to more nutritious ones. Index, 258pp. EvC 75

CLEAVE, T.L. *THE SACCHARINE DISEASE,* 4.95. Saccharine means related to sugar. Subtitled *The Master Disease of Our Time,* this book discusses illnesses resulting from the taking of sugar or via the digestion of starch in white flour, white bread and rice or other refined carbohydrates. And this includes coronary disease, diabetes, obesity, ulcers, and bowel disorders. This book by a British physician, must rank along with Dr. Yudkin's book as must reading for anyone seeking further information about America's number one form of drug addiction: sugar. Index, 216pp. Kea 74

DUFFY, WILLIAM. *SUGAR BLUES,* 1.95. Duffy was a pudgy sugarholic until he met Gloria Swanson. She set him on the right path and he not only swore off sugar but got into macrobiotics as well. This is a fascinating account of the history of sugar consumption and including as much data as the author (a journalist) could find in a pretty extensive research of the subject. If you are already anti-sugar you'll love it. If you are not, we hope you won't be put off by Duffy's slam bang, hyped-up style of writing or his somewhat unnecessary (from our point of view) plugging of macrobiotics at the end of the book. Duffy himself had a happy ending. He looks years younger than he did ten years ago, and after travelling around the country to plug the book, he and Gloria Swanson got married. 194pp. Faw 75

FREDERICKS, CARLTON and HERMAN GOODMAN. *LOW BLOOD SUGAR AND YOU,* 2.95. Dr. Fredericks is currently President of the International Academy of Preventive Medicine and one of the best-informed nutritional experts in the business. Dr. Goodman is a practicing physician who has written a score of books and several hundred medical and scientific articles. In this book they present the basic material on hypoglycemia in a well written and detailed form, suitable to an educated layman or an M.D. who wants to find out what this disease—belittled by the AMA—is all about. If your doctor pooh-poohs hypoglycemia, maybe you can get him to dip into this book and become aware of the facts his journals aren't giving him. No index, unfortunately. 190pp. G&D 69

HURDLE, J. FRANK. *LOW BLOOD SUGAR—A DOCTOR'S GUIDE TO ITS EFFECTIVE CONTROL,* 2.95. This is quite a comprehensive treatment. Dr. Hurdle deals with control of low blood sugar through diet, exercise and mind control. He also goes into a host of related conditions: heart disease, alcoholism, digestive problems, etc., showing their relationship to blood sugar and how they can be controlled or helped through blood sugar control. Index, 224pp. PrH 69

MARTIN, CLEMENT. *LOW BLOOD SUGAR: THE HIDDEN MENACE OF HYPOGLYCEMIA,* 1.65. Hypoglycemia is a condition resulting from an insufficiency of sugar in the bloodstream, the opposite of diabetes. It is hard to detect and it most frequently produces exhaustion and mental confusion and may lead to chronic alcoholism and heart attacks. Dr. Martin is a physician who has treated many hypoglycemic patients. In this book he discusses how you can determine whether hypoglycemia is the cause of your fatigue problems. He also outlines a diet and gives the rationale behind each of his suggestions. 185pp. Arc 69

SCHWANTES, DAVE. *THE UNSWEETENED TRUTH ABOUT SUGAR,* 2.95. This brief review by a journalist gives, in easy to read fashion, the basic information about the growth in sugar consumption, how it acts in the body, its harmful effects, and how you can cut down and substitute honey, maple syrup, and fruit. Lots of recipes. Not a very deep book, but useful to give to a friend or relative who needs to be led gently into better eating habits. Index, 96pp. DTP 75

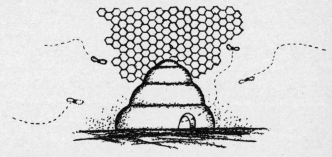

YUDKIN, JOHN. *SWEET AND DANGEROUS,* 1.95. This is *the* book about sugar. Dr. Yudkin, M.D., PhD, is Professor of Physiology at the University of London and has devoted much of his career to research on the connection between sugar and heart disease, diabetes, ulcers, and many degenerative conditions. Here he reports many of his findings as well as the pressures brought to bear by the sugar interests to see that these findings are not widely understood. Our favorite quote: "If only a fraction of what is already known about the effects of sugar were to be revealed in relation to any other material used as a food additive, that material would promptly be banned." Index, 209pp. Ban 72

SZASZ, THOMAS. *THE THEOLOGY OF MEDICINE,* 3.95. *The essays in this volume are all animated by the aim to explore the ceremonial or religious aspects of various medical practices. Formerly, people victimized themselves by attributing medical powers to their priests; now, they victimize themselves by attributing magical powers to their physicians. Faced with persons endowed with such superhuman powers, ordinary men and women are inclined to submit to them with that blind trust whose inexorable consequence is that they make slaves of themselves and tyrants of their "protectors."* . . .*People should respect physicians for their skill, but should distrust them for their power.*—Thomas Szasz. Notes, index, 192pp. H&R 77

SZEKELY, EDMUND. *THE HEALING WATERS,* 3.00. A guidebook to fifty European water cures. 57pp. Aca 73

THAKKUR, CHANDRASHEKHAR. *INTRODUCTION TO AYUR- VEDA,* c10.00. Ayurvedic Medicine is the traditional medicine practiced in India. The system is derived from the Vedas, the most ancient Indian religious writings. Basically illness is attributed to disorder in one of the four humors (air, water, phlegm and blood) and the treatment recommended basically utilizes medicinal plants. This is a comprehensive text citing the modern practices and the teachings of the most noted ancient Ayurvedic physicians. Index, 196+pp. ASI 74

THEOSOPHICAL RESEARCH CENTRE. *THE MYSTERY OF HEALING,* 1.25. This book presents an approach to healing based on esoteric teachings, especially as promulgated in theosophy. Various unorthodox treatments and diagnostic methods are discussed at length and there is also information on self healing, on the energy centers, on the power of thought, and on the human constitution. It's an excellent overview of the whole field and is well written. Notes, index, 102pp. TPH 58

THIE, JOHN and MARY MARKS. *TOUCH FOR HEALTH,* 8.95. *In the early 1960's, Dr. George Goodheart came up with a new idea in working with muscles. People talk about muscles being tight or in spasm, causing pain and pulling the spine out of line. Goodheart concluded that it wasn't muscle spasm that was causing the trouble, but rather weak muscles on the opposite side which caused the normal muscles to seem to be or to become tight. From this basic idea,* *using the techniques of early chiropractic work and the ancient Oriental practices in the activation of energies in the body, he developed* [a technique] *using muscle testing to determine the need for and effectiveness of treatment, and applying various techniques of kinesiology, the science of muscle activation, to restore muscle balance which is essential to good posture and health.* —from the introduction. In this book Dr. Thie details an unusual compendium of techniques, aiming at the restoration of wholeness and balance to the body. For each muscle or muscle group there are pictures illustrating the testing positions and treatment areas, as well as information on the functions of the muscles and their related organs. The book is spiral bound, 11½"x11½", and is fully indexed by ailment and by parts of the body. 108pp. DeV 73

THOMAS, LEWIS. *THE LIVES OF A CELL,* 1.95. Subtitled *The Notes of a Biology Watcher,* this is an exploration of man's being— his health, germs, and interior organism. Dr. Thomas is a noted physician and researcher and he expresses himself in a clear, engaging manner. Geared toward the general reader. Notes, 153pp. Ban 74

THOMPSON, PAUL. *HEALTH AND HEALING IN THE NEW AGE,* 2.95. The Association for Documentation and Enlightenment is a group of individuals—whom we presume came out of the A.R.E.— working toward the creation of a total healing center. This is a collection of psychic readings which have come through members of the group. Many specific topics are discussed and the information is well organized. 150pp. ADE 76

THOMPSON, R. WILLIAM. *LIVING WITH ANGINA,* 1.50. Angina pectoris is a heart ailment. The term is used to describe a pain which results from the heart muscle receiving less blood than it needs for the work which it is being asked to do. The major symptom is a sharp pain in the chest. This pamphlet suggests methods of coping with angina, advice on diets and treatment, and a variety of other suggestions. 64pp. TPL 76

TILDEN, JOHN. *TOXEMIA,* 1.65. One of the basic principles of natural hygiene is that disease is caused not by the invasion of germs against an innocent body, but by toxemia of the body, which makes it attractive to germs, which act as nature's scavengers. The solution, of course, is to watch what we put into our bodies and cleanse them as necessary. Dr. Tilden, who died in 1940, was one of the most eminent of the natural hygienists, and his book still says much of value. Index, 119pp. ANH 74

TURNER, R. NEWMAN. *FIRST AID NATURE'S WAY,* 1.70. Ailments such as colds, influenza, acute indigestion, and headache are dealt with here in addition to cuts, sprains, bruises and other minor accidents. The injuries and ailments have been grouped together in chapters according to the system of the body affected. There is also a chapter of miscellaneous conditions. Bibliography, 93pp. TPL 69

VALENTINE, TOM. *PSYCHIC SURGERY,* 1.50. Valentine is a reporter who spent two years in the Philippines examining the phenomenon of psychic surgery and observing and photographing operations. He also interviewed many surgeons and patients and in a number of cases also interviewed the patient's physician. This book presents the results of his study and includes photographs. 221pp. S&S 73

VALNET, JEAN. *HEAL YOURSELF WITH VEGETABLES, FRUITS, AND GRAINS,* 2.95. This is a wonderful encyclopedic discussion of the medicinal uses of vegetables, fruits, and grains. The selections are topically arranged and each entry includes a listing of the principal known constituents, natural benefits, therapeutic benefits, ways to use it, and additional notes and tips. This is a fascinating study written by a French physician who is one of France's leading authorities on natural medicine. We have found this one book more informative than countless longer tomes. And it's easy to find exactly the information you are interested in because the book is so well organized. Glossary, 224pp. S&S 75

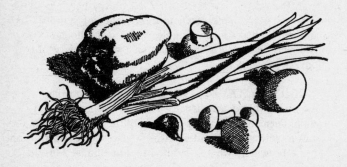

Vision

In the early years of the present century Dr. W.H. Bates, a New York oculist, became dissatisfied with the ordinary symptomatic treatment of eyes. Seeking a substitute for artificial lenses, he set himself to discover if there was any way of re-educating defective vision into a condition of normality.

As the result of his work with a large number of patients, he came to the conclusion that the great majority of visual defects were functional and due to faulty habits of use. These faulty habits of use were invariably related, he found, to a condition of strain and tension. As was to be expected from the unitary nature of the human organism, the strain affected both the body and the mind.

Dr. Bates discovered that, by means of appropriate techniques, this condition of strain could be relieved. When it had been relieved—when patients had learned to use their eyes and mind in a relaxed way—vision was improved and refractive errors tended to correct themselves. Practice in the educational techniques served to build up good seeing habits in place of the faulty habits responsible for defective vision, and in many cases function came to be completely and permanently normalized.

Now, it is a well-established physiological principle that improved functioning always tends to result in an improvement in the organic condition of the tissues involved. The eye, Dr. Bates discovered, was no exception to this general rule. When the patient learned to relax his tenseness and acquired proper seeing habits, the *vis medicatrix naturae* was given a chance to operate—with the result that, in many cases, the improvement of functioning was followed by a complete restoration of the health and organic integrity of the diseased eye.

Dr. Bates died in 1931, and up to the time of his death he continued to perfect and develop his methods for the improvement of visual function. Furthermore, during the last years of Dr. Bates' life and since his death, his pupils in various parts of the world have devised a number of valuable new applications of the general principles which he laid down. By means of these techniques large numbers of men, women and children, suffering from visual defects of every kind, have been successfully re-educated into normality or towards normality. For anyone who has studied a selection of these cases, or who has himself undergone the process of visual re-education, it is impossible to doubt that here at last is a method of treating imperfect sight which is not merely symptomatic, but genuinely aetiological—a method which does not confine itself to the mechanical neutralization of defects but aims at the removal of their physiological and psychological causes. And yet, in spite of the long period during which it has been known, in spite of the quality and quantity of the results obtained through its employment by competent instructors, Dr. Bates' technique still remains unrecognized by the medical and optometrical professions.—from **The Art of Seeing** by Aldous Huxley

AGARWAL, J. *CARE OF EYES*, 1.50. This small pamphlet, illustrated with many photographs, contains a lot of good, practical advice on eye exercises and proper use of the eyes as developed by the author's father, Dr. R.S. Agarwal at his Eye Institutes in Delhi and Madras and his School for Perfect Eyesight in Pondicherry. It also provides an introduction to Agarwal's ideas. 33pp. AAP 62

AGARWAL, R.S. *MIND AND VISION*, c6.00. Subtitled *A Handbook for the Cure of Imperfect Sight without Glasses*, this book first reviews the way the eye sees, the cause of errors of refraction, and then goes into detail regarding care of the eyes and treatment methods such as eye baths, many relaxation methods, and diet suggestions. These natural methods have become quite popular in India and this book can be used by any individual who wants to try them out for himself. Illustrated with photographs, diagrams, and eye charts. 269pp. AAP 72

AGARWAL, R.S. *SECRETS OF INDIAN MEDICINE*, c6.00. This book is primarily about the eyes, drawing upon principles of allopathic and ayurvedic medicine. It will be of interest to people who want to know more about Indian medicine and nonphysical concepts of healing, but is not for general readers since much of what it says is fairly specific to Indian culture. Dr. Agarwal has lived at the Sri Aurobindo Ashram in Pondicherry since 1955 and his ideas should appeal to many spiritual seekers. Illustrations, 240pp. AAP 71

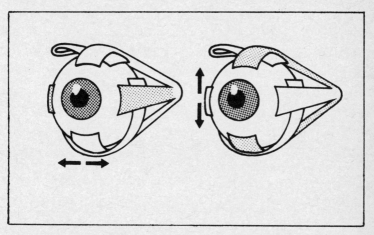

AGARWAL, R.S. *YOGA OF PERFECT SIGHT,* c5.45. This is the most recent of Dr. Agarwal's books and the one we would recommend to most general readers. It's not really about yoga, but about improving your eyesight. Covers the whole range of theory and exercises. Some of the basic principles (taken from Bates) are: (1) reading fine print is beneficial while reading large print is not; (2) reading in a dim light or in candle light is very useful; and (3) reading at a closer distance is beneficial. Includes eye charts and a series of letters to and answers from Sri Aurobindo about Dr. Agarwal's work. 223pp. AAP 74

BATES, W.H. *BETTER EYESIGHT WITHOUT GLASSES,* 1.75. This is the classic book on the use of various eye exercises to improve eyesight without glasses, originally published in 1920. Dr. Bates was the pioneer in developing methods of mental relaxation, focusing techniques and other aids that many since then have continued to promote. This book explains how the eye works, the cause and treatment of errors of refraction, and then runs through the methodology in such fashion that the reader can apply it himself. A large foldout eye chart is included. 175pp. Pyr 75

BENJAMIN, HARRY. *BETTER SIGHT WITHOUT GLASSES*, 1.70. This is another exposition of the Bates method, by a well known English naturopath. Clearly and simply written and nicely illustrated. 106pp. TPL 29

CORBETT, MARGARET. *HELP YOURSELF TO BETTER EYE-SIGHT*, 3.00. Margaret Corbett was perhaps the best known American disciple of Dr. Bates and she herself taught many eye teachers through her Los Angeles School of Eye Education. Covers the basic principles of the Bates method with a number of additional drills of her own. Nicely illustrated. 217pp. Wil 49

CORBETT, MARGARET. *HOW TO IMPROVE YOUR SIGHT*, c1.69. A collection of simple daily drills in eye relaxation based on the techniques propounded by Bates. Very clearly presented. 94pp. Crn 53

DEIMEL, DIANA. *VISION VICTORY*, 3.00. This book goes considerably beyond the usual Bates method exercise books, to cover also nutrition in relation to eyesight, homoeopathic remedies for the eyes, the effect of light on the eyes and the glandular system, iridology, chiropracty and the eyes, and much else. It includes a number of articles by others. A good round up. 193pp. ChP 72

HUXLEY, ALDOUS. *THE ART OF SEEING*, 4.95. In 1939, with eyes rapidly worsening, Aldous Huxley came in contact with the Bates method. He undertook the retraining, was able to do away with his glasses, and wrote this book in appreciation. Huxley presents a good review of the scientific arguments pro and con and then explains the various exercises. 158pp. Mnt 75

JACKSON, JIM. *SEEING YOURSELF SEE*, 3.95. An oversize book which presents a series of eye exercises designed to help the individual become more conscious of his visual processes and the functions of his eyes. The exercises are easy to follow and are fully illustrated. They are not specifically aimed at improving poor vision—although Jackson discusses this area. Visual care exercises and massage techniques are included to aid alertness, sharpen responses, and soothe tired eyes. An excellent work which everyone should find useful, no matter how bad or good their eyes are. Bibliography, 125pp. Dut 75

PEPPARD, HAROLD. *BETTER SIGHT WITHOUT GLASSES,* c3.95. Another variation of the Bates method. Illustrations, including foldout eye exercise chart. 153pp. Dou 36

ROSANES-BERRETT, MARILYN. *DO YOU REALLY NEED EYEGLASSES?* 2.45. This is generally considered the best of the recent books on eyesight improvement. The author is well known in the human potential movement and she has conducted many workshops throughout the country. Her techniques are practical and are very clearly presented. The method is somewhat similar to Bates', but is refined and new ideas are included. Index, 126pp. Har 74

SCIENCE OF LIFE BOOKS. *IMPROVE YOUR SIGHT WITHOUT GLASSES,* 1.35. This book first analyzes the causes of optical defects and then outlines a new optical science which treats the causes of the defect, cleanses the body of the toxic matter which is poisoning the blood flowing to the eyes, strengthens the eye muscles, and generally aims at giving the eye every chance to function as a healthy organ in a healthy body. 64pp. SLB 75

SIMPKINS, BROOKS. *OCULOPATHY,* 4.45. In this work, Mr. Simpkins argues against the theory that longsight, shortsight, and astigmatism are incurable visual defects, portraying how refractive errors develop and how the eye actually adjusts its focus. Diagrams are included which explain to those who prescribe glasses the irregular activity of the intracranial processes of vision primarily responsible for the external refractive error. Remedial methods of treatment, other than glasses, are indicated. This is a technical book for professionals. Illustrated with many diagrams, 105pp. HeS 63

VOGEL, VIRGIL. *AMERICAN INDIAN MEDICINE,* c12.50. *To American Indians the term medicine embraced much more than the cure of disease and the healing of injuries, but the focus here is on these aspects, and particularly those that we have borrowed.* —from the introduction. Vogel is a historian rather than a medical doctor and he presents a comprehensive historical account. Every aspect of the subject is thoroughly discussed and extensive notes and a long bibliography are also included. Illustrations, index, 578pp. UOk 70

WADE, CARLSON. *ALL NATURAL PAIN RELIEVERS,* c7.95. A copious grab bag of useful suggestions for relief from headaches, backaches, muscle pains and most every other kind of pain and ache. Wade covers herbal and nutritional remedies, exercises of many kinds, use of ice, water, sun, heat, and much else. While we don't care for Wade's hype, or agree with the claim in the foreword that the book *is the most treasured and desired reference manual for physicians, scientists, nutritionists. . .,* if you are trying to kick the drug habit you can doubtless find many ideas here worth trying. Pain locator index, 227pp. PrH 75

WADE, CARLSON. *FACT BOOK ON HYPERTENSION (HIGH BLOOD PRESSURE) AND YOUR DIET,* 1.50. A useful compendium of information for the twenty-three million Americans who suffer from high blood pressure. Begins with a detailed explanation of the heart and circulatory system, and statistics about cardiovascular diseases. The bulk of the book discusses why and how to avoid salt, sugar, caffeine and fats, how to control stress and how to reduce. Glossary, 158pp. Kea 75

WAERLAND, ARE. *HEALTH IS YOUR BIRTHRIGHT,* 2.50. Waerland devoted most of his life to turning people in Scandinavia on to natural healing and especially the Waerland System—a systematic nutritional diet designed both to cure illness and to prevent any further deterioration of the human organism. He studied medicine in London, Paris, and Sweden for almost thirty years and carried out extensive experiments in nutritional physiology before beginning to spread his findings to the European populace. He was extraordinarily successful at spreading the word and was publicly hailed by the greatest scientists and authorities of his day. This book is a detailed presentation of the Waerland System and its underlying philosophy—including sample menus. The second half of the book contains an essay entitled *Waerland Diet in the Treatment of Disease* by Ebba Waerland. Here the principles are systematically applied to various ailments and detailed menus, diets, and remedies are given. 88pp. Hum nd

WAERLAND, EBBA. *REBUILDING HEALTH,* 1.45. This is the most detailed account of the Waerland System. It includes many case histories and outlines the nutritional program of treatment for various diseases. 252pp. Arc 61

WALKER, N.W. *BECOME YOUNGER,* 4.30. Dr. Walker is a naturo-path who emphasizes simple eating habits and bodily purification. This is his most complete philosophical work. Suggestions for the health of each part of the body are offered along with a discussion of what to eat and not to eat. Many anatomical drawings are in-cluded. Dr. Walker's writing style is inspirational and a bit old fashioned; nonetheless, a great deal of important information is presented. Index, 204pp. NoP 49

WARMBRAND, MAX. *THE ENCYCLOPEDIA OF HEALTH AND NUTRITION,* 1.95. Dr. Warmbrand is a naturopath and doctor of osteopathy. In this fat book he has collected a wealth of informa-tion about natural healing methods for a wide variety of conditions, among them: respiratory diseases, stomach ailments, diabetes, arth-ritis, rheumatism and gout, heart trouble, constipation, ulcers, liver problems, asthma, nervous tension, infectious diseases and allergies. He ranges from folk medicine to modern health science and his dis-cussion is woven around the proposition that the human body has its own natural curative powers and the goal is to find ways to help it maximize these powers without resorting to harmful drugs. A good value. Index, 496pp. Pyr 62

WELL-BEING: A HEALING MAGAZINE, 1.00/issue. **Well-Being** (833 W. Fir, San Diego, CA 92101) is a monthly magazine devoted to articles on healing. The focus at its inception was on herbs, and articles on herbs still predominate. It's not a slick magazine, and the selections are often homey. Nonetheless, a great deal of useful information is offered in its pages. Each issue is about 50 pages and a yearly subscription is $10.00.

WHITE EAGLE. *HEAL THYSELF,* c2.50. For nearly half a century White Eagle, through Grace Cooke, has been healing the sick in mind and body, as well as teaching others how to heal. This is a general, inspirational treatise on healing by letting the universal love emanate from one's being. 61pp. WEP 62

WHITEHOUSE, GEOFFREY. *EVERYWOMAN'S GUIDE TO NATURAL HEALTH,* 4.70. Despite the title, this is more of a guide for mothers-to-be than a general study of ailments pecu-liar to woman. Nonetheless, there is a great deal of information on specific female ailments, including woman's hormones, vari-cose veins, cervicitis, polyps and pruitus, ailments of the urinary system, prolapse of the uterus, breast disorders, menopause and the pill. The material is presented in a straightforward manner and the suggestions are clearly put. Index, 159pp. TPL 74

WIGMORE, ANN. *NATURAMA LIVING TEXTBOOK,* 12.00. This is a large three-ring notebook filled with a wide assortment of Ann Wigmore's views and publications on many aspects of healing and health, as well as spirituality, the New Age, and much else. It is not well organized or edited, and not something to sit down with and read through. Nevertheless, for followers of Dr. Ann, nuggets of gold are to be found amidst the sand. Major categories are tabbed and there is a listing of topics under each one, but no pagination or proper index. HHI 77

WINTER, RUTH. *TRIUMPH OVER TENSION,* 3.95. A collection of *100 Ways to Relax.* Each of the suggested remedies is briefly explained and the causes of tension are examined. Bibliography, index, 106pp. G&D 76

WORRALL, AMBROSE and OLGA. *THE GIFT OF HEALING,* 3.95. The simple and factual account of the experiences of two spiritual healers. 220pp. H&R 65

WORRALL, OLGA. *OLGA WORRALL,* c7.95. Ms. Worrall is one of America's most renowned spiritual healers. Her ministry has mainly been in Christian circles and she often refers to the Bible in her healings. This is a moving biographical study of her life and ministry by Edwina Cerutti and many case studies are included. 169pp. H&R 75

YALLER, ROBERT and RAYE. *THE HEALTH SPAS,* 2.95. This guidebook to the health spas, clinics and sanitariums in the U.S., Mexico, Europe, Israel and Japan, begins with several brief chapters discussing types of institutions, what they do and what they are like. It pays special attention to fasting spas, special food spas, and the Ringberg Cancer Clinic in Germany. Then follow the country chapters with some general information, plus a listing of many of the more important spots. It is a useful guide for anyone who has the desire (or need) to visit such spas. Illustrations, glossary, 158pp. WoP 74

YESUDIAN, S. and ELISABETH HAICH. *YOGA AND HEALTH,* 1.50. See the Yoga subsection of Body Work.

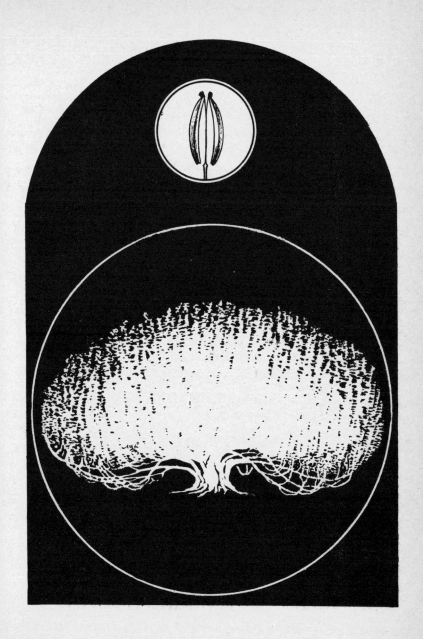

Herbs

T he employment of herbal remedies as healing agents has been practiced by the forbears of every race and land upon earth. Though separated by the vast expanse of oceans, continents, impenetrable jungles, or deserts, primitive people everywhere possessed a remarkable knowledge of plant medicine. Early mankind, by means of trial and error, accidents, etc., found that certain roots, plants, barks and seeds possessed medicinal properties. These remedies were handed down from one generation to the next. The astonishing fact is that later, when man developed sufficient modes of travel enabling him to establish contact between the various lands, it was learned that in many instances the claims made regarding the particular healing properties of a certain herb found in one area were identical with those claimed for the same herb in another.

A series of medical papyri have been discovered in Egypt over a period of years. One of the longest and most famous, dating from the 2nd century B.C., is called the Papyrus Ebers. These scrolls or documents are reputed to be the world's oldest medical literature. Descriptions of the various ailments suffered by the people of those times were given, and among the herbs employed as remedial agents were myrrh, cummin, peppermint, caraway, fennel, and the oil from olives, to name just a few. Licorice was especially esteemed among the Egyptians, and archaeologists found great quantities of this botanical stored among the fabulous jewelry and art treasures in the 3000 year old tomb of King Tut. Licorice was also one of the first herbs used in China, and is mentioned in their herbal writings as being beneficial to the lives of men in numerous ways.

The earliest Chinese book on medicinal herbs was written by Emperor Shen-ung about 3000 years B.C. In this monumental work, ginseng is regarded as the most potent of the thousands of herbs mentioned. Ginseng is also listed in the ancient medical book of India, the **Atherva Veda**, and described as beneficial in preserving youth and strength.

The Persians, Romans, Greeks, Babylonians, Hebrews, Arabs and other races were all familiar with the use and practice of herbal medicine. In our own country, we are reminded of the fact that the American Indian placed his reliance on the products of forest and field to alleviate his ills. The early colonists were also well-acquainted with the use of herbs, and brought with them to the New World the simple plant remedies that had been used for generations before them. Contact with the Indians gradually added to their medicinal knowledge the qualities and power of many new botanicals gained from the experience of the Red Man's close association with nature. Families freely exchanged this information and almost every individual joined in the search for some new herb or herbs that would prevent or relieve disease.

In many parts of the world today, herbs are still used as remedial agents. The natives in the interior part of Africa possess a knowledge of the medicinal properties of plants that astonishes the European and American. The art of healing in Sumatra consists in the application of the botanicals with which they are expertly skilled. At an early age they become acquainted with the names, qualities and properties of every shrub and herb among the variety with which their country abounds. In Brazil it is said that certain natives are able to run 100 miles at a steady pace, through jungles and over mountains with just a stick of guarana as their only food. Guarana sticks somewhat resemble licorice, while the fruit resembles the hazelnut. According to South American folklore, the stimulating and nutritious quality they claim for guarana was discovered by the Incas 300 years before the white man appeared in the Western hemisphere.

In the vast subcontinent of India, about 2000 plants are listed in the Ayurvedic, Unani and Tibbi systems of medicine, and these herbal remedies provide the most widely used treatment for the people of that area.

Formerly rather contemptuous of herbal folk medicine, modern science is today doing a startling turnabout, and has undertaken a world-wide search for old-time herbal remedies so common to the earlier periods of history as well as the plants currently used among the jungle natives of Africa and Latin America. Botanists and chemists are re-reading old books on herbs which give their medicinal uses and properties, while other medical teams are exploring tropical jungles for roots, leaves, barks, and seeds. This search is carried on chiefly by the large drug firms of the United States and Europe.

There are many reasons for the new scientific change of attitude toward herbal medicine. One of the most significant was the discovery of the medicinal value of snakeroot (Rauwolfia) which came from the botanical pharmacopoeia of ancient India. For thousands of years, the natives of India had chewed the root for its calming effects. Ciba Pharmaceutical Company isolated a tranquilizing agent from the root which proved valuable in the treatment of high blood pressure and some types of insanity. This sparked a world-wide search by the various drug firms for other botanicals that may also possess worthwhile medicinal merit.

The results realized so far from this extensive scientific program appear to be very rewarding. The head of one research team has stated that, *We've never had so much success with chemicals invented by man as we're having with plant extracts.* A top researcher comments: *We've come full circle. Back in the 1800's, fully 80 percent of the medicines were plant derived. Gradually, researchers turned more and more to chemicals, both organic and inorganic. Today, half the curatives in the average family's medicine cabinet are products of somebody's test tube. And only 30 percent are plant based. Now, almost out of desperation, we're going back to nature—back to plants. For good as the test tube is, it hasn't cured man's greatest cripplers—arthritis, heart trouble, insanity, asthma and cancer.*

Just how the researchers know where to look for possible healing plants is often started by a rumor somewhat like the following: *From the milk-white sap of a jungle herb, a witch doctor has been extracting a potion that cures insanity.* When the medical expert finally locates the witch doctor and comes to terms, he recognizes the plant he is shown as one that grows in almost every back yard in America. North Chicago's big Abbott Laboratories announced discovery of a drug which is effective against hardening of the arteries (arteriosclerosis) in 1957, and the basis for the new drug was . . .*oil pressed from the seeds of the East Indian safflower, a thistlelike herb whose American relative is the common garden aster.*

Curare, long used as a poison on the arrows of the jungle savages of the Amazon, was discovered by modern science only in 1938. Curare is now considered a *top rate anesthetic (particularly in abdominal surgery), a muscle relaxer and a "standard" for treating some victims of mental disorders, including manic-depressives.* The extract from the leaves of the foxglove plant used in the treatment of certain types of heart trouble was an old time European folk remedy. This extract is commonly known as digitalis. Seaweed-derived iodine, an old Polynesian antiseptic, is a staple in your medicine cabinet and mine.

All were discovered often by accident, when skeptical researchers decided to test the truth of an ancient remedy. It can be clearly seen that we are steadily gaining scientific proof that man's medicine is exactly where the Bible has always said that it was—in the plant kingdom. From the many facts existing, we may well believe that there is not a single disease in man that may not have its remedy or cure in some herb or other, if we but knew *which* plant and where to find it. For who has not often seen, not only our own domestic animals, but many of the untamed creatures of forest, field, and sky, seek out some one particular herb when laboring under sickness or some derangement of its organism? Nature has, of course, wisely implanted a definite instinct in these creatures, in order to serve for its health or restoration to health from disease. In man, however, such instinct is not so plainly marked, but to him has been given reason and judgment and a disposition to investigate the laws and mysteries of creation in order to secure his own highest health and perfection.

—from **Nature's Medicines** by Richard Lucas

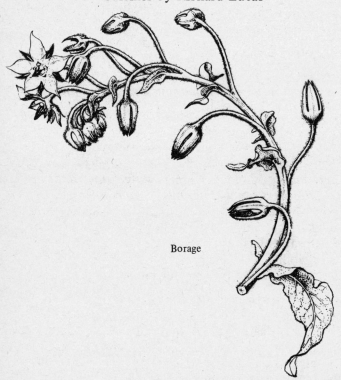

Borage

BECKETT, SARAH. *HERBS FOR CLEARING THE SKIN,* 1.30. Alphabetically organized, arranged according to herbs, with a line drawing of each herb, description, part used, and directions for use. Also includes some general information and a therapeutic index. 64pp. TPL 73

BECKETT,SARAH.*HERBSFORFEMININEAILMENTS,*1.30.Same format and content as **Herbs for Clearing the Skin.** 63pp. TPL 73

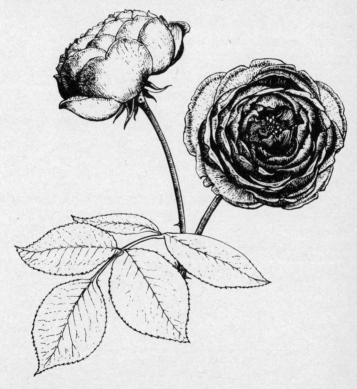

BECKETT, SARAH. *HERBS FOR PROSTATE AND BLADDER TROUBLES,* 1.35. An alphabetically arranged discussion of twenty-five herbs. Ms. Beckett also includes some general information, a therapeutic index, and a line drawing of each herb. 63pp. TPL 73

BECKETT, SARAH. *HERBS FOR RHEUMATISM AND AR-THRITIS,* 1.35. Same format as Ms. Beckett's other herbals. 59pp. TPL 75

BECKETT, SARAH. *HERBS TO SOOTHE YOUR NERVES,* 1.20. A useful, practical compendium, including description (with line drawings) and directions for use. Also includes some background information on the effects of each herb along with an introduction explaining how herbs can heal. Alphabetically arranged by herb. 64pp. TPL 72

BERGLUND, BERNDT. *THE EDIBLE WILD,* 3.45. Includes descriptions (with line drawings) of over fifty wild plants, trees, and shrubs that provide edible food, with recipes that have been adapted from those of the pioneers, early settlers and the Indians. Geared toward those whose knowledge of these plants is small. The authors are considered two of Canada's leading authorities on wilderness survival. Alphabetically arranged, index, 188pp. Scr 71

BETHEL, MAY. *THE HEALING POWER OF HERBS,* 3.00. An excellent book tracing uses of herbs and the properties of various herbs. Various diseases are discussed in detail and there are chapters on pregnancy and child care. 160pp. Wil 74

BIANCHINI, FRANCESCO and FRANCESCO CORBETTA. *HEALTH PLANTS OF THE WORLD: ATLAS OF MEDICINAL PLANTS,* c19.95. This beautiful book contains descriptions and color paintings of eighty-two medicinal plants. A full range of information is included on each: folklore, usage by old time herbalists, and modern medicinal uses. An appendix gives detailed information on the chemical action and pharmaceutical constituents of each plant, with botanical descriptions. This is the best book of type we have ever seen. Glossary, bibliography, index, 8¼"x12", 242pp. Nsw 77

CERES. *HERBS AND FRUIT FOR VITAMINS,* 1.25. Same format as Ceres' other books. 64pp. TPL 75

CERES. *HERBS FOR ACIDITY AND GASTRIC ULCERS,* 1.35. Acidity is a stress condition which can appear as indigestion, ulcers, rheumatic and arthritis complaints, skin disorders, and some forms of cystitis. The twenty herbs discussed in this book have been successful in alleviating these ailments because of their different alkalizing, sedative, tonic, or blood-purifying properties. Each herb is individually discussed and Ceres provides a line drawing of each. The arrangement is alphabetical and there is a therapeutic index. 63pp. TPL 76

CERES. *HERBAL TEAS FOR HEALTH AND HEALING,* 1.30.
Index, 63pp. TPL 76

CERES. *HERBS AND FRUIT FOR SLIMMERS,* 1.20. Twenty
plants, alphabetically arranged, with information on their nutritive
and healing properties and line drawings. 64pp. TPL 75

CERES. *HERBS FOR FIRST-AID AND MINOR AILMENTS,* 1.25.
A useful compendium, alphabetically arranged by the herbs (with
line drawings of each) and including a therapeutic index. Includes
information on usage as well as folklore. 64pp. TPL 72

CERES. *HERBS TO HELP YOU SLEEP,* 1.30. A descriptive selection of herbs which help induce sleep, including line drawings of
each one and a concise statement of the properties of the herb and
the folklore surrounding it. Alphabetically arranged, and including
a therapeutic index. 62pp. TPL 72

CHRISTOPHER, JOHN R. *SCHOOL OF NATURAL HEALING,*
c39.95. Dr. Christopher is a naturopath who has been working in
natural healing and herbalogy for over thirty-five years. He is well
known as a teacher and a practitioner on the west cost and is universally respected. This book is an edited, bound version of his correspondence course in herbal medicine which originally cost $100.
It is the most comprehensive work we can imagine. It's organized
according to the action of the herbs (i.e., alterative herbs, anthel-
mintic herbs, astringent herbs, cathartic herbs, diuretic herbs, etc.)
and is fully cross-referenced. An abundance of background information is provided in each instance and the following specific topics
are covered for each herb: common names, identifying characteristics, parts used, therapeutic action, medicinal uses, preparation,
dosage, administration. Detailed instructions for specific healing
preparations are also offered and their possible benefits are examined.
Additional chapters discuss collecting herbs and present a cleansing
program and a regenerative diet. There's also a section of herb alternatives to the ones suggested in the book. A massive volume
which is a must for all who practice herbalogy or want to be extremely well informed on the subject. Glossary, bibliography, indices of diseases, herbal preparations and formulas, and variant
names, 654pp. Crs 76

COON, NELSON. *THE DICTIONARY OF USEFUL PLANTS,*
c10.95. A compendium of information on hundreds of plants found

in the U.S. Each plant is featured in an entry, arranged alphabetically within botanical families. Each entry describes the plant and its habitat, and discusses the fact and folklore behind current and historic uses. Many practical details are included and most of the individual listings include line drawings. A clearly written account. Coon also includes a long introduction covering the main uses of plants and a special section on American Indian uses of plants. Long bibliography, index, 304pp. Rod 74

CROW, W.B. *THE OCCULT PROPERTIES OF HERBS,* 1.25. An overview of the use of herbs in areas such as astrology, alchemy, magic, and religion. Also includes material on herbs in healing and the symbolism of herbs. 64pp. Wei 69

CULPEPER, NICHOLAS. *COMPLETE HERBAL,* c6.70. A comprehensive description of many herbs with their medicinal properties. Includes color pictures of many of the herbs, descriptions of all of them, places they are found, and very complete directions for use. Includes a listing of diseases and the herbs that will cure them. This herbal is over 250 years old and has remained consistently popular. 430pp. Fou nd

CULPEPER, NICHOLAS. *CULPEPER'S HERBAL REMEDIES,* 2.00. An adaptation of Culpeper's **Complete Herbal,** intended for modern use. Includes over 100 herbs, their descriptions, and modern uses. 128pp. Wil 73

ELBERT, VIRGINIE and GEORGE. *FUN WITH GROWING HERBS INDOORS,* 4.95. This is by far the best book on indoor herb growing we have seen. The Elberts tell how to select the right plants and how to care for the seedlings. Through excellent how to illustrations, the authors demonstrate the step-by-step methods of growing a herb garden, including informative directions for quarantining, potting, repotting, decanting the plant, pot binding, cleaning the roots, multiplying plants, cutting, and growing the cuttings. The second half of the book is devoted to detailed growing instructions for many herbs. Exotic varieties are included (ginger, for example) along with the more well known ones. Some color plates, index, oversize, 192pp. Crn 74

EMBODEN, WILLIAM. *BIZARRE PLANTS,* c10.95. Folklore and descriptions of many highly unusual plants, illustrated with photographs. Index, 214pp. McM 74

226

FLUCK, HANS. *MEDICINAL PLANTS,* c8.60. Each of the more than 150 plants discussed in this volume is illustrated in color and fully described. The text includes information on the parts used, habitat and collection, constituents and actions, and usage. Glossary, index, 188pp. Fou 76

FOLEY, DANIEL, ed. *HERBS FOR USE AND FOR DELIGHT,* 3.50. A collection of articles by amateurs and scientists, this book covers an extremely wide range of material from popular historical accounts of herb usage to personal accounts of cultivating herbs to analyses of specific herbs to scientific papers on the latest research. The articles were selected from **The Herbalist,** the annual publication of The Herb Society of America. In all sixty-four different articles are presented, with illustrations and tables. 323pp. Dov 74

FOSTER, GERTRUDE. *HERBS FOR EVERY GARDEN,* c7.50. Ms. Foster and her husband have been publishing **The Herb Grower Magazine** for over twenty-five years. The articles in the magazine derive mainly from the Fosters' own herb garden in Connecticut, where they grow over 300 species of herbs, gathered from all parts of the globe. Ms. Foster is recognized nationwide as an authority on the history, cultivation, and use of herbs. She has organized and presented her knowledge very well in the volume. The contents include all the information necessary to start a successful herb garden indoors or outside, and special sections describe the use of herbs for pest control in the garden and the preparation of herbs for culinary and medicinal usage. A definitive volume. Illustrations, bibliography, index, 256pp. Dut 73

FURLONG, MARJORIE and VIRGINIA PILL. *WILD EDIBLE FRUITS AND BERRIES,* 3.95. This book depicts forty-two wild fruit and berries common to the Pacific Northwest. Each description includes a color photograph. Almost all of the plants are also found in most parts of the U.S. Glossary, index, 62pp. Nat 74

GABRIEL, INGRID. *HERB IDENTIFIER AND HANDBOOK,* c6.95. Over 100 herbs are described and pictured (many in full color). Each entry includes the following material: scientific name, popular names, where found, description, elements contained, medicinal use (with detailed instructions), and culinary use. Indexed by ailments, scientific names, popular names, and geographic locations. The pictures—line drawings and color plates—are about the clearest we've seen. 256pp. Str 75

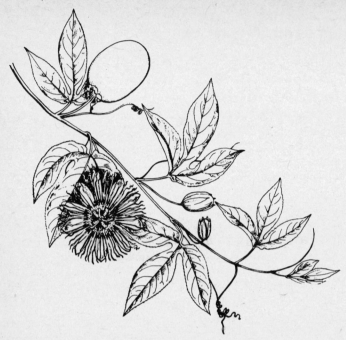

GEOGRAPHIC HEALTH STUDIES PROGRAM. *A BAREFOOT DOCTOR'S MANUAL,* 5.95. See the Oriental Medicine section.

GERARD, JOHN. *THE HERBAL OR GENERAL HISTORY OF PLANTS,* c50.00. **Gerard's Herbal** has long been the most famous English herbal. First published in 1597, it was republished in 1633 in an edition in which Thomas Johnson revised and enlarged the original text. This is a photographic reproduction of the 1633 edition which describes 2850 plants and has about 2700 illustrations. In both text and illustrations, it is a monument of Renaissance botany and at the same time it remains a remarkable compendium of Elizabethan folklore and naturalistic description. 8½"x12", 1723pp. Dov 1633

GIBBONS, EUELL. *STALKING THE HEALTHFUL HERBS,* 3.95. A discussion of many of the culinary and medicinal herbs native to North America—kinds that were well known to the Indians and early settlers. Gibbons' intimate knowledge of these plants is based on countless field studies as well as on painstaking research. Includes line drawings, descriptive and usage material. 303pp. McK 74

Ginseng

Throughout its long and honorable history in East and West, the ginseng root...has never ceased to fascinate those people who have known it. It was the most important drug possessed by the Chinese for two millenia: the essence of the perfect *yin,* the spirit of the soil, a potent restorative and tonic. Their neighbors, from whom the Chinese bought ginseng, the Tartars (Manchurians) and the Koreans, believed the root could work magic in men and that it was itself magic; ginseng in these countries was the object of a veneration just short of worship.—from **Tale of the Ginseng** by Andrew Kimmens

FULDER, STEPHEN. *ABOUT GINSENG,* 1.35. An introductory discussion, including information on the plant itself and its medicinal benefits. 64pp. TPL 76

HARDING, A.R. *GINSENG AND OTHER MEDICINAL PLANTS,* 7.00. This was the first discussion of ginseng and it remains one of the most comprehensive. It offers extremely complete cultivation instructions, including material on diseases and marketing. The same information is presented for other medicinal plants including golden seal. Many illustrations, spiral bound, 367pp. HeR 08

HARRIMAN, SARAH. *THE BOOK OF GINSENG,* 1.50. Presents ancient lore, recent discoveries, and information on buying, growing, and using ginseng. Bibliography, notes, 157pp. Pyr 73

HEFFERN, RICHARD. *THE COMPLETE BOOK OF GINSENG,* 3.95. A comprehensive presentation, divided into the following sections: botany, history, legends, grades, comparative values of Asiatic and North American varieties, early and contemporary research, cultivation and marketing, collection of the wild plant. Illustrations, bibliography, index, 127pp. CeA 76

KIMMENS, ANDREW, ed. *TALES OF THE GINSENG,* 3.95. Folklore about ginseng, mainly from Confucian and Taoist sources, in the form of stories. Annotated bibliography, index, 218pp. Mor 75

LUCAS, RICHARD. *GINSENG, THE CHINESE WONDER ROOT,* 2.15. A short treatise. 57pp. R&M 72

VENINGA, LOUISE. *THE GINSENG BOOK,* 4.95. This is the most comprehensive guide to ginseng. The author has travelled in the U.S. speaking to cultivators, importers, exporters, doctors, pharmacologists, Chinese herbalists, and numerous ginseng enthusiasts. This book represents an encyclopedia of their knowledge. Beautifully illustrated and well laid out. Appendix includes a resource section and a comprehensive bibliography. 152pp. Ruk 73

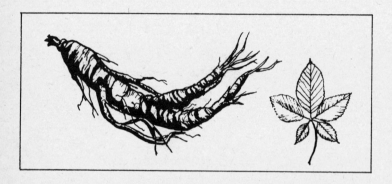

GOSLING, NALDA. *HERBS FOR COLDS AND FLU,* 1.30. Dr. Gosling is a medical herbalist, naturopath, and osteopath. Here she describes and explains how to use twenty-five different herbs to treat colds and influenza. Illustrations, index, 64pp. TPL 76

GRIEVE, M. *A MODERN HERBAL,* c21.50/set/5.00/ea. The most comprehensive herbal imaginable. Two large volumes containing the medicinal, culinary, cosmetic and economic properties, cultivation and folklore of herbs, grasses, fungi, shrubs and trees with their uses. Detailed descriptions as well as drawings of many of the plants. Unbelievably thorough and still it's enjoyable reading. Index, 888pp. Dov 71

HARPER-SHOVE, LT.-COL. F. *PRESCRIBER AND CLINICAL REPERTORY OF MEDICINAL HERBS,* 3.60. Provides leading symptoms of diseases and ailments, together with the corresponding herb or herbs for treatment by homoeopathic medicine, and the exact dosage to be prescribed in each case. The book is arranged according to parts of the body and further subdivided into ailments. Also includes a list of herbal remedies, abbreviations, and exact dosages (including time). Additionally, there's a section listing synonyms, common, and local names of herbs. 240pp. HSP 52

HARRINGTON, H.D. and L.W. DURRELL. *HOW TO IDENTIFY PLANTS*, 3.95. A scholarly text on plant identification, identifying each part of the plant and giving many guidelines. Questions following each section. Each topic is extensively illustrated throughout. Only recommended to those who are very serious about learning the subject. Seems to be quite good of type. 203pp. Swa 57

HARRIS, BEN. *BETTER HEALTH WITH CULINARY HERBS*, 3.95. A detailed survey of domestic and wild culinary herbs, their cultivation, collection, and uses. Also includes recipes and formulas for home remedies. Harris identifies the nutritive and salutary ingredients in each herb and offers some dietary tips. Index, 163pp. BaP 71

HARRIS, BEN. *EAT THE WEEDS*, 1.50. Detailed descriptions and recipes for 150 common plants, including information on habitat, part used, preparation, and synonyms in addition to the more general material. There's also a long introduction incorporating Harris' many years of experience. The herbs described are especially prevalent in the northeastern United States. Bibliography, index, 240pp. Kea 73

HARRIS, BEN. *THE COMPLEAT HERBAL*, 3.95. Harris is best known for his books on edible plants. In this volume he deals with medicinal herbs. He traces the origins of herbal remedies, offers various methods of identification and prescription—including an intriguing *doctrine of signatures*—and discusses preparation. The core of the book is a 200 plant herbal, alphabetically arranged. It is a summary survey which includes folklore. Glossary, bibliography, index, 240pp. BaP 72

HARRIS, LLOYD. *THE BOOK OF GARLIC*, c10.00. This is a humorous, comprehensive book on garlic which includes sections on the history and folklore of garlic, a garlic herbal (with many Russian remedies), and a scientific survey of garlic's composition and healing ingredients. There's also a section of garlic culinary recipes. Extensively illustrated, bibliography, oversize, 237pp. HRW 74

HEFFERN, RICHARD. *THE HERB BUYER'S GUIDE,* 1.25. The only available guide to the purchase, processing and use of herbs. The appendix contains addresses of sources for additional information. 187pp. Pyr 73

HEFFERN, RICHARD. *SECRETS OF THE MIND-ALTERING PLANTS OF MEXICO,* 1.50. A detailed study of a great number of plants, including line drawings, description, and information on their properties, uses, and the research that has been done with them. Also there's some folklore and background information. The text includes material from ancient Mayan and Aztec sources in addition to contemporary material. Index, 204pp. Pyr 74

HEFFERN, RICHARD. *THE USE OF HERBS IN WEIGHT RE-DUCTION,* 1.50. This is a better book than you would think from its title. There's a good discussion of why obesity occurs and a descriptive listing of related herbs and natural sweetening agents. Glossary, index, 141pp. Pyr 75

HERB AND AILMENT CROSS REFERENCE CHART, 4.50. A massive 30"x40" chart containing an abundance of information on well over 100 herbs. The presentation is somewhat overwhelming and the chart is not recommended to those who have problems with their eyes. Nonetheless it is far and away the best visual source of herbal remedies that we know of. UnC

HEWLETT-PARSONS, J. *HERBS, HEALTH AND HEALING,* 1.70. A well presented synopsis of herbal uses for various ailments, with specific remedies and directions for their preparations and background information on each ailment. Includes chapters on the circulatory system, digestive system, skin, respiratory system, nervous system, liver and gall bladder, urinary system, and women's complaints. Recommended as a good overview. Hewlett-Parsons is a naturopath. 94pp. TPL 75

HUSON, PAUL. *MASTERING HERBALISM,* 4.95. Huson has written extensively on witchcraft and his herbal emphasizes the folklore and traditional uses of herbs in witchcraft and astrology. There's also a great deal of material on herbal perfumes and incense and on herbal beauty secrets along with more traditional sections on herbal remedies and culinary herbs. In addition, there are chapters on growing herbs and planting and harvesting by the moon. Huson also provides an excellent annotated listing of mail-order herbal sources. A well written, unusual account. Illustrations, tables of weights and measures, glossary, index, 371pp. S&D 74

HUTCHENS, ALMA. *INDIAN HERBALOGY OF NORTH AMER-ICA,* c10.00. This is the definitive work on the subject. There's not another book that even comes close to presenting the wealth of material contained here. The material comes from the author's years' long study of Anglo-American, Russian, and Oriental literature on Indian medical botanics. The textual order is alphabetical, according to the common name of the herb. All of the proper names are also included along with a drawing of the plant and the following information: features (what the plant looks like), medicinal part, solvents, bodily influence, uses (internal and external), dose, homoeopathical clinical uses, and uses throughout the world. The information is concise, with no unnecessary verbiage. There's also a thirty-three page bibliography, very well annotated, and a twenty-nine page detailed index. Highly recommended for the serious student. 382pp. Mer 74

HYLTON, WILLIAM, ed. *THE RODALE HERB BOOK,* c12.95. Over half of this weighty volume is devoted to an herbal encyclopedia, discussing more than 150 herbs, with many entries illustrated with photographs. The unique contribution of this volume though is not the herbal encyclopedia—helpful though it is—but the specialized chapters. Each is written by an expert and the material is covered in depth. Chapters include: *The Healing Herbs* by Nelson Coon (a disease by disease discussion), *The Culinary Herbs* by Louise Hyde, *The Aromatic Herbs* by Bonnie Fisher, *The Colorful Herbs* by Barbara Foust (dyeing with herbs), *Cultivating the Herbs* by Heinz Grotzke (Heinz runs the Meadowbrook Herb Garden, source of some of the best quality herbs available), and *The Companionable Herbs* by William Hylton. Also includes a list of sources, glossary, bibliography and index. 653pp. Rod 74

JACOBS, BETTY. *PROFITABLE HERB GROWING AT HOME,* 5.95. This is the most comprehensive manual on herb growing we have ever seen. Ms. Jacobs describes how to prepare the soil, how to lay out the herb beds, and how to grow sixty-four different herbs. Subsequent chapters explain how to dry, store, and freeze herbs. Lovely full page line drawings of each herb are included. An appendix lists herb growers and suppliers. Index, 235pp. Gar 76

KADANS, JOSEPH. *ENCYCLOPEDIA OF MEDICINAL HERBS,* 1.75. Information on the preparation and uses of hundreds of herbs. Gives alternate names of the herbs (there are many) and a unique "herb-o-matic" locator index which gives many ailments and the herbs which treat them. Very clearly presented. 256pp. Arc 73

KERR, RALPH. *HERBALISM THROUGH THE AGES,* c6.55. Legends and folklore from antiquity to contemporary times. 225pp. Amo 69

KEYS, JOHN. *CHINESE HERBS,* c15.00. A technical investigation of the botany, chemistry, and pharmacodynamics of Chinese herbs, illustrated with line drawings. Technical appendices contain a collection of Chinese prescriptions, a discussion of supplementary botanical drugs, listings of mineral drugs and drugs of animal origin, and a table of toxic herbs. Glossary, notes, index, 388pp. Tut 76

KLOSS, JETHRO. *BACK TO EDEN,* c7.95/2.25. The most popular herbal—over one million copies sold. It's not our favorite, but this is the bible for many. There is material on all kinds of natural cures, a long section of diseases and suggested remedies, information on preparation, foods and a potpourri of much else. The organization leaves something to be desired, but there's certainly a lot of information here. 700pp. WoP 72

KROCHMAL, ARNOLD and CONNIE. *A GUIDE TO THE MEDICINAL PLANTS OF THE UNITED STATES,* 4.95. Dr. Krochmal has a PhD in Economic Botany and is an expert on medicinal plants. This is a well organized account, profusely illustrated with line drawings and photographs. Each entry (organized alphabetically by the common name) includes alternate names, plant description, where it grows, what is harvested and when, and uses. Appendices cite sources of botanical supplies and meanings of plant names. Fully indexed and cross-referenced, bibliography, 259pp. NYT 73

LAW, DONALD. *THE CONCISE HERBAL ENCYCLOPEDIA,* 4.95. This is an excellent compendium which is easy to use, well illustrated, and very complete. The first half of the book is devoted to an alphabetical discussion of virtually every herb which we have ever heard of, accompanied by line drawings and color plates of most of the herbs. The bulk of the rest of the book is devoted to an analysis of ailments and specific herbal remedies—all very clearly presented. There are also sections on herbal wines, making cosmetics from herbs, herbs in cooking, and veterinary herbs. Recommended. 258pp. SMP 73

LAW, DONALD. *HERB GROWING FOR HEALTH,* 1.65. Law is an authority on botanic medicine. Here he tells how to grow, use and recognize over 150 healing herbs. He includes information on growing herbs indoors and a section on the medicinal value of the bark of over forty kinds of trees. 223pp. Arc 72

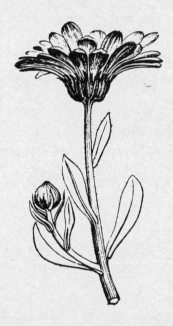

LEVY, JULIETTE. *COMMON HERBS FOR NATURAL HEALTH,* 2.45. This is an excellent herbal, one of our favorites. The author is a practicing herbalist and botanist (and some say a gypsy). A long section is devoted to herbal materia medica, there are original cosmetic and curative recipes, a chapter on the uses of certain plants for the benefit of others, notes on herb preservation, planting with the moon, and much else. The material is alphabetically arranged by the common name of each herb and each entry includes an illustration, the Latin name, where found, use, and dosage, along with a bit of folklore. Two indices: names of herbs and recipes for herbal treatments, and disorders and diseases amenable to herbal treatment. 200pp. ScB 74

LEVY, JULIETTE. *THE COMPLETE HERBAL FOR THE DOG,* 3.95. A revised edition of this definitive handbook on natural care and rearing. Index, 224pp. Arc 75

LEVY, JULIETTE. *HERBAL HANDBOOK FOR FARM AND STABLE,* 3.95. Contains sound advice on the general management of livestock and wisdom on herbal remedies. Ms. Levy gives useful information about the many herbs she lists and then sets out cures and preventions for ailments of sheep, goats, cows, horses, poultry, and sheepdogs. The text begins with a general materia medica, geared toward livestock, and then goes on to specific sections on each of the animals discussed, subdivided into ailments pertinent to each animal. Index, 320pp. Rod 73

LI, C.P. *CHINESE HERBAL MEDICINE,* 2.40. This book is the result of research conducted by Dr. Li, a Chinese born scientist. He received a grant from a U.S. government agency and the approval from the People's Republic of China to examine the use and research on herbs by the medical community in China. This is a detailed, technical report of his findings, incorporating illustrations and technical drawings. Notes, index, 128pp. GPO 74

LIGHTHALL, J.I. *THE INDIAN FOLK MEDICINE GUIDE,* 1.25. This survey was written by a lifelong student of the roots, flowers, barks, leaves, and herbs that comprise the Indian pharmacopaeia. Over 100 remedies are discussed. A big drawback is the lack of a coherent organization in the volume. 158pp. Pop 1883

LOEWENFELD, CLAIRE and PHILIPPA BACK. *THE COMPLETE BOOK OF HERBS AND SPICES,* 4.95. This is a nicely produced, well written herbal which includes medicinal and culinary information along with folklore. Each of the herbs is illustrated with a clear line drawing and the entry on each is divided into the following sections: general, description and habitat, cultivation, flavor and storage, uses, and recipe suggestions. The botanical name is also given and additional sections cover the herb garden, harvesting, and drying and storing herbs. There's also a series of charts. The herbs are discussed in alphabetical order and the book is fully indexed. We recommend this book to those who want a good general introductory survey. Glossary, bibliography, 131pp. LBC 74

LOEWENFELD, CLAIRE. *HERB GARDENING,* 2.95. An extremely complete practical compendium which includes information

236

on indoor and outdoor propagation of all the major herbs. Ms. Loewenfeld also discusses the medicinal, culinary, and cosmetic properties of the herbs and she includes a number of excellent tables and charts. Index, 256pp. Fab 64

LUCAS, RICHARD. *COMMON AND UNCOMMON USES OF HERBS FOR HEALTHFUL LIVING,* 1.65. Lucas has the wonderful gift of taking a subject and bringing it to life. This is a comprehensive treatise which includes specific chapters on a number of herbs and medicinal plants such as dandelion, elder, nettle, sage, mistletoe, parsley, sassafras, and rosemary. He also discusses healing plants from the sea, herbs for bathing and beauty, American Indian herbal lore, and herbs and their effect on emotions. Herb lore and remedial suggestions are interspersed throughout. This is the best book to read if you want to get a feeling of what herbs can do and don't want to get bogged down in technical details. Lucas' information seems to be accurate. Glossary, index, 256pp. Arc 69

LUCAS, RICHARD. *THE MAGIC OF HERBS IN DAILY LIVING,* c8.95. Lucas describes the use of herbs in the following conditions: to tone the sex organs, to restore digestive powers, strengthen vision, build blood, promote hair growth, sharpen memory, aid sleep, relieve headaches and tensions, ease foot trouble, help shed weight, improve skin and complexion, increase longevity. Also includes a section on the legendary occult powers of herbs. Glossary, index, 263pp. PrH 72

LUCAS, RICHARD. *NATURE'S MEDICINES,* 2.00. A fascinating account of the folklore and value of herbal remedies. Chapter headings include: *The Intriguing Herb that Hides from Man, Strange and Mystic Plants, The Favorite of the Pharaohs, The Secret of Perpetual Youth.* Includes practical information. 224pp. Wil 74

LUCAS, RICHARD. *SECRETS OF THE CHINESE HERBALISTS,* c8.95. This is the best book on Chinese herbs we have ever seen. The herbs themselves are fully discussed and both medicinal information and folklore are offered. The bulk of the book is devoted to an in depth analysis of the remedial effects of specific herbs for a variety of ailments. Lucas writes clearly and well and has a thorough knowledge of his material. Illustrations, index, 244pp. PrH 77

LUST, JOHN. *THE HERB BOOK,* c12.95/2.50. This is the most comprehensive and best written of all the contemporary herbals and our favorite for the general reader. Centering on a long section describing medicinal uses for more than 500 plants—nearly 300 of them illustrated—the book combines traditional herbal knowledge with the latest information from current research, especially research carried out in Europe where herbal medicine is still a vital branch of the medical profession. Special sections on botany, obtaining and keeping herbs, and making and using herbal preparations help you understand and use what you learn. There's also an extensive glossary of medicinal effects and herbs that produce them, a listing of plants applicable to various conditions and body organs, and three separate indices along with the most comprehensive bibliography we've seen. A final section discusses herbal mixtures, drinking herbs, natural cosmetics, and plant dyes—along with material on plant legend and lore. 659pp. Ban 74

MEDSGER, OLIVER. *EDIBLE WILD PLANTS,* 3.95. A classic work which has guided several generations of nature lovers. Detailed line drawings of over 150 species, along with information on where to find the plants, how to recognize them, and what parts to eat. Included are fruits and berries, salad plants and herbs, roots and tubers, nuts, beverage and flowering plants, seeds and seed pods. Plants are listed by type and species as well as by region; descriptions include characteristics, when each is in season, and scientific and common names. Index, 342pp. McM 72

MESCHTER, JOAN. *HOW TO GROW HERBS AND SALAD GREENS INDOORS,* 1.50. A good account, profusely illustrated with line drawings and photographs and step-by-step instructions. The material on salad greens is hard to find elsewhere in as clear a form. For the price the book is the best value we know of. Index, 176pp. Pop 75

MERCATANTE, ANTHONY. *THE MAGIC GARDEN,* 5.95. This is an illustrated discussion of the folklore and mythology of flowers, plants, trees, and herbs. Index, 8"x9¼", 206pp. H&R 76

MEYER, JOSEPH. *THE HERBALIST,* c5.95. This is one of the best regarded older herbals. This is a revised and enlarged edition prepared by the author's son. The herbal materia medica is one of the most complete we've seen and includes a shaded line drawing of each plant along with information on the botanic and common names, medicinal part, description, properties and uses, and dosage.

There are also over 400 color illustrations of various plants. In addition, the book has the following special features: a section detailing medicinal uses of certain classes of herbs, a section on teas, and one on culinary herbs, material on potpourri, sachets, plant dyes, and wines. Index, 304pp. Str 60

MILLSPAUGH, CHARLES. *AMERICAN MEDICINAL PLANTS,* c15.00/10.00. This is an unabridged reproduction of the 1892 edition considered the definitive herbal of its day. After general descriptions of the order and genus, every plant is presented in botanical sequence. Common and scientific names are given. Then follows a detailed description of the plant with full information on its size, color, shape, range, habitat. The medicinal uses of the plants are equally detailed, citing observations from the time of the Greeks to the end of the nineteenth century. Each disease or ailment it is reported to have an effect on is noted, and methods of preparation are given along with the chemical constituents extracted from each. Altogether 180 plants are covered—each with a full page illustration. There's also a therapeutic index which keys over 1000 ailments to herbs. Many indices, 828pp. Dov 74

MUIR, ADA. *THE HEALING HERBS OF THE ZODIAC,* 1.00. In ancient times all herbalists studied the zodiacal sign and planetary ruler of each herb and saw that it was gathered under the most favorable planetary conditions. Ms. Muir feels that today herbs are often combined irrespective of planetary laws and the active principle of one counteracts the active principle of another. This is a study of the herbs pertaining to each of the twelve signs of the zodiac, with descriptive material on each one. Some medical astrology, as it pertains to each sign, is also included. Illustrations, index, 63pp. Llp 59

NATIONAL ACADEMY OF SCIENCES. *HERBAL PHARMACOLOGY IN THE PEOPLE'S REPUBLIC OF CHINA,* 8.00. In June 1974 twelve U.S. specialists in chemistry, medicine, pharmacology, pharmacognosy, pharmacy, and Chinese culture visited a series of Chinese cities to assess the current status of herbal pharmacology (both basic and clinical) in the People's Republic of China. Their Trip Report is contained in this volume. Almost half of the book is devoted to an analysis of 248 plant and animal drugs used in China. This is a highly technical volume. 8½"x11", 269pp. NAS 75

PAGE, NANCY and RICHARD WEAVER. *WILD PLANTS IN THE CITY,* 3.95. A useful, color coded guide to the most common wild plants found in abandoned lots and parks in eastern U.S. cities. The authors have described each plant and include photographs and line drawings of each. Bibliography, index, 127pp. NYT 75

PALAISEUL, JEAN. *GRANDMOTHER'S SECRETS,* 2.50. The author's grandmothers were French herbalists and Ms. Palaiseul has recorded the folklore and remedies which they passed down to her. Over 150 plants and their medicinal properties are discussed in detail and some inadequate line drawings are interspersed. Glossary, indices of botanical and common names and of remedies, 364pp. Pen 73

RAU, HENRIETTA. *HEALING WITH HERBS,* 1.50. An encyclopedic guide to the healing properties of a large number of herbs. The information on each herb is extremely complete and is also quite approachable. All the possible uses are detailed and the usable parts of each are noted. A final section lists the herbs which are useful in over three hundred ailments. An excellent all around presentation which we recommend highly. The author is a naturopath who has worked extensively with medicinal herbs. Fully indexed, 235pp. Arc 68

ROSE, JEANNE. *HERBS AND THINGS,* 3.95. A very popular herbal which is attractively designed and clearly written. It's one of our favorites. The first part consists of an alphabetical list of human conditions and the herbs that affect them. The second part is a very well done materia medica. There's also a glossary, a table of weights and measures and their equivalents, and a listing of where to purchase botanicals. Various recipes for all types of things (including beautifying oneself) are also included and there's a good bibliography and a long index. 323pp. G&D 74

ROSE, JEANNE. *JEANNE ROSE'S HERBAL BODY BOOK,* 4.95. As the title suggests, this herbal is devoted to recipes for cosmetic herbal preparations of all types. Each topic is fully covered and the instructions are clear and often humorous. About 100 pages are devoted to descriptions of plants. There's also a cosmetic glossary and information on where to buy the herbs. This is far and away the best book of type we know of. Illustrations abound throughout. 400pp. G&D 76

240

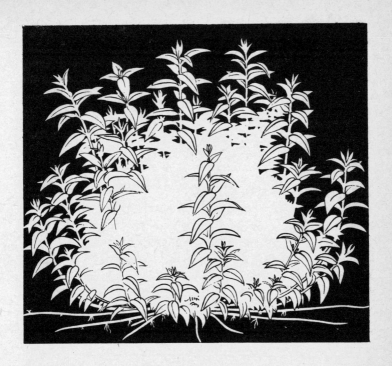

ROSE, JEANNE. *KITCHEN COSMETICS: USING PLANTS AND HERBS IN COSMETICS,* 3.95. This is Ms. Rose's most intimate guide to natural beauty. She presents over sixty recipes and formulas for the hair, hands, legs, feet, and face using common kitchen and garden herbs, flowers, and fruit. Shampoos, moisturizers, facial masks, bath oils, and other products are all described. It's not as encyclopedic a work as the **Herbal Body Book** and it covers somewhat different ground. Photographs, illustrations, 140pp. PjP 77

RUTHERFORD, MEG. *A PATTERN OF HERBS,* 2.95. This book has far and away the nicest illustrations of any volume we know of. The line drawings are clear and well made and often sections of the flowers and stems are shown in detail. The descriptions of each herb are adequate, although we do not care for many of the suggested culinary recipes. The emphasis is not on the medicinal qualities—in fact this feature is hardly mentioned. Bibliography, 157pp. Dou 76

SANECKI, KAY. *THE COMPLETE BOOK OF HERBS,* c9.95. This is a comprehensive account for the general reader, emphasizing the culinary properties and the folklore of each herb. Each entry is accompanied by an illustration, including some color photographs. The material is more extensive and better presented than most books of this type. Includes an index of common and botanical names. 8½"x11", 247pp. McM 74

SHEPHARD, DOROTHY. *PHYSICIANS POSY,* c6.60. See the Homoeopathy section.

SHIH-CHEN, LI. *CHINESE MEDICINAL HERBS,* 5.00. This work was originally published in 1578. The complete herbal comprises 1892 species of drugs, includes 8160 prescriptions, and was the product of twenty-six years of research. Two American physicians translated this massive work, added their personal observations, and annotated their translation. This is a new edition with additional references. The Latin name as well as the Chinese and English are given for each entry. 467+pp. GeP 73

SILVERMAN, MAIDA. *A CITY HERBAL,* 5.95. Subtitled *A Guide to the Lore, Legend, and Usefulness of Thirty-four Plants That Grow Wild in the City. With recipes for breads, jams, salads, teas, dyes, potpourris, cosmetics, seasonings, etc., etc.* Line drawings of each plant, 7½"x9½", 192pp. RaH 77

SIMMONS, ADELMA. *HERBS TO GROW INDOORS,* 3.50. A comprehensive, illustrated text. 146pp. Haw 69

SIMMONS, ADELMA. *THE ILLUSTRATED HERBAL HANDBOOK,* 2.50. Large line drawings are the chief feature of this handbook. The text includes folklore, a detailed description of uses, and the culture of the herb. The presentation is geared toward the general reader. Different varieties of each herb are discussed, giving the botanical names. Index, 124pp. Haw 72

SMITH, WILLIAM. *HERBS FOR CONSTIPATION,* 1.35. Dr. Smith begins with some general advice and goes on to describe a series of herbs and their usage. Line drawings accompany each selection. A handy little book. 64pp. TPL 76

SWENSON, ALLAN. *MY OWN HERB GARDEN,* c5.95. This is a beautifully illustrated book on herbs written for younger readers.

Every step of the growing, harvesting, and storing process is explored at length. The writing style is lucid and Swenson makes herb gardening sound like a fun thing to do. We like this book a lot and we heartily recommend it for young people. Many color drawings. Index, 8¼"x9½", 98pp. Rod 76

SZEKELY, EDMUND. *THE BOOK OF HERBS,* 2.25. A brief compendium of diseases and remedies as well as a herbal materia medica. 46pp. Aca 75

THE HERBALIST: MAGAZINE OF HERBAL KNOWLEDGE, 1.00/each. A slick monthly put out by students of Dr. Christopher. A number of herbs are discussed at length in each issue and there are other special features. Many photographs and line drawings. Each issue is about 40 pages and yearly subscriptions are available for $9.00 from Bi-World Publishers, Inc., 224 N. Draper Lane, P.O. Box 62, Provo, Utah 84601.

TOBE, JOHN. *PROVEN HERBAL REMEDIES,* 1.50. Includes a complete disease by disease listing of ailments and their remedies, discussions of herb teas, and information on gathering and preparing herbs. 176pp. Pyr 73

TOGUCHI, MASARU. *ORIENTAL HERBAL WISDOM,* 1.25. This is a good presentation of oriental herbalism for the general reader. The author begins with an excellent section on the oriental system of observing conditions and determining remedies—specific diseases are cited as examples and all the terms used are thoroughly explained. The second section, *Applications of the Herbal Way,* discusses ailments and the specific herbal treatments pertinent to each. A long glossary and many cross-referenced indices are included. 151pp. Pyr 73

TWITCHELL, PAUL. *HERBS: THE MAGIC HEALERS,* 1.95. A compendium of hundreds of herbs giving their ancient and modern uses, their health-giving and occult powers. A very complete account which relates herbs to the philosophy of Eckankar. 189pp. IWP 71

VENINGA, LOUISE and BEN ZARICOR. *GOLDENSEAL/ETC.,* 3.95. The first part of this study focuses on goldenseal and the rest of the volume discusses a variety of other wild American herbs. The authors entitle their study a *pharmacognosy*—which they define as the simultaneous study of the history, distribution, cultivation, collection, preparation, preservation, and therapeutics of medicinals. This is the most complete book of type that we know of. Many of the plants which are discussed are not mentioned in depth in any other book that we know of. Line drawings of all the plants accompany the text. Bibliography, 193pp. Ruk 76

WEINER, MICHAEL. *EARTH MEDICINE–EARTH FOODS,* 4.95. An illustrated disease by disease listing of plant remedies, drugs, and natural foods of the North American Indians. 8½"x11", 214pp. McM 72

WESLAGER, C.A. *MAGIC MEDICINES OF THE INDIANS,* c8.00. This is a well written comprehensive survey of the herbal treatments and folklore used by the Indians of New Jersey, Pennsylvania, Delaware, and Maryland. It includes material on the plants and trees and specifics on various cures. The book seems to be a good research project, but a bit hard to use since it is a narrative rather than an organized manual. Bibliography, index, 262pp. MAP 73

WESLEY, JOHN. *PRIMITIVE REMEDIES,* 2.25. Recent reprint of an eighteenth century herbal manual by the noted Methodist reformer. The material is alphabetically arranged according to diseases and is mainly interesting because of its archaic nature. 142pp. WoP 73

WREN, R.W., ed. *POTTER'S NEW CYCLOPEDIA OF MEDICINAL HERBS AND PREPARATIONS,* 4.95. A very scholarly reference book prepared for practitioners. Hundreds of plants are listed and the following information is given for each one: synonym, habitat, description, medicinal use, preparations. There are appendices on the forms of medicinal preparations, herbal compounds, a glossary of botanical and medical terms, and a descriptive listing of plant families. Illustrations, index, 402pp. H&R 72

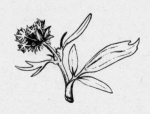

Homœopathy

T here exists in the world today a force which heals the body and the mind of man: it is so powerful, so magnificent, that our only attitude towards it can be one of awe and reverence. This force is homoeopathy. Homoeopathy is a medical system which successfully treats all man's diseases, whether acute or chronic, whether of the body or of the mind. As Dr. J.H. Clarke has put it: "It is the most complete and scientific system of healing the world has ever seen." So writes George Vithoulkas of Athens, Greece.

Homoeopathy is like a bad joke. In the beginning it appears so straightforward, so easy. But the more you study, the more difficult it becomes for you, until in the end it may seem altogether impossible! So says Miestro Flores Toledo of Mexico City.

What are we to make of such contradictory statements by two of the masters? What is homoeopathy? How does it fit into our understanding of the healing arts?

Briefly put, homoeopathy is a complete system of medicine whose masters have learned how to observe and treat the totality of a person's morbid symptoms with one nontoxic therapeutic agent. Those remedies, originally of vegetable, mineral or animal sources, are administered in a diluted form on a neutral sucrose base. Hence they have become known as sugar pills. In 1900, 20% of all American doctors were homoeopaths and homoeopathy enjoyed great popularity with the people and in the press. Concerted attacks by the AMA over licensing standards, with the help of the Flexnor Report in 1910 (which also outlawed midwives, female and non-white doctors), led to the forced closing of all American homoeopathic medical schools. Today homoeopathy is taught and practiced legally in Europe, Mexico, South America and India, where differing schools of thought have proliferated several versions of its therapeutic.

It is important to realize that 1) homoeopathy is as curative today as it was before the advent of the "wonder drugs;" 2) homoeopathy is a very difficult medical discipline requiring years of supervised study; 3) no American homoeopath is adequately trained; 4) any homoeopathic booklist will be primarily composed of Indian reprints from nineteenth century British and American works of widely varying quality. I recommend the following books as essential to an understanding of homoeopathy, as the principal works in the pure (Hahnemannian) tradition and as the basis of any self-study program:

Introductory
Coulter: Homoeopathic Medicine
Vithoulkas: Homoeopathy, Medicine of the New Man
Hubbard-Wright: A Brief Study Course in Homoeopathy

Essential
Hahnemann: Organon of the Healing Art
Hahnemann: The Lesser Writings
J.T. Kent: Lectures on Homoeopathic Philosophy
J.T. Kent: Lectures on Homoeopathic Materia Medica
J.T. Kent: Repertory of the Homoeopathic Materia Medica

Beware those homoeopathic books which seem pathological in orientation and those which compromise or violate these basic principles:

1) Simila — any substance which will produce morbid symptoms in a healthy person will cure a sick person with similar symptoms.
2) Single remedy — give only one therapeutic agent

at a time.

3) Minimum dose — give only the minimum amount of therapy necessary to cure.

4) Wait — until the action of the remedy is completely exhausted before administering another, or even the same one again.

Further, there are two levels of treatment in homoeopathy, acute and chronic. Acute or first-aid homoeopathy is harmless, inexpensive, relatively simple to administer properly and should be the common knowledge of every mother in America. Acute prescribing in the household is a gratifying demonstration of the power of similia. To obtain a homoeopathic kit, write to:

National Center for Homoeopathy
6231 Leesburg Pike
Falls Church, VA 22044

Chronic prescribing for the deepest levels of illness is the province of accomplished homoeopathic physicians. In their hands, amazing cures can occur. At present there is no homoeopathic medical school offering its own M.D. degree in the Western world. However, there is a homoeopathic community in California working for the development of such a school in Greece around the master George Vithoulkas. If you wish information about this school, or are willing to contribute time or money toward its development, write to:

International Foundation for the Promotion of Homoeopathy and Alternative Medicine
628 Vincente
Berkeley, CA 94707

How is a study of homoeopathy useful to humanistic medicine or holistic practitioners? Homoeopathy has developed the science of treating the whole person to very sophisticated levels and homoeopaths are able to judge the process of a case toward cure according to changes in the patient's mental, emotional and physical symptoms as interrelated parts of the whole organism. These same criteria can be applied in any curative process originating from any therapeutic agent. Patient study will yield many valuable principles to any student of holism.

If the physician clearly perceives what is to be cured in diseases, that is to say, in every individual case of disease; if he clearly perceives what is curative in medicines, that is to say, in each individual medicine, and if he knows how to adapt, according to clearly defined principles, what is curative in medicines to what he has discovered to be undoubtedly morbid in the patient, so that recovery must ensue. . .then he understands how to treat judiciously and rationally and he is a true practitioner of the healing art. —from **Organon**, section 3.

Sounds simple at first, doesn't it? Read on!

Vithoulkas once asked me if I understood the true power of healing. When after a few fumbling attempts I admitted I did not, he replied: *True healing—a cure— is an event no amount of money on earth can buy. To be able to truly heal is to hold a power above all others on earth. People will bring stacks of money. The healer must reject that, or he is finished. The physician who does not heal from compassion is finished.*

—Don Gerrard

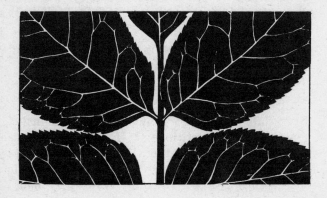

ALLEN, H.C. *KEYNOTES AND CHARACTERISTICS OF THE MATERIA MEDICA WITH NOSODES,* 3.75. A keynote is something that specifically identifies a particular remedy. This is the definitive work on keynotes and it is indispensable for physicians. Dr. Allen continued to expand his original work to the end of his life, incorporating later findings of his own and his colleagues. This is a reprint of the sixth and final edition. Index, 388pp. JPC 75

ALLEN, H.C. *MATERIA MEDICA OF SOME IMPORTANT NOSODES,* .50. A very complete account. 67pp. JPC nd

ALLEN, H.C. *THE MATERIA MEDICA OF THE NOSODES AND PROVING OF X-RAYS,* c9.50. This is a classic work which should be in the library of all practitioners. This edition includes a supplement containing materia medica and therapeutics of the new nosodes—mainly extracted from Dr. Clarke's **Dictionary of Medicine**. 584pp. SeD 42

ALLEN, J.H. *CHRONIC MIASMS,* 5.75. Rin

ALLEN, J.H. *DISEASES AND THERAPEUTICS OF THE SKIN,* c3.50. An extremely complete study, generally considered the best book available on the subject. Indices of diseases and therapies, 331pp. SeD 51

ALLEN, J.H. *INTERMITTENT FEVER,* 6.15. Rin

ALLEN, J.H. *PRIMER OF MATERIA MEDICA,* 3.85. Rin

ALLEN, J.H. *THE THERAPEUTICS OF FEVER,* 7.75. Rin

ALLEN, TIMOTHY FIELD. *BOENNINGHAUSEN'S THERAPEUTIC POCKET BOOKS,* c4.15. This book has long been considered a classic. In addition to Allen's edition of the work, this version includes a long, detailed introduction by H.A. Roberts and Annie Wilson. The book includes information on specific remedies for conditions and an analysis of the effects of a number of remedies. Index, 579pp. JPC 72

ALPH, TESTE. *A HOMOEOPATHY TREATISE ON THE DISEASES OF CHILDREN,* 2.30. Rin

BERJEAU, J. *THE HOMOEOPATHIC TREATMENT OF SYPHILIS, GONORRHOEA, SPERMATORRHOEA, AND URINARY DISEASES,* c2.75. This edition includes many revisions and additions by J.H.P. Frost. The information is topically arranged. Index, 224pp. SeD 52

BHATTACHARJEE. *FAMILY PRACTICE,* 3.25. Rin

BHATTACHARJEE. *FIRST AID,* .75. Rin

BLACKIE, MARGERY. *THE PATIENT, NOT THE CURE,* c15.00. Dr. Blackie was appointed physician to the Queen of England in 1969. She is also Dean of the Faculty of Homoeopathy and Honorary Consulting Physician to the Royal London Homoeopathic Hospital. This is a well written discussion of the basics of homoeopathic practice. Dr. Blackie begins with a summary of the concepts of homoeopathy and goes from there to a discussion of Samuel Hahnemann and his contemporaries. The next part of the book discusses homoeopathy in practice and includes sections on taking the case, types of remedies, and the materia medica. After this she discusses homoeopathy in a number of specific areas and gives a number of case histories. There's also a survey of the contemporary homoeopathic scene. A final section illustrates *the homoeopathic bouquet.* Index, 247pp. MCD 76

BLACKWOOD, A.L. *DISEASES OF THE LIVER, PANCREAS AND DUCTLESS GLANDS,* c3.25. A concise discussion which reviews many specific conditions and gives a variety of therapeutic indications. Fully indexed, 166pp. SeD 07

BOENNINGHAUSEN, C. VON. *MATERIA MEDICA AND REPERTORY,* c17.00. Rin

BOENNINGHAUSEN, C. VON. *SIDES OF THE BODY,* .85. Rin

BOENNINGHAUSEN, C. VON. *THERAPEUTIC POCKET BOOK,* c9.50. Rin

BOERICKE, WILLIAM. *A COMPENDIUM OF THE PRINCIPLES OF HOMEOPATHY,* 3.50. *This little book is intended to be an introduction and an aid to a fuller study and wider acceptance of Hahnemann's doctrines. It does not pretend to be more than an attempt to elucidate the salient and vital points often abstrusely*

250

and always metaphorically treated by Hahnemann, and thus to familiarize the student with the fundamental groundwork of our school.—from the preface. Index, 159pp. HeP 1896

BOERICKE, WILLIAM. *MATERIA MEDICA WITH REPER-TORY,* c6.40. This is a reprint of the ninth edition which includes a comprehensive repertory, revised and updated by Oscar Boericke. The main part of the text analyzes the preparations as used in specific ailments. This book is considered one of the best materia medicas available and is an essential aid to all practitioners. Includes many indices, 1105pp. JPC 27

BOGER, C.M. *ADDITIONS TO KENT'S REPERTORY,* .80. 105pp. JPC 72

BOGER, C.M., tr. and ed. *BOENNINGHAUSEN'S CHARACTER-ISTICS AND REPERTORY,* c17.60. This is generally considered the most authoritative work available. *It has been universally acclaimed to be the nearest approach to perfection in finding the correct similimum and so the work presented to the profession embodies all the essentials of his masterpieces, being most comprehensive in logic, philosophy, applicability and far reaching in influence.*—from the acknowledgement. Index, 1091pp. JPC 36

BOGER, C.M. *A SYNOPTIC KEY OF THE MATERIA MEDICA,* c3.95. As the title suggests, this is a detailed guide to the use of various preparations intended for the serious practitioner. Also includes an index of symptoms and the related preparations. 350pp. JPC 31

BORLAND, DOUGLAS. *CHILDREN'S TYPES,* 1.00. This is an in depth discussion of the five principal types of children. Dr. Borland reviews the remedies that are especially efficacious for each type. 66pp. BrH nd

BORLAND, DOUGLAS. *HOMEOPATHY FOR MOTHER AND INFANT,* 1.00. A useful discussion which considers the mental health and development of the infant (up to two years of age) and pregnant mother as well as their physical health. Specific remedies are provided. 20pp. BrH nd

BORLAND, DOUGLAS. *INFLUENZAS,* .80. Transcription of a series of lectures discussing eight remedies. 20pp. BrH nd

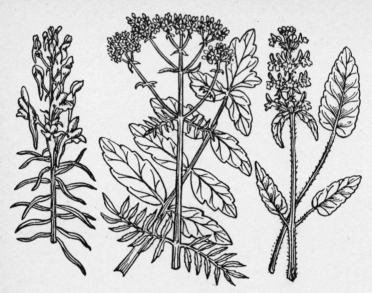

BORLAND, DOUGLAS. *PNEUMONIAS,* 1.80. A discussion of prescribing for acute pneumonia divided into sections on the incipient stage, fully developed pneumonia, complicated pneumonia, and late pneumonia. Specific remedies are advanced and discussed in each case. The appendix, which contains a repertory for pneumonia-related conditions, is topically arranged and exceedingly helpful. 76pp. BrH nd

BOSE, S.K. *MIDWIFERY,* c1.10. A homoeopathic treatise. The first chapter surveys the anatomical structures and functions of the male and female reproductive organs. The second discusses the maladies to which these organs are susceptible and suggests treatments. The third looks at midwifery and childbirth at length, and the final chapter contains therapeutic indications for all infant diseases. 190pp. Bha 66

BRITISH HOMEOPATHIC ASSOCIATION. *A GUIDE TO HO-MEOPATHY,* 1.20. A small pamphlet prepared by the British Homeopathic Association containing articles on the history of homoeopathy and a short review of several topics in homoeopathic practice. 25pp. BrH 75

BURNETT, J. COMPTON. *CATARACT,* 2.70. Rin

BURNETT, J. COMPTON. *CHANGE OF LIFE IN WOMEN,* 1.45. Rin

BURNETT, J. COMPTON. *DELICATE AND BACKWARD CHIL-DREN,* 1.90. Rin

BURNETT, J. COMPTON. *LIVER,* 1.50. Rin

BURNETT, J. COMPTON. *ORGAN DISEASES OF WOMEN,* 1.50. Rin

BURNETT, J. COMPTON. *SKIN,* 1.50. Rin

BURNETT, J. COMPTON. *TONSILS,* .75. Rin

BURNETT, J. COMPTON. *VACCINOSIS,* 1.10. *By vaccinosis Burnett means the disease known as Vaccinia, the result of vaccination plus that profound and often long lasting morbid constitutional state engendered by the vaccine virus. To this state Thuja is homoeopathic, and therefore curative of it.* This is a very complete discussion. 93pp. HSP 60

Cell Salts

Tissue salts, also known as the Schuessler biochemical cell salts, named after the physician who discovered their value many years ago, are not drugs. They are tiny, sweet-tasting, white tablets about twice as thick as the head of a pin. They contain inorganic minerals which, on analysis, have been found already to exist in the body. These tissue salts are not new, but merely forgotten in favor of drugs. W.H. Schuessler, M.D., isolated them as early as 1873. He analyzed human blood and found these important minerals in it, as well as in the ashes of humans after death, proving that they are an integral part of the body.

In countless experiments, Dr. Schuessler learned that if

the body became deficient in these precious minerals, the deficiency caused an abnormal or "diseased" condition. By studying various symptoms he ascertained which minerals were lacking in his patients, and supplied them. He found that if diseases were curable at all, and the proper cell salt were chosen and given in the correct amount, the deficiency which caused the abnormality was corrected and the body healed itself. Thus the tissue salts are not used to "cure" anything. They are merely supplied to the body to remedy a deficiency so that health can return to the cells and thus to the body, which is made up of cells. —Linda Clark

BOERICKE, WILLIAM and **WILLIS DEWEY.** *THE TWELVE TISSUE REMEDIES OF SCHUSSLER,* c4.80. This volume includes a comprehensive discussion of each of the cell salts, accompanied by an alphabetical analysis of ailments and their corresponding remedies. Case histories are presented throughout and there's also a complete repertory. Index, 450pp. JPC 14

CHAPMAN, ESTHER. *HOW TO USE THE TWELVE TISSUE SALTS,* 1.25. Gives specific instructions in tissue salt therapy for a large number of illnesses, details each salt's role, and shows how an imbalance in one or more can lead to persistent, troublesome illness. Also includes sections on the body's need for various vitamins and minerals along with many tables. 140pp. Pyr 60

CHAPMAN, J.B. *DR. SCHUESSLER'S BIOCHEMISTRY: A MEDICAL BOOK FOR THE HOME,* c3.25. The author of this work was regarded by Dr. Schuessler as one of the most capable exponents of his therapy. This is an excellent, comprehensive disease by disease text, with information on causes and symptoms, treatment, and suggestions. Glossary, fully indexed, 185pp. TPL 61

JANSKY, ROBERT. *HOW TO USE THE CELL SALTS,* 1.50. Jansky is an astrologer and a biochemist. He is most noted for his work with nutritional and medical astrology. Here he presents the general reader with an introduction to the cell salts, discusses how they should be taken, and reviews the physiological use of each of the twelve cell salts together with the common ailments that they seem to influence most strongly. 10pp. AsA 74

NEW ERA LAB. *THE NEW BIOCHEMIC HANDBOOK,* 1.50. Subtitled *An introduction to the cellular therapy and practical application of the twelve tissue salts in accordance with the Biochemic System of Medicine.* Includes descriptions of the salts, information on selecting a remedy, and specific remedies for many ailments. 127pp. FoI nd

POWELL, ERIC. *BIOCHEMISTRY UP-TO-DATE,* 2.40. In addition to listing and explaining the use of Schuessler's original twelve biochemical salts, Powell also provides details of thirty more elements now employed by modern biochemists. A quick-reference treatment guide is given for over 250 disorders. Notes of potencies, frequency of doses, and examples of dosage are presented. 66pp. HSP 63

SCHUSSLER, W.H. *ABRIDGED THERAPEUTICS,* 5.00. An in depth discussion of the tissue salts and their uses in various ailments. Includes material on the theory and function of the salts, an extensive glossary, and an index. 226pp. HeR 74

CHAVANON, PAUL and RENE LEVANNIER. *EMERGENCY HOMOEOPATHIC FIRST AID,* 5.20. This is the most complete book on emergency homoeopathic first aid. The authors are French homoeopaths and they have culled their suggestions out of long experience. The ailments are arranged alphabetically, and remedies are given for each along with details of dosage and frequency of administration. Often a series of remedies are suggested. The authors also provide thirty-five pages of explanatory material, although this information is not terribly clear. 159pp. TPL 77

CLARKE, JOHN H. *CATARRH, COLDS AND GRIP,* 1.30. A discussion of the ailments, symptoms, and appropriate remedies. A materia medica is appended. 122pp. JPC 1899

CLARKE, JOHN H. *CLINICAL REPERTORY,* c9.60. This is an excellent supplement to the larger materia medicas. Part I gives clinical information such as the remedies for many disorders, alphabetically arranged by ailment. Part II deals with causation, i.e., bee stings, anxiety, acid food, cold air, etc., also alphabetically arranged by cause. Part III examines temperaments, dispositions, constitutions, and states, i.e., agitation, angry and excited persons, chubby children, peevishness, etc., again, alphabetically arranged. Part IV indicates clinical relationships, naming, when known, complementary remedies, what the remedy follows well, what the remedy is followed well by, compatible remedies, incompatible remedies, remedy antidotes, what the remedy is antidoted by, and duration of action. This is one of the most useful comprehensive books for the layman and is certainly a necessity for all practitioners. 346pp. HSP 71

CLARKE, JOHN H. *COLDS,* 3.80. Rin

CLARKE, JOHN H. *CONSTITUTIONAL MEDICINE,* 3.25. Includes a general discussion, examples, and information derived from the experiences of Grauvogl and Bojanus. Index, 182pp. JPC 74

CLARKE, JOHN H. *DICTIONARY OF PRACTICAL MATERIA MEDICA,* c120.00/set. This is far and away the most comprehensive materia medica available. It includes thousands of references and quotations and is considered a remarkably precise work. It is also the most clearly presented and well written of the materia medicas. Both the characteristics of the remedy and the symptoms are discussed in great detail. Highly recommended to all who are serious about homoeopathic study and practice. Three volumes, 2585pp. HSP 77

CLARKE, JOHN H. *HEART,* 1.15. Rin

CLARKE, JOHN H. *HOMOEOPATHY EXPLAINED,* 1.30. As the title suggests, this is an introductory book covering the careers and achievements of the major homoeopathic doctors, and general material on what homoeopathy is and how it works. The organization is a bit scattered and the writing style not as flowing as in some of the other books, so this is not an ideal introduction but it can serve as a good supplement to some of the other introductory works. Index, 212pp. JPC 71

CLARKE, JOHN H. *INDIGESTION,* .95. Rin

CLARKE, JOHN H. *NON-SURGICAL TREATMENT OF DISEASES OF THE GLANDS AND BONES,* .65. Index, 170pp. JPC nd

CLARKE, JOHN H. *THE PRESCRIBER,* c4.80. This is the definitive prescriber, alphabetically organized by symptom or part of the body affected. Includes material on using the preparations and specific advice on the potency of each medicine and the dosage. Edward Cotter, a practitioner with wide experience, has thoroughly revised and added to the treatment section of this edition. Also includes Clarke's treatise, *How to Practice Homoeopathy*. 382pp. HSP 72

COULTER, HARRIS. *HOMOEOPATHIC MEDICINE,* 1.65. An introductory discussion which presents the basic principles of homoeopathy in a highly intellectual fashion. 73pp. FoI 72

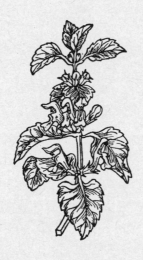

COWPERTHWAITE, A.C. *A TEXT BOOK OF GYNAECOLOGY,* c5.15. This is the most complete account of homoeopathic gynaecology that we know of. The material is very well organized and is illustrated throughout. All aspects of the subject are fully covered. Index, 549pp. JPC 1888

COWPERTHWAITE, A.C. *A TEXT-BOOK OF MATERIA MEDICA AND THERAPEUTICS,* c8.00. This is generally considered one of the most valuable materia medicas available and is recommended to all practitioners. This is a well bound reprint of the eleventh edition. Index, 886pp. JPC 76

257

COX, DONOVAN and JONES. *BEFORE THE DOCTOR COMES,* 1.30. Although homoeopathic treatment for serious illness requires the attention of a homoeopathic physician, there are a number of simple and safe remedies for the relief of everyday ailments. This guide tells you what to buy and all you need to know to deal with minor illnesses and accidents. It contains an alphabetical list of ailments, along with appropriate remedies. Index, 48pp. TPL 76

DEWEY, W.A. *ESSENTIALS OF HOMEOPATHIC MATERIA MEDICA,* 3.60. Rin

DEWEY, W.A. *ESSENTIALS OF THERAPEUTICS,* 2.70. Rin

DEWEY, W.A. *PRACTICAL HOMOEOPATHIC THERAPEUTICS,* c3.50. This text is devoted exclusively to homoeopathic prescribing. The indications for the remedies have been culled from the experience of many noted homoeopathic prescribers. The book is topically arranged by ailments and each section is further divided into an analysis of the preparations efficacious for each ailment. Indices of ailments and subindices of remedies for each ailment plus a listing of the authorities quoted, 479pp. JPC 34

FARRINGTON, E.A. *CLINICAL MATERIA MEDICA,* c9.60. This is one of the classic materia medicas and is often used as a text in college courses. Each of the major remedies is extensively discussed. Dr. Farrington expresses himself clearly and covers a great deal of material which is not available elsewhere. Indices of remedies and therapies, 826pp. JPC 08

FARRINGTON, E.A. *THERAPEUTIC POINTERS AND LESSER WRITINGS WITH SOME CLINICAL CASES,* c6.00. A collection of articles originally published in British and American professional journals in the late nineteenth century. The first part of the book is devoted to a series of therapeutic pointers, alphabetically arranged by ailments. The second, and largest section, contains "lesser writings" on a wide number of subjects. The third part relates some clinical cases. 454pp. SeD nd

FERGIE-WOODS, H. *ESSENTIALS OF HOMOEOPATHIC PRESCRIBING,* 3.00. A discussion of eighty-one remedies which the author has found most generally useful in his homoeopathic practice, with their most characteristic symptoms. The second half of the book contains a "rapid repertory," indicating the most likely remedies for various symptoms. 78pp. HSP 70

FORMUR, INC. *THE LUYTIES REFERENCE HANDBOOK,* 1.25. Presents basic information on the homoeopathic combinations, a condensed materia medica, and a therapeutic index. Geared toward the layman and written in a somewhat archaic style. FoI nd

GIBSON, D.M. *ELEMENTS OF HOMEOPATHY,* 1.05. *This short text-book has been prepared primarily for the information of doctors and medical undergraduates who are interested in exploring the possibilities of homoeopathy. It is intended as an introduction to the subject and is offered as such.* The text is divided into the following chapters: basic principles, materia medica, diagnosis, remedy selection, small dose and potencies, the single remedy, and administration of the remedy. 38pp. BrH nd

GIBSON, D.M. *FIRST AID HOMEOPATHY IN ACCIDENTS AND AILMENTS,* 3.25. **A very clearly written discussion of some of the most prevalent conditions resulting from accidents and injuries. All the relevant remedies are discussed and programs of usage are outlined. This is one of the most useful homoeopathic books for the general reader and if you are interested in homoeopathic treatments we suggest you buy this book. Index, 84pp. BrH 75**

GUERNSEY, H.H. *OBSTETRICS AND DISORDERS PECULIAR TO WOMEN AND YOUNG CHILDREN,* c11.20. This is the most comprehensive work on the subject. The organization is according to ailments and conditions and there is also a great deal of background information. The book is very fully indexed and there's also a glossary. 1004pp. SeD 34

GUERNSEY, JOSEPH, ed. *KEYNOTES TO THE MATERIA MEDICA AS TAUGHT BY HENRY N. GUERNSEY,* c5.40. This book consists of a series of lectures delivered to students of the Hahnemann Medical College of Philadelphia in 1871-3. Dr. Guernsey's aim was to present enough of the outline and the leading characteristics of each remedy to help the student ascertain the proper remedy. A repertory is appended. Index, 263pp. SeD 39

GUERNSEY, W.J. *THE HOMOEOPATHIC THERAPEUTICS OF HAEMMORRHOIDS,* c3.75. A comprehensive study, including a section on comparative therapeutic indications and a chapter on external therapeutics. The bulk of the book is devoted to detailed information on the remedies and their indications. Index, 152pp. SeD 44

GUERNSEY, W.J. *MENSTRUATION*, .80. Rin

HAEHL, RICHARD. *SAMUEL HAHNEMANN—HIS LIFE AND WORK*, c12.80/set. This is the definitive study (in two volumes) of Hahnemann's life and work. There's probably more information here than most people would like to know about his personal life but also a great deal of material on how he developed his theories. Bibliography, index, 958pp. JPC 22

HAHNEMANN, SAMUEL. *THE CHRONIC DISEASES*, c16.00. Hahnemann (1755-1834) was educated as a physician and a linguist. Rejecting contemporary medicine for doing more harm than good, he translated chemical and medical works until he began to evolve the homoeopathic principles that eventually spread all over the world. He treated numerous patients, educated homoeopathic physicians, and developed an extensive set of principles. This is the most comprehensive text available. 160 pages are devoted to an exposition of the *Nature of Chronic Diseases* and the rest of the book is a detailed analysis of fifty of the major medicines, including material on how to use them and what kind of reaction to expect. The latter section also includes a listing of most of the symptoms which are treated with each preparation. Index, 1620pp. JPC 1898

HAHNEMANN, SAMUEL. *THE CHRONIC DISEASES—THEORETICAL PART*, c2.50. The theory of *chronic diseases* explicated in this volume was something that came to Hahnemann late in his career after he found that the principles he outlined in the **Organon** did not always effect a permanent cure. The approach given here to the treatment of psora, syphillis, and syeosis serves as a guideline to the treatment of all types of chronic diseases. The material presented here is considered an invaluable aid to all practitioners. 269pp. JPC 72

HAHNEMANN, SAMUEL. *THE LESSER WRITINGS*, 10.00. A reprint of all of Hahnemann's important homoeopathic articles originally published between 1789 and 1834. They clearly reveal the development of his conceptual thinking and therapeutic ex-

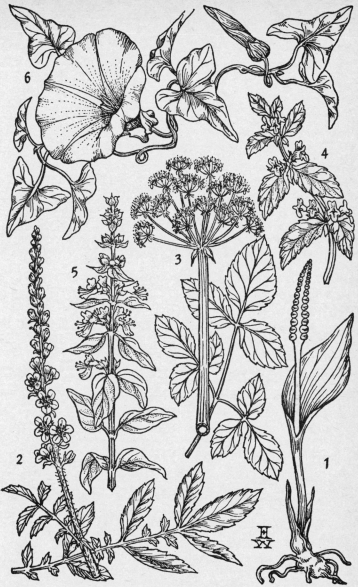

Plate 1. 1. Adder's Tongue 2. Agrimony 3. Angelica
4. Balm   5. Basil   6. Bindweed

perimentation. The articles give the student the necessary perspective on the evolution of homoeopathic principles from which a deeper understanding of Hahnemann's work will grow. We recommend that students read these articles in conjunction with their study of the *Organon*. 850pp. Hrm 77

HAHNEMANN, SAMUEL. *MATERIA MEDICA PURA,* c23.50/set. Rin

HAHNEMANN, SAMUEL. *THE ORGANON OF MEDICINE,* c2.90/4.00. Any true understanding of homoeopathy must be based on the principles set forth in the *Organon*. It presents Hahnemann's most developed philosophical insights into the practice of homoeopathic medicine and incorporates his vast experience in the treatment of both acute and chronic diseases. It is written in a highly condensed epigrammatic style, and it is hard to understand without a great deal of study. The *Organon* was printed in five editions during Hahnemann's lifetime, each one extensively revised by him. In addition, revisions for a sixth were left at his death. Two versions are available today—both incorporating these revisions: a translation by William Boericke, a noted homoeopath, which is generally known as the sixth edition is available in a cheaply made Indian hardcover (c2.90, 314pp.); and the Dudgeon translation, available in a quality, stitched American paperback (4.00, 210pp.). There is some controversy as to which is the more desirable edition. Hrm 77

HAHNEMANN, SAMUEL. *SPIRIT OF HOMEOPATHY,* .80. SeD

HAHNEMANN, SAMUEL. *THERAPEUTIC HINTS,* 1.80. SeD

HANSEN, OSCAR. *A TEXTBOOK OF MATERIA MEDICA AND THERAPEUTICS,* 3.50. This is designed as a supplement to Dr. Cowperthwaite's text. The stress is on rare homoeopathic remedies. 121pp. HeR 1899

HERING, CONSTANTINE, ed. *DR. H. GROSS' COMPARATIVE MATERIA MEDICA,* 6.40. In his introduction Dr. Gross discusses the difficulty of knowing the results of provings which the homoeopathic physician has not personally participated in. His goal in this volume is to exhibit *the differential diagnosis of such remedies as are similar in their effects.* He compares the effects of the remedies and furnishes proof that the collective effects of a remedy agree with each other. Each of the remedies is very fully surveyed. 552pp. JPC nd

HERING, CONSTANTINE. *GUIDING SYMPTOMS OF THE MA-TERIA MEDICA,* c128.00/set. This is one of the most valuable of all homoeopathic books for the practitioner and it has long been out of print. This new ten volume set is relatively low-priced and is well printed and bound. Each volume is over 500 pages. JPC 1879

HOBHOUSE, ROSA. *CHRISTIAN SAMUEL HAANNEMAN,* 1.70. A biography. 55pp. Dan 61

JAHR, G.H.G. *FAMILY PRACTICE OR SIMPLE DIRECTIONS IN HOMOEOPATHIC DOMESTIC MEDICINE,* c2.10. As the title suggests, this is a discussion of the remedies which can most usefully be applied in the home. The arrangement is alphabetical, according to symptoms and ailments. Both medicinal and accessory treatments are suggested and the discussion of each remedy includes dosage suggestions. Index, 276pp. JPC nd

JAHR, G.H.G. *THERAPEUTIC GUIDE,* c5.75. SeD

KAUFMAN, MARTIN. *HOMEOPATHY IN AMERICA: THE RISE AND FALL OF A MEDICAL HERESY,* c14.75. An academic history of the homoeopathic movement in America which focuses on the relationship between homoeopaths and the traditional medical establishment. Bibliography, notes, index, 215pp. JHU 71

KENT, J.T. *LECTURES ON HOMOEOPATHIC MATERIA MEDI-CA,* c15.30/c7.05/10.00. Kent (1848-1916), an outstanding American physician and master homoeopath, developed, clarified, and systematized the work of Hahnemann, von Boenninghausen, Hering, and others into the structure of contemporary homeotherapeutics. In this revised and edited transcription of his lectures Dr. Kent presents and discusses 180 remedies, showing how the materia medica can be evolved and used. They constitute the proper focus of study for the student, since a working knowledge of their symptomatology will be broad enough to cover almost all of the cases any practitioner will treat in his career. An indispensable volume, available in three versions: a quality Indian hardcover (c15.30), a cheaply produced Indian hardcover (c7.05), and a quality, stitched American paperback (10.00). Index, 1031pp. SeD 71

KENT, J.T. *LECTURES ON HOMOEOPATHIC PHILOSOPHY,* c4.45/c2.90/4.00. These lectures were originally delivered in the Post-Graduate School of Homoeopathy as a commentary on Hahnemann's *Organon.* Each one elucidates and develops the principles of natural healing promulgated in the *Organon.* A clear, useful work which is essential reading for all who seek a thorough understanding of homoeopathic principles. Three versions are available: a quality Indian hardcover (c4.45), a cheaply produced Indian hardcover (c2.90), and a quality, stitched American paperback (4.00). 276pp. SeD 74

KENT, J.T. *NEW REMEDIES: CLINICAL CASES, LESSER WRITINGS, APHORISMS AND PRECEPTS,* c10.00. This volume is composed of a materia medica of several new remedies, Kent's lectures, his directions on choosing medications, and a selection of his aphorisms and precepts. Index, 544pp. SeD 58

KENT, J.T. *REPERTORY OF THE HOMOEOPATHIC MATERIA MEDICA,* c28.90/c12.50. This is considered the definitive general repertory of the homoeopathic materia medica. Kent compiled it from many sources—both previous books and the experiences of practitioners. This is a reprint of the sixth American edition, edited, revised, and updated by Dr. Clara Kent, J.T. Kent's wife. The text is topically arranged by the parts of the body and within each section, further broken down into symptoms and remedies. Includes a seventy-seven page index. The more expensive edition is beautifully bound, printed on good quality paper, and thumb indexed. It is published by Sett Dey. 1516pp. JPC 74

KENT, J.T. *USE OF THE REPERTORY,* .55. Includes Kent's essay, *How to Study the Repertory* and *Repertorising* by Margaret Tyler and John Weir. 36pp. JPC nd

KENT, J.T. *WHAT THE DOCTOR NEEDS TO KNOW IN ORDER TO MAKE A SUCCESSFUL PRESCRIPTION,* .85. Index, 35pp. SeD 57

LILIENTHAL, SAMUEL. *HOMEOPATHIC THERAPEUTICS,* c16.00. This is generally considered the most complete guide to therapeutics available. It was originally published at the end of the nineteenth century and it has been revised a number of times since then. The information is arranged according to ailments. This is a reproduction of the fifth edition. Index, 1154pp. JPC 25

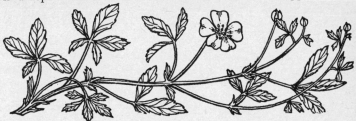

MAURY, E.A. *DRAINAGE IN HOMEOPATHY (DETOXIFICA-TION),* c3.00. *In brief,* [drainage] *is an organic cleansing process brought about by means of homoeopathic remedies indicated according to the law of similars and preparing the ground for the more effective action of constitutional remedies.* Dr. Maury's discussion is divided into the following chapters: *What is Drainage, Reasons for Drainage, How Drainage Acts,* and *How to Practice Drainage.* A materia medica of drainage remedies closes out the book. 60pp. HSP 65

MORGAN, W. *PREGNANCY,* c2.05. The full title of this small book gives as good idea of its coverage as anything we can say. It is **The Signs and Concomitant Derangements of Pregnancy, Their Pathology and Treatment to Which is Added a Chapter on Delivery; the Selection of a Nurse; and the Management of the Lying-In Chamber.** Glossary, index, 132pp. SeD 66

MUZUMDAR, K.P. *PHARMACEUTICAL SCIENCE IN HOMEO-PATHY AND PHARMACODYNAMICS,* c3.40. A detailed study for the practitioner which explains potentization and includes instructions for the preparation of a wide number of remedies. 176pp. JPC 74

NASH, E.B. *HOW TO TAKE THE CASE AND FIND THE SIMIL-LUM.* .35. 24pp. JPC nd

NASH, E.B. *LEADERS IN HOMOEOPATHIC THERAPEUTICS,* c4.10/c2.70. An in depth discussion of the leading preparations. Each entry begins with a detailed listing of the symptoms related to each preparation. This is followed by a lengthy discussion of the effects of the preparation, with citations of related preparations. All of the material comes from the author's extensive experience as a homoeopathic physician and the text is written in an informal style. Two indices, therapeutic and remedies. The more expensive edition is published by Sett Dey and is far better bound and is printed on good paper. 493pp. JPC 72

NASH, E.B. *LEADERS IN RESPIRATORY ORGANS,* c2.90. A discussion of specific respiratory conditions which includes a detailed repertory and the indications for various drugs. Nash emphasizes the importance of selecting the proper remedy for each condition and he gives a number of useful suggestions. Index, 168pp. SeD 62

NASH, E.B. *REGIONAL LEADERS,* c3.25. A summary of the most important remedies for all the areas of the body and for a variety of ailments and conditions. 148pp. SeD 50

NASH, E.B. *RESPIRATORY ORGANS,* c2.90. Rin

NASH, E.B. *SULPHUR,* c2.30. Rin

NASH, E.B. *THERAPEUTICS,* c4.55. Rin

NORTON, A.B. *ESSENTIALS OF DISEASES OF THE EYE,* c2.90. A concise discussion, including information on causes, symptoms, and treatment. Index, 325pp. SeD 04

PELIKAN, WILHELM. *THE ACTIVITY OF POTENTIZED SUBSTANCES,* 2.45. This is a very detailed statistical analysis of experiments on plant growth using certain remedies. Includes many charts and graphs and an analysis of this material. 33pp. PAV 65

PERRY, EDWARD. *LUYTIES HOMEOPATHIC PRACTICE,* 1.65. An easy to read, very popular home handbook, alphabetically arranged by ailments and suggesting both remedies and general treatment as well as giving symptoms for each ailment. This is the most accessible of all the practical books for the layman. 158pp. FoI 74

POWELL, ERIC. *THE GROUP REMEDY PRESCRIBER,* c4.70. Indicates treatment for a great variety of diseases by combinations of homoeopathic and biochemic remedies, supplemented by homoeopathic remedies in higher potency. The right potency and the correct remedy are ascertained through radionic testing. Includes some explanatory material, many examples and formulae, and a therapeutic guide. 144pp. HSP 70

PUDDEPHATT, NOEL. *PUDDEPHATT'S PRIMERS,* **3.00.** Three of Puddephatt's popular books bound into one: *First Steps to Homoeopathy, How to Find the Correct Remedy,* and *The Homoeopathic Materia Medica, How It Should Be Studied.* This is an excellent first book to read for all who are interested in becoming practicing homoeopaths. Puddephatt writes well and expresses himself clearly. 68pp. HSP 76

PUDDEPHATT, NOEL and **MARJORIE KINCAID-SMITH.** *SIGN POSTS TO THE HOMEOPATHIC REMEDIES,* 3.60. In the introduction Puddephatt writes, *The dictionary tells us that a sign post is a post supporting a sign; especially as a mark of direction at cross roads. It is at the cross roads where the student is most likely to go astray. The well proved remedies in the homoeopathic materia medica I have likened to cities and towns which may look superficially very similar to the novitiate; but to the experienced and the shrewd their essential dissimilarities are known and recognised.* Seventy-two homoeopathic remedies are written up with this in mind. An excellent book for the beginning practitioner. 132pp. HSP nd

QUAY, G.H. *DISEASES OF NOSE AND THROAT,* c2.75. The discussion is arranged according to ailments and each entry is broken down into the following sections: synonyms, etiology, symptoms, diagnosis, prognosis, and treatment. The presentation is not strictly homoeopathic. 197pp. SeD 54

ROBERTS, HERBERT. *ART OF CURE BY HOMOEOPATHY,* c10.20/c4.00. This is a well written basic text for the beginning student. It includes introductory material, chapters on vital force and vital energy, remedies and why they act, analyses of sample cases, the law of cure, the dosage and dynamic action of the drugs, and a great deal of specific material on disease classification. The more expensive edition is from Health Science Press in England, the cheaper one is from India. Needless to say, the paper, printing, and binding on the English edition are far superior to the Indian book. 286pp. HSP 42

ROBERTS, HERBERT. *SENSATIONS AS IF,* c3.80. This is the most comprehensive index available of remedies for use in individual cases. The text is divided into major parts of the body and within these divisions specific, very detailed symptoms are listed and further subdivided, with remedies for each aspect of the symptom listed. An invaluable aid for all practitioners. 519pp. JPC 37

ROSS, A.C. GORDON. *HOMEOPATHY: AN INTRODUCTORY GUIDE,* 1.30. This study begins with a survey of homoeopathy and then goes on to compare homoeopathy with allopathy. This is followed by a discussion of potency and the minimum dose and of the vital force and chronic disease. Another chapter reviews the procedure for taking the case and assessing symptoms. 64pp. TPL 76

ROYAL, GEORGE. *HANDY BOOK OF REFERENCE,* c5.75. Rin

ROYAL, GEORGE. *HOMOEOPATHIC THERAPY OF DISEASES OF THE BRAIN AND NERVES,* c3.20. A discussion of the indications for homoeopathic remedies for patients suffering from mental and nervous diseases, arranged according to specific diseases. Indices of diseases and remedies, 360pp. JPC nd

ROYAL, GEORGE. *TEXTBOOK OF HOMOEOPATHIC THEORY AND PRACTICE OF MEDICINE,* c5.15. This is a very comprehensive text for the practitioner. Dr. Royal was a Professor of Homeopathic Materia Medica and Therapeutics at the University of Iowa for thirty years and President of the American Institute of Homoeopathy. The book covers blood and infectious diseases, diseases of the bones, the muscles, the mucous and serous membranes, the heart, arteries, and veins, the brain and nervous systems, the urinary, digestive, and respiratory organs, the glands, and miscellaneous conditions. The section on each specific ailment is divided into the following parts: synonym, description, etiology, symptoms, complications and sequelae, etiology, prognosis, treatment, diet, remedies, and pathology. Separate comprehensive indices for both diseases and remedies. 688pp. JPC 23

RUDDOCK, E. HARRIS. *THE COMMON DISEASES OF CHILDREN,* c1.25. This is an abridgment of the author's manual **The Diseases of Infants and Children.** Dr. Ruddock's expectation was that this book could be used in the home and he has tried to make the contents easily comprehensible to the nonprofessional. The book is topically arranged by diseases and it begins with a section explaining many of the terms used. Each listing includes material on causes, symptoms, remedies, and accessory treatments. Index, 168pp. JPC nd

RUDDOCK, E. HARRIS. *THE POCKET MANUAL OF HOMO-EOPATHIC VETERINARY MEDICINE,* 2.00. Contains the symptoms, causes, and treatment of the diseases of horses, cattle, sheep, swine, and dogs as well as information on the general management of animals. This is a reprint of the third edition, revised and enlarged by Dr. George Lade. Index, 166pp. JPC nd

RUSHOLM, PETER, ed. *COUNTRY MEDICINES,* 1.10. A listing of over 100 ailments, with herbal and homoeopathic remedies. All the ailments are common ones and the remedies are ones that can be applied by the nonprofessional. 64pp. HSP 71

SHADMAN, ALONZO. *WHO IS YOUR DOCTOR AND WHY,* c10.00. This is the only comprehensive book on homoeopathy written for the general reader which does not employ technical terms. It includes chapters on Hahnemann, the history of homoeopathy and the reasons behind its decline in the U.S., and material on the following areas as they relate to homoeopathy: vaccination, the common cold, arthritis, food and drink, constipation, eczema, injuries and burns, the heart, cancer, smoking, having a baby. The final 200 pages are a reprint of **Pointers to the Common Remedies** by M.L. Tyler, revised by D.M. Borland, and a descriptive listing of remedies for frequent household ailments. Bibliography, 446pp. Mey 58

SHARMA, C.H. *A MANUAL OF HOMOEOPATHY AND NATURAL MEDICINE,* 2.95. *This is no ordinary book. . . .Dr. Sharma is far more than a successful homoeopathic physician. He has penetrated deeply into the medical systems of East and West. This combined with his own original research work and his vast clinical experience has given him a rare insight into the bases of health and disease that he seeks in this book to share with others. He has not written a treatise on homoeopathy for the practising physician, but rather an introduction to the fundamentals of natural healing addressed as much to the interested layman as to the specialist. It is also a work book that everyone can use.*—J.G. Bennett. Divided into two sections: *The Essentials of Homoeopathic Therapy* and *Catalogue of Remedies.* Bibliography, 154pp. Dut 75

SHEPHERD, DOROTHY. *HOMOEOPATHY FOR THE FIRST AIDER,* 2.40. Easily understandable homoeopathic remedies for pain, aches and bruising, wounds, hemmorhage, burns and scalds, poisons, boils, carbuncles, and other medical emergencies. Also includes material on potencies and an index. Dr. Shepherd writes very well; we enjoy reading her books. 72pp. HSP 45

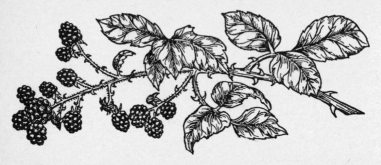

SHEPHERD, DOROTHY. *HOMEOPATHY IN EPIDEMIC DISEASES,* c5.40. This book has been edited from a series of papers written by Dr. Shepherd. It begins with a general discussion of epidemics and prophylaxis and then goes into a survey of homoeopathic remedies for a variety of epidemic diseases. Index, 100pp. HSP 67

SHEPHERD, DOROTHY. *THE MAGIC OF THE MINIMUM DOSE,* 5.40. A collection of case histories taken from Dr. Shepherd's own experience. These cases feature many disorders and diseases, including arthritis, bronchitis, the common cold, epilepsy, influenza, kidney trouble, pneumonia, rheumatism, tonsilitis, and whooping cough. She also discusses homoeopathy in dentistry, obstetrics, first-aid, veterinary medicine, and women's ailments. The book is very clearly written. Index, 214pp. HSP 64

SHEPHERD, DOROTHY. *MORE MAGIC OF THE MINIMUM DOSE,* 7.00. Additional cases from Dr. Shepherd's wide experience, topically arranged by types of ailments (i.e., skin diseases, eye infections, etc.) along the lines of her earlier book, **Magic of the Minimum Dose,** with a glossary and a comprehensive index. 286pp. HSP 74

SHEPHERD, DOROTHY. *A PHYSICIAN'S POSY,* c7.70. Homoeopathic treatments utilizing herbs in addition to the more traditional remedies. 256pp. HSP 69

SHEPPARD, K. *TREATMENT OF CATS BY HOMOEOPATHY,* 1.95. A detailed discussion, arranged according to ailment, with an additional section on general hints. 62pp. HSP 60

SHEPPARD, K. *THE TREATMENT OF DOGS BY HOMOEO-PATHY,* 3.00. Sheppard is an experienced practitioner. Here he indicates proven remedies for common ailments to which dogs are prone. The material is topically arranged by ailment. Index, 96pp. HSP 72

SMITH, DWIGHT. *HOMOEOPATHY,* .80. A general introduction by a noted homoeopath. Includes chapters on pediatrics, dentistry, childbirth, and allergies. Very clearly written. 64pp. JPC 71

STEPHENSON, JAMES. *A DOCTOR'S GUIDE TO HELPING YOURSELF WITH HOMEOPATHIC REMEDIES,* c8.95. This is the only homoeopathic text we know of which is specifically geared toward home use. Dr. Stephenson is a homoeopath with over two decades of experience and he presents his treatment suggestions and the philosophy of homoeopathy in a clear, simple manner. Many case histories are included which show the efficacy of the remedies. This is not a terribly complete or fine book, but it does give some useful household hints for those who want to learn about homoeopathic medicine. A materia medica and a symptom guide are included. 198pp. PrH 76

TYLER, M.L. *HOMOEOPATHIC DRUG PICTURES,* c20.50. Dr. Tyler is one of the most noted female homoeopathic teachers and practitioners and this is considered her finest book. She presents essential details of the leading 125 remedies for the guidance of students who wish to learn the basic characteristics. Successful prescribing depends on a knowledge of the difference—often very slight—between remedies, and it is this area that Dr. Tyler emphasizes. The text includes material from the author's own practice along with many case studies. Topically arranged by remedy. 885pp. HSP 52

TYLER, M.L. *POINTERS TO COMMON REMEDIES,* c4.35. Nine books bound in one: (1) *Colds, Influenza, Sore Throat, Coughs, Croup, Acute Chest, Asthma;* (2) *Stomach and Digestive Disorders, Constipation, Acute Diarrhoea, Acute Intestinal Condition and Colic, Epidemic Diarrhoea of Children, Acute Dysentery, Cholera;* (3) *Dentition, Rickets, Malnutrition, Tuberculosis, Diseases of Bones and Glands;* (4) *Convulsions, Chorea, Rheumatism of Children and of Adults, Common Heart Remedies;* (5) *Chicken Pox, Diphtheria, Erysipelas, Herpes Zoster, Measles and Mumps, Scarlet Fever,*

Smallpox, Typhoid, Vaccination, Whooping Cough; (6) *Some Drugs of Strong Mentality, Fears with their Dreams, Indices;* (7) *Nephritis and Suppression, Renal Calculi and Renal Colic, Cystitis, Enuresis, Retention;* (8) *Vertigo, Headache, Apoplexy, Sleeplessness, Collapse, Sun-Stroke;* and (9) *Organ Remedies.* Also available in separate pamphlets, for $1.25 each. 337pp. JPC nd

TYLER, M.L. and JOHN WEIR. *SOME OF THE OUTSTANDING HOMOEOPATHIC REMEDIES FOR ACUTE CONDITIONS, INJURIES, ETC.—WITH SPECIAL INDICATIONS FOR THEIR USE,* 2.25. In two parts, the first covering a series of conditions and ailments and the second discussing remedies and their uses. 44pp. BrH nd

VANNIER, LEON. *HOMOEOPATHY: HUMAN MEDICINE,* 2.80. This is an interesting philosophical discussion of homoeopathy by one of the foremost European homoeopaths. Dr. Vannier presents both his specific techniques and his philosophical outlook. He also discusses the human conception of medicine, the different constituents and temperaments, and various aspects of homoeopathic therapeutics. 231pp. HSP nd

VERMA, S.P. *PRACTICAL HANDBOOK OF GYNECOLOGY,* 3.10. This is an excellent illustrated account, written for both the student and the practitioner. The material is clearly presented and the coverage is comprehensive. 255pp. JPC 73

VERMA, S.P. *PRACTICAL HANDBOOK OF SURGERY,* 3.70. A comprehensive analysis including introductory material, sections on preoperative and post-operative care, and a descriptive listing arranged topically by diseases. 567pp. JPC 74

VERMA, S.P. *TEXTBOOK OF GYNECOLOGY,* c5.75. JPC

VOEGELI, ADOLPH. *HOMEOPATHIC PRESCRIBING,* 4.55. An excellent home manual for those who want to use homoeopathic remedies in the home. Dr. Voegeli discusses common illnesses such as influenza, head colds, sore throats, gastric complaints, and so on, and describes the remedies suitable for each ailment, matching them to the characteristics of different types of individuals. A listing of remedies at the end of the book introduces a comprehensive selection of treatments, with pointers for matching them to individual cases. The book is well organized and clearly written. 94pp. TPL 76

WEIR, JOHN. *THE SCIENCE AND ART OF HOMOEOPATHY*, .50. Transcription of a talk. 14pp. BrH 27

WHEELER, CHARLES. *AN INTRODUCTION TO THE PRINCIPLES AND PRACTICE OF HOMOEOPATHY*, c7.80. This is one of the newest major books on homoeopathy available, written by the past president of the British Homoeopathic Society. Topics include a discussion of the principles of homoeopathy, the structure of homeopathic materia medica, homoeopathic pharmacy, potentization, dosage, the choice and mode of administration of the remedy, a therapeutic index and repertory, and a materia medica of thirty-one leading remedies. Therapeutic index and general index, 371pp. HSP 48

WILLIAMSON, WALTER. *DISEASES OF FEMALES AND CHILDREN AND THEIR HOMOEOPATHIC TREATMENT*, c2.40. A detailed account including a description of the diseases, their symptoms, mode of administration of remedies, and the doses and repetitions according to Hahnemann's *Law of Similars*. Divided into three sections: diseases of females, treatment of children, and general diseases. Topically arranged by the ailment. Index, 256pp. JPC 74

WOODS, H. FERGIE. *HOMOEOPATHIC TREATMENT IN THE NURSERY*, 1.00. Includes some general information as well as specific sections on the ailments and the remedies. 12pp. BrH nd

YINGLING, W.A. *ACCOUCHEUR'S EMERGENCY MANUAL*, c3.40. This handbook is designed to aid physicians and especially obstetricians in bedside treatment during childbirth. It is short and to the point and is organized both topically by conditions and by remedies. 303pp. SeD 36

Life Energies

To the extent that we can comprehend the difference between a living organism and that same organism after life has departed from it, we realize that the difference lies in the presence or absence of certain energy manifestations. Take, for example, a human body five minutes before death and five minutes after death. What is the difference? Size, weight and chemical constituents are virtually the same. Yet in the living body we have many manifestations of energy.

To name a few: flow of nerve currents; contraction of muscles; circulation of the blood; generation of heat; movement of food through the alimentary system; movement of liquid through the urinary system; movement of air through the respiratory system; production of matter to repair the various cellular structures. None of these manifestations of energy are found in the dead body.

Except in cases of sudden death through accident, the transition from the living to the non-living state is simply the last step of a prolonged deterioration of the energy processes of the body. For example, as a person ages, the blood circulation diminishes, muscular contractions lessen in amplitude, until locomotion becomes more and more difficult—generation of heat lessens (old people feel colder than younger ones), production of material for cellular repairs becomes inadequate, so the organism deteriorates, and there is a corresponding diminution of every energy process in the body.

It would seem appropriate to express life in a quantitative

as well as in an absolute manner—i.e., there is in general more life in a young person than in an older person, which is another way of saying that in a young person the energy processes take place at a higher level of amplitude.

One of the most common symptoms of illness is a feeling of weakness, which is simply a lessening of energy available for muscular contraction. Ageing can be expressed as a progressive deterioration of the energy processes of a living organism, and illness can be expressed as a disturbance of the energy processes. The disturbance can be temporary, as in acute illness, or more lasting, as in chronic illness. Whether illness is the cause or the effect, of the energy disturbance, is a controversial point. . . .Death occurs with the cessation of the energy processes of the living organism.

In view of the foregoing, it is not surprising that there has been a great deal of research on therapeutic methods using various forms of energy. Human thought tends to run in cycles or epochs, and we have been undergoing an epoch in which the main emphasis in therapeutics has been placed on the chemical aspects of the human organism—hence the wide use of drugs and the prolific discoveries and synthetization of new drugs. Yet, superimposed on what might be termed the chemical epoch, we can see at least the start of an energy one.

The concepts of scientific research as developed by the Western world in recent centuries, with the emphasis on established principles and the efforts to fit newly observed facts into those principles insofar as possible, has had the effect of encouraging the study and use of certain types of energy—namely, those with widespread uses in material or non-organic science, such as heat, steam, shortwave, etc. and has had the effect of discouraging the study and use of other types of energy. Physics has dealt mainly with non-organic uses of energy, and has attempted to explain organic application of energies in the light of the principles of non-organic uses of energy. It is our view that this has led to many misconceptions and blind spots in the study of the energy aspects of human and animal organisms.

It is becoming apparent, from research in various fields, that the characteristics of the living organism embrace more types of energy than has previously been realized, and include some energy types that have not entered into the field of non-organic science. Also, it is found that there are ways of applying conventional energies (i.e., energies widely used in non-organic sciences) to living organisms to produce effects that are not known in the non-organic or strictly material field.

It is a truism that the unconventional discoveries of today often become the accepted or conventional principles of tomorrow. However, this is not an automatic process. If discoveries of new and valuable facts are to be incorporated into the accepted scheme of things, they must be met with an open mind and adequate attention or consideration. Unfortunately these conditions frequently are lacking.

There are many causes for this lack. Among these causes we may mention: economic restrictions; psychological inertia; vested interests; institutional politics; and the general concepts of current scientific research previously mentioned.

These facts tend to favour the development and use of certain types of discoveries and to ignore or suppress the development and use of other types of discoveries. In the search for means to combat illness an to prolong the useful and satisfactory portion of life, we can learn much from a deeper research into the energy complex which is an integral part of the living human body.

—from **New Light on Therapeutic Energies** by Mark L. Gallert

ABRAMS, ALBERT. *NEW CONCEPTS IN DIAGNOSIS AND TREATMENT,* 12.00. A detailed study of the practical applications of Dr. Abrams' electronic theory in the interpretation and treatment of disease. This is an invaluable work for all those who are interested in radiesthesia and in the potentials of energy for healing and health. Many specific ailments are covered. Almost one hundred illustrations, notes, spiral bound, 431pp. HeR 22

ARCHDALE, F.A. *ELEMENTARY RADIESTHESIA AND THE USE OF THE PENDULUM,* 3.00. A short treatise by a practicing radiesthesist discussing the medical and geological possibilities of radiesthesia and offering suggestions on practical experiments. Stapled, 8½"x11", 33pp. HeR 50

ASKEW, STELLA. *HOW TO USE THE PENDULUM,* 3.00. This is a clear instruction manual, including a great deal of background material, explaining the process of dowsing, and giving various examples and illustrations. Stapled, 8½"x11", 38pp. HeR 55

BARRETT, WILLIAM and **THEODORE BESTERMAN.** *THE DIVINING ROD,* c10.00. Sir William Barrett was a physicist and chemist and Theodore Besterman served for many years as Investigations Officer of the Society for Psychical Research, London. This is a recent reprint of the first major experimental and psychological study of dowsing. The authors made a thorough study of contemporary dowsers under closely controlled conditions. One of their most notable contributions is to show that the two main theories about dowsing—a straight physical explanation and a psychical one—can be fused into a unified theory solidly grounded in scientific procedure. Leslie Shepard's foreword to this edition reviews the recent literature on the subject. Extensive bibliography, notes, index, 361pp. UnB 68

BEARNE, ALASTAIR. *ENERGY, MATTER AND FORM,* 10.00. An overview of the whole area of paranormal phenomena and perception, especially as it interfaces with the life forces and energies of the universe. The first section discusses the use of energies and vibrations by psychics, and the second surveys more directly energies and vibrations and their effects. Many graphic examples are incorporated into Bearne's exposition. The final section (about half the book) is devoted to detailed instructions on using the techniques introduced earlier. The book is self published and is not laid out very clearly. There's a great deal of good material, but the presentation is often hard to follow. Illustrations, bibliography, 8"x11", 143pp. UTP 76

BEASLEY, VICTOR. *DIMENSIONS OF ELECTRO-VIBRATORY PHENOMENA,* 10.00. *The accounts presented in this volume are concerned with the possible influence which certain radiational or "electro-vibratory" forces might exert upon human behavior. The term "electro-vibratory" is meant to have a generic application. We might have substituted in its place, the standard term, "electromagnetism," but electromagnetism, as understood by science, refers only to a definite spectrum of what is probably an infinite range of vibrations occurring in nature.*—from the preface. This is a fine work, which, while it reads like a PhD dissertation (which it is), clearly summarizes a great body of information. A scientific account, illustrated with many excellent charts and drawings. Bibliography, notes, 8½"x11", 106pp. UTP 75

BEASSE, PIERRE, et al. *A NEW AND RATIONAL TREATISE OF DOWSING,* 5.00. This is a practical textbook which explains all aspects of dowsing and details how to dowse for a variety of things including subterranean springs, buried treasures, coal fields, ores, oil, and much else. Line drawings throughout illustrate the instructions. The second half of the book surveys medical dowsing and astro dowsing and again gives clear practical techniques. Many case studies are also cited and examined. A very complete work. Spiral bound, 214pp. HeR 41

BENDIT, LAWRENCE and PHOEBE. *THE ETHERIC BODY OF MAN,* 2.75. A clairvoyant and a psychiatrist study the health aura and the vital etheric body of man. There's some interesting material here, but it's not presented in a manner that draws us. It's a hard book to pinpoint; the Bendits discuss consciousness, the process of incarnation, the stages of growth from infancy to manhood, death, and health and disease. They do not delve deeply into any area. Originally entitled **Man Incarnate**. 127pp. TPH 57

BLAIR, LAWRENCE. *RHYTHMS OF VISION,* 5.25. This is an important new book which falls outside a restricted category and encompasses many disciplines. Dr. Blair is basically discussing energies in all forms of life and the correspondences between man and the natural world. He analyzes many of the phenomena generally classified under the rubric of the occult and shows how similar the ancient teachings are to the discoveries of scientists over the ages. Perhaps the most illuminating section of the book is Blair's extensive discussion of number and form, most of which is based on Rudolf Steiner and his disciples. There are also many beautiful illustrations. While Blair has done a fine job of researching and compiling a great deal of material, his presentation is scattered and not nearly as clearly written as we would like. 244pp. ScB 76

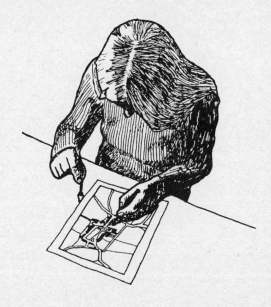

BORDERLAND SCIENCES. *THE LAKHOVSKY MULTI-WAVE OSCILLATOR,* 3.55. A detailed study of the material related to the MWO, with diagrammatic instructions. Also includes summary studies of Mark Clement's *The Waves That Heal* (a review of Lakhovsky's work), John O'Neill's *Nikola Tesla's Giant Oscillator,* and Lakhovsky's *Curing Cancerous Plants With Ultra Radio Frequencies.* Stapled, 8½"x11", 42pp. BSR nd

BOYLE, JOHN. *THE PSIONIC GENERATOR PATTERN BOOK,* 5.95. Plans and diagrams for constructing a dozen psi-activating devices, including a pyramid, an "occult illuminator" that you can use like a crystal ball, a cone cluster generator that rotates with the energy from your body, dowsing rods, various other kinds of generators, aurameters, and much else. 8½"x11", 89pp. PrH 75

BROWN, JOHN. *I DISCOVER THE IMMORTAL B-CELL,* 2.00.
This is a recent reprint of Brown's pioneering study in which he
describes the finding and development of a new form of cell life—
a catalyst that releases radiant energy to all living things which can
absorb it through water. This edition includes many illustrations
and additional material by Hilary Dorey, Joe Sloan, Riley Crabb,
Henry Gallart, and Thomas David. Stapled, 8½"x11", 42pp. BSR 73

BURR, HAROLD SAXTON. *BLUEPRINT FOR IMMORTALITY,*
c5.60. A comprehensive account of Dr. Burr's discovery that all
living things are molded and controlled by electrodynamic fields
which can be measured and mapped with standard modern volt-
meters. *These fields of life, or L-fields, are the basic blueprints of
all life on this planet. . . .The Universe is an ordered system, the
human organism an ordered component. In short, the universe has
meaning and so have we.* Thousands of experiments by Dr. Burr
and his colleagues over a period of nearly forty years have confirmed that L-fields exist in all forms of life. Dr. Burr was a member of the faculty of Yale Medical School for forty-three years.
192pp. Spe 72

CAMERON, VERNE. *AQUAVIDEO,* 6.95. Subtitled *Locating
Underground Water through the Sensory-Eye of Verne Cameron,*
this is an in depth, fully illustrated study of just that. Cameron is
considered a master dowser and has been recognized and acclaimed
by many authorities as the most highly developed American dowser
ever. The book is not very well organized and the writing style is
overly adulatory; nevertheless there's a great deal of information,
including introductory and biographical material, and chapters on
locating underground water, determining water volume, reading the
geological signs, quakes and earth movement, locating geysers and
hot springs. There's also material on the phenomenon of dowsing
and Cameron's analysis of it as well as a study of dowsing devices.
Index, 158pp. ECa 70

CAMERON, VERNE. *MAP DOWSING,* 2.75. *Map dowsing is a term
applied to the locating of persons, animals, objects, and substances
from a distance, either above, in, or below, ground or water, by
means of a pointer, map, chart, photo, and dowsing instrument.*
This is a detailed, explanatory pamphlet, including illustrations and
background material. 40pp. ECa 71

CAMERON, VERNE. *OIL LOCATING,* 2.75. In the early 1950's Cameron perfected the Cameron *Aurameter* (a water-compass device), followed by his gyrating *Petroleometer.* He has located many high producing underground oil and water sites and is acclaimed for his subsurface oil and water theories. Here he relates his experiences and presents his theories on how to do it. Illustrations, 39pp. ECa 71

CAVE, FRANCIS, ed. *THE ELECTRONIC REACTIONS OF ABRAMS,* 4.00. Dr. Abrams did pioneering work in the early twentieth century in the field of radionics. *Abrams. . .takes the stand that all material things are radioactive and that if sufficiently delicate apparatus can be devised, the degree of radioactivity of all matter can be measured in such a way that when its radioactive characteristics are ascertained, it would be possible from this data to determine the actual substance being examined, without even seeing it.* –from the foreword. Abrams developed the instruments and the conceptual framework from which all the subsequent research has stemmed. Half this book is devoted to Dr. Cave's foreword and the other half is a reprint of Abrams' original paper. It includes many detailed examples and instructive material. Illustrations, stapled, 8½"x11", 36pp. HeR 22

CHRAPOWICKI, MARYLA DE. *SPECTRO-BIOLOGY,* 2.00. *Spectro-Biology is a system of cosmic correspondence, dealing with the fundamental principles of the bio-chemical relationship which binds human physiology to the whole of Nature and which offers a complete synthesis of all branches of science in their mutual relation to Life. . . .The object of this book is. . .to offer a method whereby we can calculate. . .what the normal biological factor of each individual body should be. . . .To show that health is a purely biological state and a direct result of radiation, while disease is but a relative condition. . . .To prove that there is a changeless and universal method of diagnosis whereby we can not only determine the cause of disease, but which enables us to preserve a normal state of health. . . .* –from the foreword. Stapled, 62pp. HeR 65

COOPER-HUNT, C.L. *RADIESTHETIC ANALYSIS,* 3.00. A practical handbook by a radionic practitioner covering the following topics: polarity, colors, resonant key notes, extra sensory perception, diagnosis, the etheric body, unconscious disturbing energies, and "dis-ease." Stapled, 40pp. HeR 69

CRABB, RILEY, ed. *RADIONICS,* 6.50. Crabb is the director of

281

Borderland Sciences Research Foundation. Here he gives us a detailed scientific study in three parts. Part I covers the history and development of radionics, with sections on the doctors and the equipment, techniques of diagnosis, colored light and disease, and amplification for treatment. Part II, *Radionics Instruments and How to Make Them,* includes a modified drown circuit, a diagnostic instrument diagram, and an atlas of diagnostic and treatment rates. Part III is an interview with Dr. Leonard Chapman, a radionics practitioner. Stapled, 8½"x11", 77pp. BSR nd

CRABB, RILEY. *THREE GREAT AQUARIAN AGE HEALERS,* 2.00. Crabb begins with a discussion of the work of William Lang, a surgeon who died in 1938, but who carries on his practice through the medium George Chapman at Arlesbury clinic in England. Lang (through Chapman) explains how a spirit doctor works. In the second section Crabb analyzes *New Age Color Therapy* developed by Drs. S. Pancoast and George Starr White, and explains the basic Qabalistic principles on which all successful color therapy must be established—balance and rhythm. Many illustrations and technical drawings, including the construction of a simple, duo-rhythm color machine along the lines developed by Dr. White. Stapled, 8½"x11", 62pp. BSR 68

DAKIN, H.S. *HIGH-VOLTAGE PHOTOGRAPHY,* 4.95. *High voltage photography, known also by other names including Kirlian photography, electrography, and corona-discharge photography, is a technique for making photographic prints or visual observations of electrically-conductive objects with no light source other than that produced by a luminous corona-discharge at the surface of an object in a high-voltage, high-frequency electric field.* This is the most comprehensive manual we know of, intended as a practical guide for experimenters, as well as for nonspecialists who may skip over the technical material (of which there is an abundance). Construction methods and instruction techniques are very complete in both written and diagrammatic form. Notes, 8½"x11", 65pp. HSD 76

DAVIS, ALBERT and WALTER RAWLS. *THE MAGNETIC EFFECT,* c6.00. The authors discuss biomagnetic experiments and research that has been successfully duplicated by members of the orthodox scientific community. The findings which they discuss can be applied to the treatment of such conditions as arthritis, cancer, glaucoma, sexual problems, and aging. Notes, 128pp. ExP 75

DAVIS, ALBERT and WALTER RAWLS. *MAGNETISM AND ITS EFFECTS ON THE LIVING SYSTEM,* c8.00. This is a well researched investigation into the discovery that a magnet has not one effect on the living system but two effects, each supplied by one of the two forms of energy that are transmitted from each pole of any magnet, including the earth, which itself is a giant magnet. The authors feel that this discovery (which they term biomagnetics) can alter the genetics of plants, animals, and all forms of life. Here they present the fruit of their years of intensive research, illustrated with many case studies and diagrams. Chapters include *Understanding Magnetism, The Effects of the Two Poles on the Living System, Cancers and Tumors and Magnetism, The Bioelectric Control of Nerve Pain, Magnetism and Gravity,* and *The Human Biomagnetic Aura.* Notes, 139pp. ExP 74

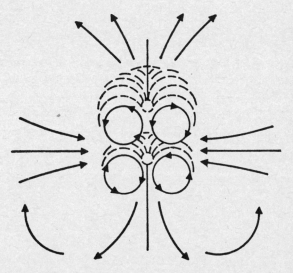

DAVIS, ALBERT and WALTER RAWLS. *THE RAINBOW IN YOUR HANDS,* c5.95. *By your very thoughts you can offer help, good will and happiness to all around you. You can live a better life. All you have to do is have an understanding about your natural energy and direct your hands toward building a more natural world. We will explain the presence and use of this energy. You will be the judge concerning its effectiveness. . . . The great healers and comforters of history used this natural healing power.*—from the introduction. 101pp. ExP 76

DAY, LANGSTON and **GEORGE DE LA WARR.** *MATTER IN THE MAKING,* c10.00. Day here describes the course of research and discovery at the Delawarr Laboratories in England during the 1955-65 period. In a previous work, *New Worlds Beyond the Atom,* the author explained that Mr. de la Warr and his staff had discovered new forms of radiation, hitherto unknown to science, which shed light on some of the enigmas of physics and biology, such as the origin of shapes and forms in nature, the means whereby vital energy passes to living things, and the mystery of the creation of matter out of an apparent void. The researchers found that we must work with nature, not against her, to discover in what forms the unifying force appears when it descends to the level of matter. The Delawarr Laboratories have been the center for all recent radionic research and this book, written for the general public, enables us to see how the discoveries can affect our daily lives. Includes chapters on the radionic box and how it works on music and color, and on thought, light, and sound. There are also many case studies and photographs and diagrams are interspersed throughout. A well written account. 161pp. Wat 66

DAY, LANGSTON and **GEORGE DE LA WARR.** *NEW WORLDS BEYOND THE ATOM,* c7.50. The new worlds beyond the atom are found in a universe of energies more primordial than those of matter and are still unexplored by mainstream science. George de la Warr's research with these energies began with increasing the growth rate of plants by using sound waves. Later he found that a plant's vibrations could be detected by a machine with aerials made to the right wavelengths, using a person as the receiver. Carrying the idea further, he learned that he could detect and treat human diseases using the same type of machine, due to the different vibrational rates of different illnesses. By tuning the frequency of a patient's blood specimen he was even able to photograph diseased tissue over long distances, showing an immediate connection between life forms beyond the vibration rate of ordinary matter. Photographs, 136pp. DAC 73

EBON, MARTIN, ed. *MYSTERIOUS PYRAMID POWER,* 1.50. A collection of essays from a wide variety of sources, mostly written in a popular vein. Bibliography, 170pp. NAL 76

EDEN, JEROME. *VIEW FROM EDEN: TALKS TO STUDENTS OF ORGONOMY,* c8.00. Eden's newest effort. The content is much the same as his other books and the material has been compiled from a number of talks. Bibliography, 208pp. ExP 76

EEMAN, L.E. *COOPERATIVE HEALING,* 1.50. Eeman, over forty years ago, demonstrated that vitality (or human ectoplasm) flows like electricity. He showed that unhealthy spiritual, mental, emotional and physical states can be brought into a healthy, balanced state by hooking up the positive and negative areas with copper screens and wires. Excerpts from Eeman's book **Cooperative Healing** (long out of print) are included here along with the results of research and testing being carried out by the Borderland Sciences researchers. Illustrations, stapled, 8½"x11", 20pp. BSR nd

ELLIOT, J. SCOTT. *DOWSING: ONE MAN'S WAY,* c9.30. Major General Scott Elliot is past president of the British Society of Dowsers, and this book is the result of twenty years of experience. He writes for both the expert dowser and the novice and he is interested in showing the wide potential of dowsing. Part I describes what can be done by dowsing, who can do it, what the tools are, and how they can be used. Part II is devoted to special applications such as archaeology, and the location of oil, water, minerals, lost objects, etc. Part III offers a number of examples of how dowsing has been used and suggests a number of potential uses. Many photographs and illustrations accompany the text. 159pp. Spe 77

FINCH, W.J. *THE PENDULUM AND POSSESSION,* 4.00. Finch is a healer who has had years of experience in the use of the pendulum. This practical instruction manual clearly covers the following areas: what a pendulum is, history of the pendulum, what makes a pendulum work, everyday uses for a pendulum, how to use a pendulum, measuring people, interpretations from irregular pendulum movements, recording your data, and making comparative measurements. The last part of the book is devoted to a section on possession. 116pp. EsP 71

FLANAGAN, G. PATRICK. *BEYOND PYRAMID POWER,* 3.95. This is a discussion of tensor fields, Flanagan's new name for the energies and forces which he discussed in previous books and referred to as pyramid power. Here he relates the results of his four years of research since his initial pyramid publications. He feels that he has made great strides and also believes that his earlier theses are no longer valid. In addition to a general discussion, Flanagan graphically details the construction of instruments which measure the tensor fields, including pyramids, spirals, and cones, and explains how and why they capture this energy. 67pp. DeV 75

FLANAGAN, G. PATRICK. *THE PYRAMID AND ITS RELATION TO BIOCOSMIC ENERGY,* 3.00. A pamphlet detailing some of Flanagan's early studies and including a cardboard pyramid. 8½"x11". LEP nd

FLANAGAN, G. PATRICK. *PYRAMID POWER,* c6.95. Flanagan is one of the best known people doing practical research on the pyramid. He discusses the most important aspects of his work in this volume and includes information on the history of pyramid energy studies and other studies of energy in recent years. The major portion of the book is devoted to pyramid research projects and measuring devices. He includes detailed instructions. Illustrations, notes, index, 173pp. LEP 75

GALLERT, MARK, ed. *NEW LIGHT ON THERAPEUTIC ENERGY,* c6.65. A detailed, advanced work which presents the wisdom and experience of many pioneers in the healing arts. Theory, equipment and instructions for practical use are all included for most of the methods presented. Includes illustrated essays by George Starr White, Wilhelm Reich, George Lakhovsky, L. E. Eeman, William Schussler, and many others. Recommended for the serious student. 256pp. Cla 66

GEORGE, KARL. *DOWSING,* 4.95. George was a dowser who felt that he has made some important advances in dowsing which he would like to pass on to others. This book consists of an autobiography and a general history of dowsing as well as a detailed description of 189 of his own dowsing cases, each one briefly evaluated. The cases are topically arranged. 140pp. Geo 74

GEORGE, KARL. *DOWSONOLOGY,* 3.30. Dowsonology is George's special healing technique. He achieves healing by positively charging dowsing rods with the positive ion structure of a healthy person. When the positively charged rods are used to treat an unhealthy person the person's ion structure is changed and his or her ailments are relieved. Practical instructions are included—although George's writing style leaves much to be desired. Stapled, 20pp. Geo 74

GEORGE, KARL. *ION SCENT,* 3.30. Presents additional research on the effects of ion on dowsing rods. Stapled, 30pp. Geo 74

GOODAVAGE, JOSEPH. *MAGIC: SCIENCE OF THE FUTURE,* 1.50. A scattered collection of information on all aspects of energy. Many case studies are included and virtually every conceivable topic is covered. Goodavage writes well and, while he often seems to be appealing to the mass market mind, a great deal of interesting phenomena is examined. And the material itself is more serious than the title of the book would have you think. Bibliography, 196pp. NAL 76

GRAVES, TOM. *THE DIVINER'S HANDBOOK,* **1.95. This is far and away the most comprehensive, practical manual on dowsing we have ever seen. Line drawings and step-by-step instructions cover every aspect of the practice. Graves outlines a variety of exercises and gives complete instructions for making all the dowsing implements. Problems that might occur are also discussed. The material is well organized and clearly written. Annotated bibliography and sources for equipment, 160pp. War 76**

HILLS, CHRISTOPHER. *NUCLEAR EVOLUTION,* 4.00. This is a strange book which contains some interesting philosophical insights. It is subtitled *A Guide to Cosmic Enlightenment* and it contains Hills' thoughts about the consciousness which will be necessary to bring in the new age. A discussion of colors and consciousness is also included. Hills' exposition is often hard to follow. Notes, 152pp. UTP 68

HILLS, CHRISTOPHER. *RAYS FROM THE CAPSTONE,* 4.95. A discussion of the *Pi-Ray Coffer which incorporates a skilful combination of pyramid energies and biomagnetics.* Construction details and suggested experiments are included along with a great deal of both extraneous and related information on energy. Illustrated throughout and, like Hills' other books, badly lacking organization and editing. 8½"x11", 155pp. UTP 76

HILLS, CHRISTOPHER. *SUPERSENSONIC INSTRUMENTS OF KNOWING,* 1.95. A catalog of "supersensonic instruments" sold by Hills' University of the Trees. Lengthy descriptions are given of each instrument. Propaganda about Hills' theories is also included. 127pp. UTP 75

HILLS, CHRISTOPHER. *SUPERSENSONICS,* 15.00. Hills defines supersensonics as the spiritual physics of all vibrations from zero to infinity. This is an incredibly detailed—albeit scattered—account of every aspect of the subject. It is oriented toward the specialist and we recommend this book only to those who are deeply interested in this area and who have a working knowledge of physics. **Supersensonics** is divided into the following general topics: the science of radiational physics, light, and supersensonic detectors. Many illustrations illuminate the text. 8½"x11", 603pp. UTP 76

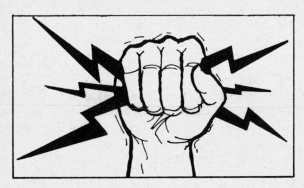

HOFFMAN, ENID. *HUNA: A BEGINNER'S GUIDE,* 3.00. Centuries ago the Kahunas (the ancient Hawaiian priests) discovered and worked with the fundamental pattern of energy flow in the universe. Max Freedom Long did pioneering work in the study of the Kahunas and in modern day applications of their theories. In this book Ms. Hoffman builds on the work of Long and others and explains the practical benefits of working with the ancient Kahuna magic. The book is written in a how to style, is packed with suggestions and exercises, and there's also a fair amount of theoretical material. Index, 118pp. PaR 76

KERRELL, BILL and KATHY GOGGIN. *THE GUIDE TO PYRAMID ENERGY,* 3.95. This is one of the most popular of the recent books on pyramid energy and it is also considered one of the best. The authors have spent many years researching the subject and, while their bias is obvious, they present their results with a fair amount of objectivity. The book begins with a general examination of pyramid energy, including directions on how to prove it and use it. The second section discusses a variety of specific topics including dowsing energies and pyramids, gems, stones and minerals, psychic healing, and the Great Pyramid. Illustrations, bibliography, 172pp. PPV 75

KING, SERGE. *PYRAMID ENERGY HANDBOOK,* 1.95. A simple survey, topically organized and written in the form of questions and answers. Annotated bibliography, 192pp. War 77

KORTH, LESLIE. *HEALING MAGNETISM.* 1.25. A general study by a British osteopath with chapters on magnetism, contact therapy and hypnotherapy, healing magnetism in practice, magnetopathic technique, examples of hand emanations, breathing, and the odic force. Bibliography, 64pp. Wei 65

KRIPPNER, STANLEY and DANIEL RUBIN, eds. *THE ENERGIES OF CONSCIOUSNESS,* c12.95. A collection of papers from the Second Western Hemisphere Conference on Kirlian Photography, Acupuncture, and the Human Aura. Includes information on the latest findings in electrophotography, as well as some of the first American research in acupuncture and auras. The papers are all fairly technical and are extensively illustrated. Notes, 252pp. G&B 75

KRIPPNER, STANLEY and DANIEL RUBIN, eds. *THE KIRLIAN AURA,* 3.95. See the Color and Aura section.

LAKHOVSKY, GEORGES. *THE SECRET OF LIFE,* 5.00. An important work on the subject of electricity and radiation in man and in the universe. The author shows that the fundamentals of electricity can be seen in the basic functions of the human body. All living entities and even the cells of which they are comprised are rapidly pulsing electrical oscillators that project streams of radiating energy throughout their environment. The quality of the radiations differs with the nature of their source. The fascinating subject of cosmic stellar radiations is discsssed as is its possible consequences for humanity. Spiral bound, 213pp. HeR 35

LANE, EARL, ed. *ELECTROPHOTOGRAPHY,* 4.95. See the Color and Aura section.

LAYNE, MEADE. *THE CAMERON AURAMETER,* 4.70. This study details the contributions of Verne Cameron to the science of dowsing for water and it describes the performance of the instrument invented by him, the aurameter (or water compass). Chapters include an introduction by Layne, Cameron's own story, delineation of the human aura, the aurameter and "vitic" (nerve energy derived from magnetic and carbon), psychic investigations, Eeman circuits, and locating underground water. Many illustrations and detailed instructions. Stapled, 8½"x11", 89pp. BSR 70

LEFTWICH, ROBERT. *DOWSING,* 1.30. This small book explains the history and present day application of dowsing and also discusses how to recognize and develop dowsing ability. In addition, Leftwich surveys the relative merits of various instruments. There are also chapters on radiesthesia and on map dowsing. 64pp. TPL 76

LONG, MAX FREEDOM. *MANA,* 2.25. This is the complete text of lessons which Max Freedom Long sent to members of the Huna Research Association for the experimental use of Huna in the early days of his research. Mana was Long's name for the vital force in humans which he discovered during his research with the Kahunas in Hawaii. Stapled, 20pp. HRA 72

MASSY, ROBERT. *ALIVE TO THE UNIVERSE,* 7.50. Massy has a degree in physics from the University of London. He studied with Christopher Hills for a number of years and has devoted over three years to putting together the material presented in this book. His goal is to simplify and modify the language of physics. The book is subtitled *A practical step-by-step guide to becoming Supersensitive Man by the techniques of Supersensonics* and it is profusely illustrated throughout. Layout skill and organization are definitely lacking in the book and it is often hard to follow Massy's discussion because of this. Nonetheless, many interesting ideas are introduced and the discussion is generally nontechnical. 8½"x11", 185pp. UTP 76

MASSY, ROBERT. *HILLS' THEORY OF CONSCIOUSNESS,* 5.95. Hills has renamed his theory of "Nuclear Evolution" the "Hills' Theory of Consciousness," and in this volume one of his leading students—who also happens to be a physicist—explores and elucidates the theory and gears his discussion toward the nonspecialist. As is usual with the books produced by Hills' group, the information is scattered throughout a badly laid out book and the illustrations are not very artistic. Our aesthetic sense is put off by the book. Nonetheless, it does contain a great deal of interesting information—all of which is oriented toward practical application. 8½"x11", 138pp. UTP 76

MEEK, GEORGE. *FROM ENIGMA TO SCIENCE,* c6.95. This is a scattered study of various facets of the paranormal, emphasizing the use of body energies. Meek has quoted and cited the studies of many of the most noted researchers in this field. Appendices list the major related organizations in the U.S. and Great Britain, publications, and an extensive subject indexed bibliography—all with full addresses. Illustrations, including color Kirlian photographs, index, 199pp. Wei 73

MERMET, ABBE. *PRINCIPLES AND PRACTICE OF RADIES-THESIA,* **7.40. This is far and away the best book on radiesthesia ever written. Abbe Mermet was both a researcher and a practitioner and he expresses his theories and techniques with extraordinary clarity. We recommend this book to all who are interested in radiesthesia. Notes, index, 230pp. Wat 35**

Franz Mesmer

Mesmer (1734-1815), the architect of modern hypnotism, is one of the most controversial and fascinating figures in medical and scientific history. He has been considered both a quack and a charlatan, and also the father of psychotherapy. Early in his study of medicine Mesmer suggested that the sun, moon, and planets might have a direct influence on human bodies by way of a subtle fluid— and that when this force (a kind of universal energy) exerts itself, the fluid expands and contracts the nervous system. Although this theory received little attention at the time, it was the forerunner of his theory of animal magnetism through which he achieved remarkable cures of functional disorders. Mesmer's experiments today remain an inspiration to all the researchers in the field of life energies.

BURANELLI, VINCENT. *THE WIZARD FROM VIENNA,* c8.95. This is a fine biographical study of Mesmer which emphasizes his psychiatric contributions. It is vividly written and both the times and the main characters come to life. Many quotations from critics of Mesmer and from Mesmer's defenses and theories are included. Annotated bibliography, 256pp. CMG 75

EDEN, JEROME. *ANIMAL MAGNETISM AND THE LIFE ENERGY,* c8.50. Over 200 years ago Dr. Franz Anton Mesmer announced his controversial discovery for treating disease which he called "Animal Magnetism"—the word "animal" in this case meaning "pertaining to the soul." Eden reviews Mesmer's discoveries and includes a great deal of material from Mesmer's own writings on his principles, methods, and some case histories. Notes, index, 221pp. ExP 74

WYCKOFF, JAMES. *FRANZ ANTON MESMER,* c8.95. This biographical study of Mesmer emphasizes his medical researches. Wyckoff has also written a biography of Wilhelm Reich and a Reichian perspective is apparent in this work. Wyckoff writes very well and his study is especially valuable for the light that it sheds on Mesmer's esoteric influences. 152pp. PrH 75

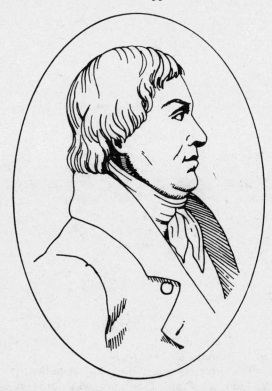

MILNER, DENNIS and EDWARD SMART. *THE LOOM OF CRE-ATION,* c14.95. Milner and Smart believe that they have discovered experimental evidence for the forces of creation described by mystics. They have spent over ten years painstakingly researching their thesis and they have drawn on a wide spectrum of data. In advancing their thesis they begin with a review of the nature of man and his development in earlier cultures. This is followed by a survey of *the experiences and viewpoint of Expanded Awareness* in which they discuss the human experience and the processes of creation and evolution. A third section details their experiments with etheric forces and a fourth is an extensive annotated bibliography. The presentation is highly esoteric and is largely based on the philosophical speculations of Rudolf Steiner and Guenther Wachsmith. A great deal of fascinating material is advanced but the book is written and organized in such a way that the authors' concepts elude the reader no matter how carefully s/he studies the material. This is another recent work which has potential, but which very often lacks clarity. Profusely illustrated in color and black and white. Index, 7½"x10", 319pp. H&R 76

NIELSEN, GREG and JOSEPH POLANSKY. *PENDULUM POWER,* 1.95. A general examination of the use of the pendulum in healing. The book is well organized and clearly written and covers a great deal of material not generally found in books of this genre. Bibliography, 190pp. War 77

OTT, JOHN. *HEALTH AND LIGHT,* 1.95. Subtitled *The Effects of Natural and Artificial Light on Man and Other Living Things.* Ott, head of the Environmental Health and Light Research Institute in Florida, is the leading researcher in this area. Here he presents some of his studies and many case histories to show the subtle effects the new light technology is having upon our physical and mental well being. Illustrations, bibliography, notes, index, 208pp. S&S 73

PARCELLS, HAZEL. *PENDULUM,* 14.50. Ms. Parcells is a noted radiesthesic practitioner and teacher. She developed and designed this pendulum. It is made of silver and stainless steel and is extremely sensitive. Many consider it the finest pendulum available. ShM

PYRAMID ENERGY GENERATOR/PYRAMID ENERGY PLATE COMBINATION. This set is based on Pat Flanagan's designs. The

Pyramid Energy Generator is designed so that energy flows from the peak of each pyramid on the generator. There's also a built in magnetic field which eliminates the necessity of aligning the pyramids along a north-south axis. The **Plate** works like a battery. It's made of anodized aluminum which soaks up the energy given off by the generator. Available in three sizes: 3"x5" generator and plate, $7.50; 4"x5" generator and plate, $10.95; 4"x5" generator and 8"x10" plate, $13.95. **LEP**

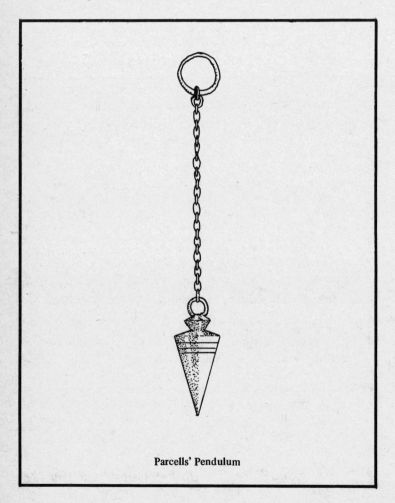

Parcells' Pendulum

Wilhelm Reich

Wilhelm Reich is a controversial figure because of the breadth and the scope of his ideas and their impact on our times. His philosophy swung the pendulum from the mechanism of the scientific approach to the functional identity of man with nature and the cosmos. . . .[His] work brings the human being back to his physical nature, and the importance it has for his life and his development. In our era, wherein scientific knowledge reigns supreme and the functions of man are further split by the exact and detailed knowledge of science and the complexity of the environment, Reich's work reverses the process of splitting and brings man back to the unity of his nature. Humanity resists this because each one of us desperately attempts to run away from the pain of the actual experience through our emotions and body. We are afraid to perceive our negativities, for fear of losing control over them, and we drive them into our unconscious, thus acting them out indirectly and in a destructive way, and by intellectualizing the basics of life. Reich recognized that the negative aspects of man as expressed in the distortion of the body and mind (his concept of character structure) prevent him from experiencing the flow of life within and outside himself, thus arresting his development. . . .

Reich came to these concepts from his extensive work in psychoanalysis, where he observed that at the beginning of therapy, there is no positive relationship with the doctor, even if the patient behaves in a positive way. That is due, he postulated, to the patient's tendency to avoid the perception of painful experiences. The patient accomplishes this by unconsciously developing physical and emotional blocks to arrest the feeling. . . .Reich postulated that the blocks to feeling developed early in life so as to avoid punishment or rejection of the child by his parents, and are actually muscular rigidities that regulate the flow of the feelings. He noticed that there is a relationship be-

295

tween the ability to flow emotionally and physically and the discharge of feeling during sex. People who are bound with blocks are unable to discharge fully, that is, to have a total orgasm, even though at times they achieve a partial release. These concepts led to the theory of the orgasm and its relationship to illness and health. . . .

At first Reich believed that this energy, *orgone,* was specific to living organisms, but later he defined it as a universal preatomic energy. . . .His work from the individual extended to the environment and the cosmos. He devised methods of weather control and change, and attempted to understand the functioning of the heavenly bodies, in terms of the concept of orgone energy. Reich's work extends to the depths of the universe, to the ramifications of the microcosm and macrocosm. He also contributed significantly to many fields of knowledge, such as psychology, sociology, medicine, biology, pathology, agriculture and meteorology. In our civilization there are few beings who, through their understanding of the life processes, become the navigators of life. Wilhelm Reich has navigated humanity to the depths of its biological existence.—from John Pierrakos' foreword to Mann's **Orgone, Reich and Eros.**

BAKER, ELSWORTH. *MAN IN THE TRAP,* 1.95. Baker, a specialist in medical orgonomy who has practiced for twenty years (eleven of which were spent in close association with Reich), presents a fascinating, in depth examination of the Reichian theory of character. Dr. Baker describes varying character types in terms of specific blockings of sexual energy at different stages of emotional development. Drawing upon many illuminating case histories, he carefully details methods of treating these various blocks and preventing neurotic development. Notes, index, 384pp. Avo 67

BOADELLA, DAVID, ed. *IN THE WAKE OF REICH,* 10.95. In the Wake of Reich *collects together in one volume a number of important papers by those of Reich's colleagues and students who wrote about their work, either during the time Reich was alive, or in the twenty years since his death. These contributions span three generations of Reichian studies. . . .All the people in this volume* *were influenced in a major way by the work of Reich, and have succeeded in developing their own style of working with the concepts, insights, and techniques that his work generated. For all but two of the contributions, this is the first time they have appeared in book form in English.*—from the introduction. Illustrations, 432pp. Asl 76

BOADELLA, DAVID. *WILHELM REICH—THE EVOLUTION OF HIS WORK,* 3.95. Based on a thorough examination of all the primary sources, including hitherto untranslated German writings and articles that have appeared only in relatively inaccessible journals, Boadella surveys the development of Reich's thought from his early psychoanalytic writings, which established him as a major revolutionary thinker, to his later innovative and controversial theories. Supplementing the main text are articles by a number of Reich's close associates. Boadella is the editor of the Reichian journal *Energy and Character: The Journal of Bio-energetic Research.* Bibliography, notes, index, 400pp. Reg 73

CHESSER, EUSTACE. *SALVATION THROUGH SEX,* 1.50. A good critical but friendly resume of Reich's life and work by an English psychiatrist. Relates Reich's ideas to more recent research and social development but includes little on the orgone period. It has been described accurately as a *layman's guide to Reich that defines, in clear and non-technical terms, the essence and meaning of his thought.* Bibliography, 172pp. Pop 72

EDEN, JEROME. *ORGONE ENERGY,* c6.00. In his famous Oranur Experiment, Reich found that the interaction of atomic energy and orgone energy as antithetical forces produced a deadly form of orgone energy called oranur or DOR. Eden believes that our atmosphere is becoming increasingly contaminated with oranur and, if allowed to proliferate, this will constitute a most serious threat to planetary life. 156pp. ExP 72

MANN, W. EDWARD. *ORGONE, REICH AND EROS,* 3.95. A fascinating study in which Mann describes Reich's theory of orgone energy and its applications, and shows how they relate to current energy theories as well as to the Hindu concepts of prana as well as to the vital force theory behind acupuncture. Mann discusses the whole range of experimentation in the area of biological rhythms, the effects of weather on health and behavior, psychic healing, and the results of his own work with orgone energy accumulators as healing devices. This work offers a rich exploration of the frontiers of the scientific and spiritual imagination. Often it's difficult reading; however, we recommend it highly to all seriously interested in the subject. Excellent bibliography, index, 382pp. S&S 73

REICH, PETER. *THE BOOK OF DREAMS*, 1.50. This book, by Reich's son, moves in a series of images, like a movie, between past and present, dream and reality. As the images interweave, layer after layer of defenses, fears, and uncertainties are stripped away until Peter is finally able to see both himself and his father with clear eyes and an open heart. 191pp. Faw 73

REICH, WILHELM. *THE CANCER BIOPATHY*, 4.95. See the Cancer subsection of Healing.

REICH, WILHELM. *CHARACTER ANALYSIS*, 6.95/2.50. First published in 1933, this has been the most influential of Reich's works in analytic circles. It is concerned with the way in which character responses are embedded in the body—the body armor which represents feelings. Notes, index, 572pp. S&S 45

REICH, WILHELM. *EARLY WRITINGS, VOLUME I*, 4.95. Included here are an important early work, *The Impulsive Character*, and a number of his other papers, all of which are an integral part of the development that led to his discovery of orgone energy. Introduction, notes, 341pp. FSG 75

REICH, WILHELM. *ETHER, GOD AND DEVIL—COSMIC SUPERIMPOSITION*, 3.45. In the first of these books, Reich describes the process of functional thinking and reveals how the inner logic of this objective thought technique led him to the discovery of cosmic orgone energy. In **Cosmic Superimposition** he shows how man is rooted in nature. The superimposition of two orgone energy systems which is demonstrable in the genital embrace is revealed as a common functioning principle that exists in all of nature. Illustrations, 308pp. FSG 49

REICH, WILHELM. *THE FUNCTION OF THE ORGASM*, 3.95/ 1.95. Possibly Reich's most important work, this is an intellectual autobiography of sorts, summarizing his medical and scientific work over a period of twenty years. Illustrations, 400pp. S&S 73

REICH, WILHELM. *THE IMPULSIVE CHARACTER AND OTHER WRITINGS,* 3.95. A selection of the full texts of some of Reich's early writings. The following works are included: *The Impulsive Character, Biophysical Papers, The Basic Antithesis of Vegetative Life Functions, The Orgasm as an Electrophysical Discharge,* and *Experimental Investigation of the Electrical Function of Sexuality and Anxiety.* The selections are a bit less analytical than those in the other collection of Reich's early writings. 211pp. NAL 74

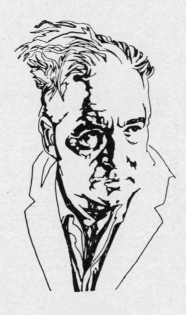

Wilhelm Reich

REICH, WILHELM. *INVASION OF COMPULSORY SEX-MORALITY,* 3.45. Growing out of his involvement with the question of the origin of sexual suppression, this attempt to explain historically the problem of sexual disturbances draws upon the ethnological works of Morgan, Engels and, in particular, Malinowski, whose studies of the Trobriand Islanders confirmed Reich's clinical discoveries. Notes, 215pp. FSG 71

REICH, WILHELM. *LISTEN LITTLE MAN,* 2.95. Tells of Reich's inner storms and conflicts as he watched, first naively, then with amazement, and finally with horror, what the *Little Man* does to himself—how he suffers and rebels, how he esteems his enemies and murders his friends, how, whenever he gains power as a representative of the people, he misuses it. More apt today than when it was written in 1945. Illustrated by William Steig. 126pp. FSG 74

REICH, WILHELM. *THE MASS PSYCHOLOGY OF FASCISM,* 3.95/2.75. Reich views fascism as the expression of the irrational character structure of the average human being whose primary biological needs and impulses have been suppressed for thousands of years. The social function of this suppression and the crucial role played in it by the authoritarian family and the church are carefully analyzed. 423pp. S&S 70

REICH, WILHELM. *REICH SPEAKS OF FREUD,* 4.95. Discusses the personally tragic but scientifically vital implication of his relationship with Freud. Based on a tape-recorded interview conducted by a representative of the Freud Archives. Illustrations, 290pp. FSG 67

REICH, WILHELM. *SELECTED WRITINGS: AN INTRODUCTION TO ORGONOMY,* 6.95. This anthology is not intended to replace any of Reich's works, but rather to serve as an introduction to them. Includes the *Oranur Experiment* and *Cosmic Orgone Engineering.* Bibliography, 560pp. FSG 51

REICH, WILHELM. *THE SEXUAL REVOLUTION,* 2.95/1.95. Reich here criticizes prevailing sexual conditions and demonstrates, by way of individual examples, the conflicts of marriage, the revolution in family life, and the problems of infantile and adolescent sexuality. Includes a detailed study of the sexual revolution that occurred briefly in Russia after its revolution. 273pp. S&S 62

RYCROFT, CHARLES. *WILHELM REICH,* 1.65. A critical analysis of Reich's work, excluding his later orgone study. Rycroft describes his life as *tormented, persecuted, and futile.* 115pp. Vik 69

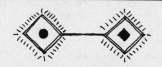

REICHENBACH, KARL VON. *THE ODIC FORCE: LETTERS ON OD AND MAGNETISM,* c5.00. Von Reichenbach was a chemist, metallurgist, technologist, and expert on meteorites. He discovered a mysterious force, named it *Od,* published his findings in Germany in 1845, and continued his study until his death in 1869. His findings were largely ignored until Wilhelm Reich rediscovered this energy and named it the *orgone.* What von Reichenbach discovered was the mysterious vital force or energy permeating nature. It is blue in color and can be demonstrated visually by heat, and by electric charge, in plants, animals and humans—but it can only be perceived by very sensitive people under careful guidance by a sympathetic scientist. This edition includes valuable supplementary material. 119pp. UnB 68

REICHENBACH, KARL VON. *RESEARCHES ON THE VITAL FORCE,* c10.00. This is the most extensive presentation available of von Reichenbach's researches in the area of magnetism, electricity, heat, light, crystallization, and chemical attraction in relation to the vital force. Illustrations, 514pp. UnB 74

REICHENBACH, KARL VON. *SOMNAMBULISM AND CRAMP,* 8.50. This translation is excerpted from a much larger work entitled **The Sensitive Man and his Relation to Od.** *Somnambulism is a peculiar abnormal fit, or temporary condition, wherein man loses his normal consciousness and gets another abnormal one, and becomes a different person, with a new memory, powers of perception, and modes of thought and action.*—from the introduction. Cramp is an opposite condition and the influences which cause one will cure the other. Reichenbach surveys these states in terms of his odic theory and cites many case histories. Introduction, spiral bound, 279pp. HeR 1860

RICHARDS, W. GUYON. *THE CHAIN OF LIFE,* c8.40. This is an interesting study by a noted radiesthesic practitioner. Richards delves far deeper into the subject than do most writers and his own personal experiences make illuminating reading. The account begins with a review of how he became interested in radiesthesia and discusses Abrams' discoveries and his own experiments with the atom. A second section surveys esoteric anatomy, with special reference to the needs of radiesthesic practitioners. The final 100 pages examine the uses of radiesthesia in a variety of specific areas including cancer and color. A technical work, illustrated with many tables and graphs. Index, 220pp. Spg 54

RUSSELL, EDWARD. *DESIGN FOR DESTINY,* c5.60. A synthesis and interpretation of the work of many scientists, providing a link between science and religion, intellect and perception, man and his universe. Russell was especially close to Harold Burr, whose pioneering work with L-Fields (the permanent electro-magnetic fields which mold the constantly changing material of the cells) is described in great detail. Other scientists discussed include L.L. Vasiliev, J.B. Rhine, and Wilder Penfield. An important book for the layman; well researched and annotated. 213pp. Spe 71

RUSSELL, EDWARD. *REPORT ON RADIONICS,* c8.70. This is the most comprehensive account of radionics available, as seen through the eyes of a reporter. Russell describes the developments over the past half century and talks about the major practitioners, many of whom he knew or knows personally. The book is well written and includes case studies from both sides of the Atlantic. This is an excellent introduction for the nonprofessional and provides a good overview for all. Illustrations, bibliography, notes, 255pp. Spe 73

RUSSELL, WALTER. *ATOMIC SUICIDE?* c10.00. After pointing out the health dangers of atomic energy, including cancers and mutations, Russell presents a view of the harmonics of energy and matter. It is a vision of the patterns making up the physical world: how the elements in atoms and stars evolve out of each other, how electricity, magnetism, and light manifest in the motion of the creative energy. Many diagrams illustrate his theory. 304pp. USP 57

RUSSELL, WALTER. *THE SECRET OF LIGHT,* c15.00. A technical examination of light and vibration in all its manifestations. Many of Russell's own complex diagrams illustrate the text. 302pp. USP 47

SCHUL, BILL and ED PETTIT. *THE PSYCHIC POWER OF PYRAMIDS,* 3.95. This seems to be the year for books on pyramid energy. The authors of this one write well and they are good at piecing together bits of information into coherent chapters. The chapters don't necessarily follow each other in logical sequence, but that's OK. This is a fine book for those who want to know some facts and suppositions about the healing benefits of pyramid energy and about the possibilities of all kinds of energy. The information here does not duplicate the material in the authors' earlier book. Bibliography, index, 224pp. Faw 76

SCHUL, BILL and ED PETTIT. *THE SECRET POWER OF PYRA-MIDS,* 1.75. A good introduction to effects of pyramids and pyramid shapes on plants and people, the history and construction of pyramids, altered states of consciousness and pyramids, and the relation of ancient earth energy grids to the pyramids. Photographs, bibliography, 223pp. Faw 75

SHEARS, C. CURTIS. *SCIENCE OF SELF-HEALING,* 4.50. This book is not so much about self-healing as it is about nutrition, metaphysical concepts of disease, and the use of radiesthesia in divining disease and nutritional imbalances. Dr. Shears has written extensively on nutrition; this book covers more metaphysical aspects of health. He calls for more radiesthetic operators who are trained in nutritional science and this combination is apparently being developed at his Nutritional Science Research Institute of England. 55pp. NuS 75

SOYKA, FRED and ALAN EDMONDS. *THE ION EFFECT: HOW AIR ELECTRICITY RULES YOUR LIFE AND HEALTH,* c7.95. Ions are tiny particles of electrically charged air, either positive or negative. When the air you breathe has too few negative ions, you suffer from ion starvation, which may make you feel anxious, tired, and unable to cope. When the atmosphere is heavy with too many positive ions, as often occurs with weather disturbances, you suffer from positive ion poisoning, which can induce heart attacks, aggravate asthma, migraines, insomnia, rheumatism, arthritis, hay fever, most allergies, and other afflictions. This is a journalistic account of how ions can affect our lives. Bibliography, index, 181pp. Dut 77

STARK, NORMAN. *THE FIRST PRACTICAL PYRAMID BOOK,* 5.95. The latest in a seemingly unending series of books on putting pyramid energy to work. This one is better than most and touches on many areas not covered in earlier books. Stark explains how to energize water, dry foods, make yogurt without a culture, energize aluminum foil, and much else. He gives instructions for building your own pyramid and provides a pattern which can be adapted to both indoor and outdoor uses. Many illustrations are included and there's an easily assembled pyramid contained in the book. 7"x10", 150pp. SAM 77

TANSLEY, DAVID. *RADIONICS AND THE SUBTLE ANATOMY OF MAN,* 4.20. Radionics is defined as a method of diagnosis and therapy which is primarily concerned with the utilization of subtle force fields and energies for the purpose of investigating and combating the causes of disease. Tansley relates radionics to laws and principles governing the etheric, emotional, and mental levels of existence. He includes valuable data on the esoteric constitution of man, the etheric body, the force centers, the chakras, vitality and prana. This is the only radionics book that deals with these areas. Many diagrams are included. 95pp. HSP 72

TANSLEY, DAVID. *RADIONICS: INTERFACE WITH THE ETHER-FIELDS,* c8.40. This is an excellent esoteric exposition of radionics, geared toward the practitioner and the knowledgable layman. The following chapter headings should give the reader a good feeling for the content and orientation: *An Esoteric Ether-Field Construct, The Connective Tissue of Space, The Geometric Etheric Link, Radionic Etheric Photography, Radionic Potentizing—Remedies from the Ether-Field, Scanning the Human Aura, The Spine and Radionic Therapy, Bio-Dynamic Rhythm,* and *Some Esoteric Aspects of Radionics.* Many examples taken from Tansley's practice are included within the body of the text. 124pp. HSP 75

Nikola Tesla

Tesla was an inventor, but he was much more than a producer of new devices: he was a discoverer of new principles, opening many new empires of knowledge which even today have been only partly explored. In a single mighty burst of invention, he created the world of power of today; he brought into being our electrical power era, the rock-bottom foundation on which the industrial system of the entire world is built; he gave us our mass-production systems for without his motors and currents it could not exist; he created the race of robots, the electrical mechanical men that are replacing human labor; he gave us every essential of modern radio; he invented the radar forty years before its use in World War II; he gave us our modern neon and other forms of gaseous-tube lighting; he gave us our fluorescent lighting; he gave us the high-frequency currents which are performing wonders throughout the industrial and medical worlds; he gave us remote control by wireless. . . .And these discoveries are merely the inventions by the master mind of Tesla which have thus far been utilized—scores of others still remain unused.—from **Prodigal Genius** by John O'Neill

O'NEILL, JOHN. *PRODIGAL GENIUS: THE LIFE OF NIKOLA TESLA*, 3.45. O'Neill was a personal friend of Tesla. This is the story of his life and work. 326pp. McK 44

TESLA, NIKOLA. *INVENTIONS, RESEARCHES AND WRITINGS OF NIKOLA TESLA*, 10.00. This volume was put together by Thomas C. Martin, an electrical engineer, with the approval and blessings of Tesla himself. It is basically a record of the pioneering work done by Tesla in the field of electrical invention. It includes his lectures, miscellaneous articles and discussions, and makes note of all his inventions up to the time of publication (1893), particularly those bearing on polyphase motors and the effects obtained with currents of high potential and high frequency. Spiral bound, 496pp. HeR 70

TESLA, NIKOLA. *NIKOLA TESLA—LECTURES, PATENTS, ARTICLES*, 35.00. The purpose of this massive volume published by the Nikola Tesla Museum is to acquaint the reader with Tesla's most important works in the numerous fields of science to which he dedicated himself. The first part contains Tesla's most important lectures in chronological order. The second part contains Tesla's patents, selected from those registered at the U.S. Patent Office. These are divided into select groups, each being arranged according to the order of registration. The third part, containing a cross section of Tesla's scientific and technical articles, is also divided into select groups. This is an unwieldy book, but it is the only source of this information. Photographs, spiral bound, 8½"x11", 833pp. HeR 73

TOMILSON, H. *MEDICAL DIVINATION: THEORY AND PRAC-TICE,* c5.25. This is an advanced study by an English physician who works with both radiesthesia and homoeopathy. Dr. Tomilson includes chapters on the absolute, the octave structure, the etheric body, the toxic effects of aluminum, water fluoridation, radiesthesic testing. Case histories are also included. Bibliography, 86pp. HSP 66

TOMPKINS, PETER and CHRIS BIRD. *THE SECRET LIFE OF PLANTS,* 1.95. An excellent, comprehensive account. The authors begin by describing the latest discoveries in plant research, including current Russian work, Cleve Backster's studies in plant communication, and the work of scientists from various disciplines. They go on from there to trace and analyze experiments and theories from the past, including extensive surveys of the pioneers of plant research. Their narrative is extensively documented. Long bibliography, 402pp. Avo 73

TOTH, MAX and GREG NIELSEN. *PYRAMID POWER,* 1.95. This is a newly revised version of one of the first books to be written on the subject of pyramid energy. It is a more serious study than most of the others and the authors begin with an excellent historical overview of the theories of pyramidologists. This is followed by diagrams, practical information and a discussion of the serious work in the area. A well written, cohesive study which includes a number of experiments readers can perform themselves. Bibliography, index, 257pp. War 76

WAYLAND, BRUCE and SHIRLEY, eds. *STEPS TO DOWSING POWER,* 4.95. A collection of articles on dowsing, illustrated with photographs and line drawings. A number of noted dowsers discuss their experiences, and practical instructional material is offered. Water and map dowsing are surveyed in separate articles and there's also an essay on dowsing living things. Despite the title, this is a serious work. 8½"x11", 68pp. LFP 76

WESTLAKE, AUBREY. *THE PATTERN OF HEALTH,* 3.95. Dr. Westlake set out to study medicine from the standpoint of health, instead of from disease. He has been studying the supersensory healing force which, under so many names, keeps on being rediscovered without the discoverer seeming to know that someone else has done so before. He discusses the discoveries of Guyon Richards, Bach, Reichenbach, Wilhelm Reich and Eeman.

He also describes his own experiences in radiesthesia and homoeopathy. A fascinating book, which we highly recommend. Illustrations, index, 214pp. ShP 73

WETHERED, VERNON. *AN INTRODUCTION TO MEDICAL RADIESTHESIA AND RADIONICS,* c6.60. An excellent technical study, written primarily for physicians, especially those interested in homoeopathy. Dr. Wethered describes radiesthesic techniques which he has developed for diagnosis and treatment which offer mathematical precision in assessing the functioning of organs, the severity of disease, and the determination of treatment. He also discusses the psychological aspect of disease from the radionic point of view. Photographs, illustrations, bibliography, index, 194pp. Dan 57

WETHERED, VERNON. *THE PRACTICE OF MEDICAL RADIESTHESIA,* c4.00. This is the latest work by Wethered, vicepresident of the British Society of Dowsers and a well known researcher in this field. It shows how the practitioner can learn simple methods of pendulum testing, and includes chapters on the psychic factor in pendulum work, energy levels in elements and people, and nuclear fall-out. It also relates radiesthesia to homoeopathic diagnosis and prescribing. 150pp. Fow 67

WHITE, GEORGE S. *THE FINER FORCES OF NATURE,* 7.00. *This handbook, explaining, describing, and illustrating my original method of using the* **Finer Forces of Nature** *for diagnosing and treating all manner of unhealth, is a condensation and revamping of voluminous literature that I have written on the subject, augmented with new discoveries gained through many additional years of study and clinical experience.* Includes many two color illustrations and photographs. Spiral bound, index, 231pp. HeR 69

WILLEY, RAYMOND. *MODERN DOWSING,* 5.00. This is a comprehensive presentation which begins with a general discussion of dowsing and then goes into a detailed study of the tools of dowsing. Willey also surveys holds and movements utilizing many types of rods. Virtually every type of rod is discussed and there's information on dowsing without devices and on using the pendulum. Map dowsing is also covered. Many case studies and explicit instructions are included. The author is a trustee of The American Society of Dowsers. This is the best overall manual to use if you want to learn how to dowse. 196pp. EsP 76

Natural Childbirth

A woman invests nine months of her life in the creation of a baby—an astonishingly long period of time. And despite outward appearances, for most women life does *not* go on as usual during these months. They are keenly aware of the new being to whom they are giving so much of themselves. They live with change. They forego many pleasures. They put up with enormous inconveniences. They plan and dream and worry. They are cautious for their baby's safety. They avoid all manner of commonplace circumstances which now become potential hazards. They eat foods which they may detest, take pills which may nauseate them, put up with unpleasant examinations at the hands of their doctors, too often after an interminable wait in his reception room, and still remain irrepressibly happy. Bravely they face the experience of birth, not without moments of fear, but bravely still. And it is well that women are brave, because both the fact and the fiction surrounding birth American style are enough to discourage the faint of heart.

The modern obstetrician invests a *total* of two to three hours in the prenatal care of a woman. For this he is most often paid whatever fee he has asked, and with far more gratitude than he probably deserves. For up to the point of labor, he is a very minor figure in the enterprise of childbearing.

The event of labor and its culmination in the incredibly beautiful act of birth are the zenith of the creative experience. Zenith, not end, for parenthood, too, is creative, and there are more satisfactions to come. But childbirth is transcendent and transfiguring—an experience shared with God. No one else can share this experience, although other mothers present may often relive briefly their own childbirths. A husband can come close to sharing, for the child is flesh of his flesh too, and for a fleeting few moments he and his wife become as one. The professionals present, doctor, nurses, anesthesiologist, would do well to maintain dignified silence and awe at the moment of birth. Their job has been to exert all the skill of which they are possessed to insure that this birth will be an act of flawless beauty.

Too often in American obstetrics, this is not what happens. We obstetricians begin to act as if we were the major concern. With vast impatience we start running the show to our own liking. Our examinations are hurried, our instructions cryptic, our orders routine, as if there were such a thing as a routine childbirth. If we are impatient, we speed things up a bit. Sometimes we even slow things down a bit for our convenience. We have persuaded ourselves that women don't really like childbirth, so we use anesthetics, then of course find it necessary to deliver the babies ourselves, our patients having been rendered incapable of using their own forces. We have become very skillful at such deliveries. Our forceps do not leave marks, and our episiotomies heal beautifully. Patients recover nicely from their anesthetics and thank us for our help. But in the 85 to 90 percent of women who are able to deliver spontaneously, we are wrong to interfere. Slowly we are learning that we have been wrong.

Women and their husbands must be trained for childbirth, a fact now taken for granted and government sponsored in much of the Western world. Husbands must be restored to a position of dignity in this event by which they become parent, no less than do their wives. It seems so obvious. The habit of separating mother and baby at birth and for most of the next several days is almost criminally neglectful of the most fundamental needs of both. Hospital personnel have a tremendous responsibility to promote the sense of family as two people become three, rather than to rupture this unit at every step of the way.

Mothers who wish to nurse their babies must be helped, not hindered. I cannot know if breast feeding will ever again become the preferred method of feeding babies in the United States. I do know that we are beginning to learn the frightful price we are paying in allowing the dairy and baby food industries to dictate custom to us in this respect. Immunity to various diseases, freedom from digestive disturbances, prevention of allergies, and avoidance of later orthodontic problems are possibly just a few of the benefits which flow from the human breast.

But far more is at stake than merely for a woman to have a joyful birth experience or a pleasant few days in the hospital. Her self-esteem is either bolstered mightily or battered badly by her experience. Her attitude toward and her relationship with her child and her husband are affected by what happens during this crucial period. She will share with the whole world that which we give her. It can be resentment, hurt, hostility, or it can be a deeper understanding, dignity, love. This is the true challenge to all of us. . . .—from John S. Miller's foreword in **Commonsense Childbirth** by Lester Dessez Hazell

ARMS, SUZANNE. *IMMACULATE DECEPTION, 6.95. This is a book about childbirth in America. It is neither a medical textbook, nor a political treatise, nor a whole birth catalog. Rather, it is a statement that grew out of my need to understand and explain my own birth experience. It is my contribution to anyone interested in the American way of birth.* This is an excellent comprehensive collection of essays on many topics related to women and childbirth in America. It is illustrated with many photographs and also quotes extensively from the experiences of individual women. Bibliography, oversize, 317pp. HMC 75

ARMS, SUZANNE. *A SEASON TO BE BORN,* 2.95. Eloquent photographs and a simple personal text create an emotional experience for the reader as s/he watches the Arms' move through pregnancy, birth, and celebration of their daughter. Oversize, 112pp. H&R 73

BEAN, CONSTANCE. *METHODS OF CHILDBIRTH,* 2.50. *I cannot praise this book highly enough. . .a trailblazing contribution toward enlightening women everywhere. Bean covers what everyone else leaves out. . . .It also drives home the message that "The woman educated for childbirth keeps her adult role." For those who wish the latest medical and statistical reasons why such a role is best for mother and baby, this is the book to turn to.*—**Ms. Magazine.** Includes chapters on childbirth and childbirth education, methods of preparation, labor and delivery, drugs and anaesthesia, father, mother, and baby, breastfeeding, and the childbirth education class. Glossary, bibliography, notes, 235pp. Dou 74

BING, ELISABETH. *MOVING THROUGH PREGNANCY,* 1.95. Presents a series of exercises which can be incorporated into the everyday schedule of a pregnant woman, including clear photographs of each exercise. The exercises themselves have been developed by Ms. Bing in her classes and have been tested extensively. 175pp. Ban 75

BING, ELISABETH. *SIX PRACTICAL LESSONS FOR AN EASIER CHILDBIRTH,* 1.50. This is one of the best of the Lamaze instruction manuals. It is written by the co-founders of the American Society for Psychoprophylaxis in Obstetrics and who was a pioneer in introducing the Lamaze method to America. The book is easy to follow, packed with information, and cheap. Even if you have a good Lamaze class, you'll find the book useful for review. 128pp. Ban 73

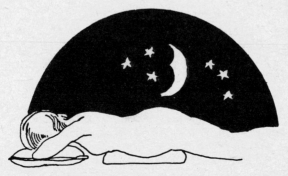

Breastfeeding

Most babies in America are bottle fed and few mothers until recently have considered breastfeeding. Breast milk is obviously the most perfect food for the human baby—a fact that formula manufacturers acknowledge when they proclaim that their product is the closest to a mother's milk. The reasons for both the lack of interest in breastfeeding and the benefits of breastfeeding are outlined in many books. There are many benefits, both nutritional and psychological, as these books point out.

EIGER, MARVIN and SALLY OLDS. *THE COMPLETE BOOK OF BREASTFEEDING,* 1.75. Dr. Eiger is one of New York's leading pediatricians and Ms. Olds is a medical writer who nursed her own three children. Their presentation is the most comprehensive one available, with clearly written material on all aspects of the subject. Recommended. Includes many photographs, a long bibliography, and an index. 208pp. Ban 72

EWY, DONNA and RODGER. *PREPARATION FOR BREAST FEEDING,* 2.95. A very full exploration of breastfeeding, with information on the physiology involved. Psychological and physical problems the mother and baby may encounter are also discussed and suggestions made. Photographs and line drawings illustrate the exposition. Very clearly written. Bibliography, index, 125pp. Dou 75

KIPPLEY, SHEILA. *BREAST FEEDING AND NATURAL CHILD SPACING,* 2.95. A dry survey backed up with case studies and reviews of the recent research. Every aspect is well covered. Index, 216pp. Vik 74

LA LECHE LEAGUE. *THE WOMANLY ART OF BREAST-FEEDING,* 4.00. The La Leche League has been one of the primary groups in the natural childbirth movement and they have been the foremost exponents of breastfeeding: *Breastfeeding gives the baby back to the mother. Her baby securely in her arms, she finds her motherly response, like her milk, is never* *measured, but ample.* This book, written by seven of the founders, was designed as the La Leche League manual, developed originally for mothers too far away from a group to attend meetings. The following topics are discussed: *why breastfeeding?, planning for baby, nutritional know-how for nursing mothers, some common worries and old wives' tales, your baby arrives, how to mother the newly-born child, special circumstances,* and *the father's role.* Bibliography, index, 166pp. LLL 63

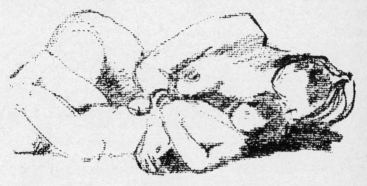

PRYOR, KAREN. *NURSING YOUR BABY,* 1.95. This is a scholarly advocacy of breastfeeding, complete with pictures and household hints. In Part I Ms. Pryor discusses the nursing relationship, how breasts function, the composition of milk, the mother instinct, doctors, milk banks, the La Leche League, and attitudes toward breastfeeding. Part II contains practical information: brassieres, diet, putting the baby to breast for the first time, leaking, night feeding, vitamins, weaning. Extensive bibliography, index, 289pp. S&S 63

RAPHAEL, DANA. *THE TENDER GIFT: BREASTFEEDING,* 3.45. This book differs from other books on breastfeeding in two ways. First, a great deal of space is devoted to a comprehensive survey of breastfeeding, past and present, in many cultures, and even among animal groups. Second, the instructional material on breastfeeding is basically devoted to suggested nursing techniques, based upon the author's extensive research and her own experience. This volume is highly recommended by the La Leche League. Glossary, bibliography, notes, index, 200pp. ScB 73

BOSE, S.K. *MIDWIFERY,* c1.10. See the Homoeopathy section.

BRADLEY, ROBERT. *HUSBAND-COACHED CHILDBIRTH,* c7.95. Since 1947 Dr. Bradley has been practicing and promoting the principles of true natural childbirth, including the concept of an active role for the husband as "labor coach." Here he gives practical pointers on what happens during the pregnancy, labor, and actual birth, psychological hints for living with a pregnant woman, and suggestions on how the man can help with exercises and diet and give the woman support during crisis periods. 224pp. H&R 74

BRADY, MARGARET. *HAVING A BABY EASILY,* c4.70. This is a recent reprint of a comprehensive 1944 English manual. The material is very British and covers areas not referred to in other books. Ms. Brady includes the following main chapters: *Diet, Sunshine, Fresh Air, Sleep, Elimination, Avoiding Morning Sickness, Physical Training, Spiritual Outlook, The Confinement, Breast Feeding, Weaning,* and *Routine and Management of the New Born Baby.* Glossary, index, 234pp. HFA 68

BRENNAN, BARBARA and JOAN HEILMAN. *COMPLETE BOOK OF MIDWIFERY,* 4.95. The author of this book runs a nurse-midwifery program. In this book she describes her personal experiences and discusses what the role of midwives can be and what a midwife can offer an expectant mother. This is the only book on midwifery written for the layperson and it is illustrated throughout with photographs. A listing of the addresses of nurse-midwifery services in the U.S. and a bibliography and index are also included. 154pp. Dut 77

BRICKLIN, ALICE. *MOTHER LOVE,* 4.95. Subtitled *The Book of Natural Child Rearing,* this is a lovely volume covering the following main topics: *Baby Closeness at Birth, Baby-Led Nursing and Nutrition, Baby and the Family.* The account is personal and the approach is positive. Annotated bibliography, notes, index, oversize, 110pp. RuP 75

BROOK, DANAE. *NATUREBIRTH: YOU, YOUR BODY, AND YOUR BABY,* 3.95. This is a comprehensive, beautifully produced volume which discusses all aspects of natural childbirth. The first section is a thorough review of the realities of childbirth today which raises important and provocative questions. The second section is a practical guide to pregnancy and labor which includes new techniques for preparation for natural birth, information on the effects of drugs, a section on the ailments common to pregnancy—with a discussion of midwifery and herbal and homoeopathic remedies, and a series of exercises. Illustrations, bibliography, 304pp. RaH 76

BURNETT, C.W.F. *THE ANATOMY AND PHYSIOLOGY OF OBSTETRICS*, 4.95. This is a short textbook for students and midwives. All the important information is included and the discussion is not as overwhelmingly detailed as the other textbooks. The material is clearly presented and excellent line drawings accompany the text. Index, 215pp. Fab 69

CLYNE, DOUGLAS. *A CONCISE TEXTBOOK FOR MIDWIVES*, 5.95. A comprehensive discussion of virtually every aspect of midwifery. The book has been used as a text for student midwives in England for many years and this fourth edition has been carefully revised. While not as complete as Myles' **Textbook**, the presentation is exceedingly clear and there are line drawings throughout. Index, 448pp. Fab 75

CRISP, TONY. *YOGA AND CHILDBIRTH*, 1.75. Despite its intriguing title this is basically just another book on childbirth with very little about yogic exercises and almost no pictures. The emphasis is on methods of relaxation through breathing and physical movement. There are also a number of hints on what to do about problems that might arise. Index, 128pp. SBL 75

DICK-READ, GRANTLY. *CHILDBIRTH WITHOUT FEAR*, 2.25. This is a classic work on natural childbirth based on the author's conclusions after many years of study and observation as an obstetrician. Dr. Dick-Read describes the development of the child from conception to birth, the anatomy and physiology of mother and child during pregnancy and delivery, the reasons for fear and the resulting painful labor when the mother has not been prepared for childbirth, and the proper place of anaesthetics in natural childbirth. He also includes a short, badly illustrated section of simple exercises. Index, 384pp. H&R 53

ELOESSER, LEO, EDITH GALT and ISABEL HEMINGWAY. *PREGNANCY, CHILDBIRTH AND THE NEWBORN: A MANUAL FOR RURAL MIDWIVES*, 4.20. **This is an excellent illustrated**

manual which was originally written to accompany courses given in China to women with no more than a primary school education and no previous knowledge of medicine or nursing. It has been considerably revised and enlarged and is today considered the finest work available for the nontechnical reader. It includes chapters on anatomy and physiology of the female reproductive organs, on the progress and conduct of pregnancy and childbirth, and on care of the newborn. The book should be of interest not only to midwives, but to all women who want a deeper understanding of what happens and what is to be done during pregnancy. Recommended. Illustrations, index, 167pp. III 73

EWY, DONNA and RODGER. *PREPARATION FOR CHILDBIRTH,* 1.75. The Lamaze method prepares a woman emotionally, psychologically, intellectually, and physically for childbirth. This book is one of the best available manuals on the method. The Ewys present exercises for body building, stretching, relaxation, and breathing and their discussion is complete with diagrams and photographs outlining each sequence from labor through delivery. The authors write well and they speak from their hearts. This is a revised edition. Bibliography, index, 220pp. NAL 76

FITZGERALD, DOROTHY, et al. *HOME ORIENTED MATERNITY EXPERIENCE: A COMPREHENSIVE GUIDE TO HOME BIRTH,* 3.75. This is an excellent, practical study of the home birth experience. The authors begin with an essay on the advantage of home birth and a discussion of parental responsibilities. Next comes a section on equipment and procedures. This is followed by a lengthy discourse on the psychological aspects of home birth and the medical considerations. There are also chapters on breastfeeding and on food for expectant mothers. Every topic we can think of is covered and notes refer the reader to more complete discussions elsewhere. Appendices discuss post-partum care and the use of herbs, and offer a lengthy bibliography. 94pp. HME 76

FLEMING, ALICE. *NINE MONTHS,* 2.50. This book is subtitled *A Practical Guide for the Expectant Mother* and that describes the contents as well as anything we can say. Many of the most common questions and concerns are discussed and important points to keep in mind during pregnancy are raised. The tone is positive throughout. Bibliography, index, 194pp. H&R 72

GLAS, NORBERT. *CONCEPTION, BIRTH AND EARLY CHILD-*

HOOD, 2.50. A sensitive, intuitive account of the soul entering into a new physical vehicle and the effects the conception process has on the mother, based on Rudolf Steiner's Spiritual Science and on Dr. Glas' own experience. As the title suggests there are chapters on conception, pregnancy and birth—all oriented around the spiritual development of mother and child. The major part of the book is devoted to an analysis of the newborn's coming into the world and developing his or her senses, will, feeling, and ego. We highly recommend this volume to all who want to understand the deeper meaning and potentiality of the birth process. 152pp. API 72

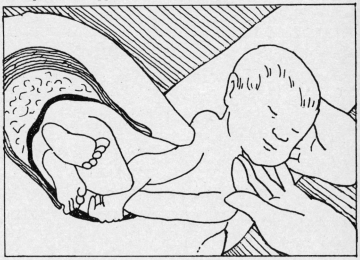

HARTMAN, RHONDDA. *EXERCISES FOR TRUE NATURAL CHILDBIRTH,* c9.95. Mrs. Hartmann is an R.N. and has been active in the American Academy of Husband-Coached Childbirth and the La Leche League. She has taught the exercises illustrated here since she had the first of her five children. Her approach is practical, including easy to follow instructions arranged under the headings how, where, and when. The photographs are not terribly helpful—they are not detailed enough and there are too few of them. The exercises are arranged in sequence so that you will have your body and muscles ready by full term pregnancy. It's not a great book—but there is so little available on the subject that anything is welcome, and the written instructions are good. Index, oversize, 139pp. H&R 75

HAZELL, LESTER. *COMMONSENSE CHILDBIRTH,* 1.95. "*Commonsense Childbirth* is one of the most important and valuable books ever written on the art and science of having a baby. It is not written by a male obstetrician, but by a mother who, because of her unhappy obstetrical experience with her first child, determined to discover for herself whether childbirth could not be a happy and rewarding experience. What she discovered is set out in her wonderful book for all prospective parents, as well as obstetricians, to read."–Ashley Montagu. This is a revised edition. Index, 281pp. Ber 76

HODSON, GEOFFREY. *THE MIRACLE OF BIRTH,* 1.75. Hodson, probably the most intuitive theosophist of this century, presents his clairvoyant study of the formation and development of the emotional, mental, and physical bodies of a being during the prenatal period. The material is based on his observation of one individual. 64pp. TPH 29

KARMEL, MARJORIE. *THANK YOU, DR. LAMAZE,* 1.95. A lucid, straightforward account of the author's experiences with the Lamaze technique, as explained to her by Dr. Lamaze himself. Ms. Karmel writes very personally, and many details of the various exercises are included. Bibliography, 195pp. Dou 59

KITZINGER, SHEILA. *THE EXPERIENCE OF CHILDBIRTH,* 2.95. This is an excellent book, designed by Ms. Kitzinger as a complete manual of physical and emotional preparation for the expectant mother. The physiology of pregnancy, the development of the fetus, and the successive stages of labor are described in detail. Moving on from the pioneering work of Grantly Dick-Read and later psychoprophylactic techniques, Ms. Kitzinger's research and teaching focus particularly on the psychological aspects of childbearing, on the preparation of both wife and husband not only for birth but for parenthood and marital adjustment, and on the woman's changing relationship with her own mother. This revised edition includes a full discussion on the touch-relaxation method which she has developed, and she also adds many personal accounts of labor recorded by some of her pupils. Recommended, Index, 280pp. Vik 72

LAMAZE, FERDNAND. *PAINLESS CHILDBIRTH: THE LAMAZE METHOD,* 1.95. Lamaze is a French physician who developed the most widely used method of natural childbirth. Much of this book is devoted to a theoretical presentation of the physiology of childbirth along with transcriptions of his lectures on various related areas. This is a reference book rather than a work designed to turn a woman on to the idea of natural childbirth. Illustrations, index, 191pp. S&S 70

LANG, RAVEN. *BIRTH BOOK,* 6.00. This is one of the best home birth books, complete with many photographs, varied experiences, and an interesting history of childbirth. Some of the information is practical: various home remedies are offered and equipment needed for home delivery is discussed. Some is a little less conventional—such as the recipe for placenta stew! Oversize. GeP 72

LEBOYER, FREDERICK. *BIRTH WITHOUT VIOLENCE,* c8.95. This is an important book that asks us to focus our attention on the infant just born—to examine and radically change what is being done in hospitals all over the world to the new human being who has just emerged, after hours of unavoidable tumult and pain, from the once-peaceful womb. The man who makes this plea is Frederick Leboyer, whose revolutionary techniques for easing the birth trauma are stirring great interest. He has himself delivered more than 10,000 babies. Of these, the last 1,000 have been brought into the world in the new way that he here fully and clearly describes. Leboyer shows us exactly what we can do to replace the ugly mask of terror that we have until now taken for granted in the newborn with the peaceful, rapt expression that is apparent in the photographs of babies delivered without violence. Many photographs, oversize, 115pp. RaH 75

LEBOYER, FREDERICK. *LOVING HANDS,* c7.95. This is a beautiful book which shows us how, in the weeks and months following a baby's birth, we can use the flowing rhythms of the traditional Indian art of baby massage to communicate our love and strength to infants in a primal language of touch and sensation. The actual techniques of this massage and the embracing vision that animates them, are seen through the person of a radiant young Indian mother, whom Dr. Leboyer met with, observed, and photographed with her babies in India. 9¾"x11", 139pp. RaH 76

LINDEN, WILHELM ZUR. *A CHILD IS BORN,* 3.50. What do we really mean when we say: *A child is born*? Dr. zur Linden is concerned with a total answer to the question. Indeed he holds that it is impossible to answer any single aspect of it without facing them all. He regards the child as a threefold being of body, soul and spirit and feels that the organism in the womb is already being prepared by the child himself as a vehicle for the expression of his soul and spirit. It must be nurtured and nourished as such a vehicle both before and after birth. Dr. zur Linden details physical treatment and environment based on Rudolf Steiner's Spiritual Science. Many practical suggestions on nutrition and childcare during pregnancy, birth, and early childhood are given. Bibliography, index, 199pp. API 73

LOVELL, PHILLIP. *PREGNANCY AND CHILD CARE THE NATURAL WAY,* 5.50. A hip but somewhat scattered manual for natural childcare and pregnancy. Many potential problem areas are discussed and advice on proper care is given. The material is oriented toward the philosophy we believe in but the tone is often a bit heavy. 252pp. NuB 72

MACFARLANE, AIDAN. *THE PSYCHOLOGY OF CHILDBIRTH,* 2.95. This volume looks at the actual birth experience as only one part of a continually unfolding relationship from conception outward, first between the baby and mother and, after birth, between the child, the parents, and the environment in general. The chapters are chronologically ordered, dealing first with the baby's experience in the uterus and with the mother's psychology during pregnancy. After this comes a discussion of the delivery and the parents' first reactions to the newborn baby. The final chapters survey the way in which the baby perceives the outside world and how s/he may influence and be influenced by her new environment. Between chapters are transcripts of actual deliveries. An excellent psychological study for those who like this sort of work. Illustrations, bibliography, notes, index, 140pp. HUP 77

MARZOLLO, JEAN, ed. *9 MONTHS, 1 DAY, 1 YEAR,* 4.95. *9 Months, 1 Day, 1 Year is one of the few books that deal with the whole period of pregnancy, birth, and that first special year as a new parent. It's a book of feelings, facts, and opinions that you can talk back to, laugh with, and share as part of your own experience. I particularly like the fact that it concentrates on both parents and not just mothers. When you are about to become a parent or have just become one, you're at your most vulnerable. This book pro-*

vides support, cheer, and companionship without the condescending and patronizing tone often found in doctors' books. The book is written by a number of mothers and is well organized. Appendices contain sources of infant paraphernalia and an excellent annotated bibliography. All in all this is an enjoyable and useful book. Index, 9"x8", 191pp. H&R 75

MAY, INA. *SPIRITUAL MIDWIFERY,* 5.95. *This is a spiritual book, and at the same time it is a revolutionary book. It is spiritual because it is concerned with the sacrament of birth—the passage of a new soul into this plane of existence. . . .This book is revolutionary because it is our basic belief that the sacrament of birth belongs to the people and that it should not be usurped by a profit-oriented hospital system. . . .We live in a self-sufficient farming community in Tennessee. . . .We deliver our own babies by natural childbirth, and some other people's too. Among us we have delivered over 350 babies at the time of this writing.* The book is divided into the following sections: *Amazing Birthing Tales, You and Your Baby,* and *Instructions for Midwives.* A profusion of photographs and drawings accompany the text. Index, 378pp. BPC 75

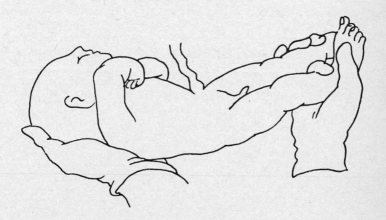

MEDVIN, JEANNINE. *PRENATAL YOGA,* 2.50. In answer to numerous requests, here finally is an excellent yogic manual for the expectant mother. The format is oversize and the postures are well described and illustrated. There are also many related line drawings and excellent general philosophical material. The explanations are very complete. 8½"x11", 55pp. FPC 75

MILINAIRE, CATERINE. *BIRTH,* 5.95. This is our most popular general book on natural childbirth. The information is plentiful and the enthusiasm catching. Some of the chapters cover prenatal care, mother's body care, birth choices, birth experiences, fathers, newborn infant care, and birth customs around the world. The text includes a lot of illustrations and photographs. There's a bit of visual chaos but when you get beyond that, there's a great deal of useful information. A good gift book for the mother-to-be (or even a good present for yourself!) Oversize, 356pp. Crn 74

MITCHELL, INGRID. *GIVING BIRTH TOGETHER,* c8.95. This is the first English translation of the leading German manual on natural childbirth. The author is one of the leaders in the movement in Europe. She has organized her presentation into six graded lessons which are designed to aid the mother-to-be in developing the capacity to stay awake, aware, and in optimal control of her body during labor and childbirth. Photographs and line drawings illustrate the exercises and some of the physiology, and there are a series of color photographs of an actual birth. Many case histories are included. All in all, this is an excellent work which complements the currently available works on the Lamaze method. Bibliography, 139pp. Sea 75

MYLES, MARGARET. *TEXTBOOK FOR MIDWIVES,* 17.65. This is the most comprehensive treatment of midwifery we can imagine. This new edition (the eighth) has been thoroughly revised and updated to ensure adequate presentation of modern thought and practice. It is also profusely illustrated with technical and more general material. The material is British but it can be applied to the American situation without any difficulty. 848pp. Lon 74

NILSSON, LENNART. *A CHILD IS BORN,* 5.95. A collection of incredible photographs which given an artistic as well as an accurate and realistic picture of a human being's physical development from the moment of conception until birth. Here, step-by-step, you can follow the stages of fetal development: when the different organs are formed, when the heart begins to beat, when the arms and legs begin to move, etc. In this way the new life, which takes shape hidden from the world, becomes vivid and more easily perceived as a new and independent individual. Oversize, with many full color photographs. Index, 160pp. Del 66

NOBLE, ELIZABETH. *ESSENTIAL EXERCISES FOR THE CHILD-*

BEARING YEAR, 4.95. Ms. Noble is an Australian physical therapist specializing in obstetrics and gynecology. Her exercise program stresses an understanding of the biomechanics of the entire maternity cycle and the rationale for, and against, certain exercises. She shows how to recognize weakness and dysfunction and offers therapeutic exercises for conditions arising from the burdens of pregnancy on the average woman. Post-partum restoration is also discussed. Line drawings illustrate the text and illustrated, one page summaries of prenatal, post-partum, and Caesarean exercises provide handy references. Annotated bibliography and list of resources, index, 8"x9¼", 192pp. HMC 76

NULL, GARY and STEVE. *SUCCESSFUL PREGNANCY*, 1.50. Suggestions on diet and on things to watch out for and take care of during the period of pregnancy. The presentation is often overly detailed and scattered—but there is material here that is not available elsewhere. The Nulls are good researchers, and the book is filled with tables, charts, and the latest medical information. Notes, index, 208pp. Pyr 76

ROSEN, MORTIMER. *IN THE BEGINNING*, 3.95. A nontechnical study of the development of intelligence and the nervous system during the months between conception and birth. Illustrations, index, 143pp. NAL 75

SALK, LEE. *PREPARING FOR PARENTHOOD*, 1.95. Dr. Salk is the director of pediatric psychology at New York Hospital and professor of pediatrics and psychology at Cornell University Medical College. While Dr. Salk has not been at the forefront of the recent boom in interest in natural childbirth, he is sympathetic to its main tenets. This is a useful guide which offers practical suggestions on preparing psychologically and physically for parenthood. Index, 211pp. Ban 74

SCIENCE OF LIFE BOOKS. *BEFORE AND AFTER BABY COMES*, 1.35. Details a diet rich in vitamins and minerals for building up the health of expectant mothers and their babies. 62pp. SLB 75

SOUSA, MARION. *CHILDBIRTH AT HOME*, 2.25. This is the most comprehensive, unified manual on childbirth at home yet produced. The author provides practical information on how to prepare for the home birth. Recommended prenatal nutrition, exercises, and classes are discussed along with descriptions of equipment and bedding. Ms. Sousa also tells how to recruit experienced medical supervision in the case of an emergency. Bibliography, notes, index, 221pp. Ban 76

THOMPSON, JUDI. *HEALTHY PREGNANCY THE YOGA WAY,* 3.95. Judi Thompson is a yoga teacher and a mother of four. She believes that "Pregnancy is the perfect time in which to practice Yoga. These slow-motion exercises. . .relieve tension, strengthen and stimulate vital muscles, organs, and glands, and conserve rather than dissipate energy. Through the performance of Yogasanas, muscles are stretched, strengthened, and firmed while the joints utilized in the birth process become flexible. There is no strain or enervating exercise involved in performing the Asanas." This is an excellent, fully illustrated manual which includes a philosophical discussion and step-by-step instructions. There are also chapters on special problems and on post-natal asanas. Photographs, 7"x10", 157pp. Dou 77

URBANOWSKI, FERRIS. *YOGA FOR NEW PARENTS,* 6.95. A personal portrayal of the author's experience of birth and its aftermath. The photographs of Ms. Urbanowski while pregnant do not show her exercising, which is a pity. The exercises are all demonstrated in a non-pregnant state. The photographs are not terribly clear, but the accompanying instructions are quite complete. The many photographs all have captions stating the author's philosophy. Bibliography, 9½"x8½", 126pp. H&R 75

WALTON, VICKI. *HAVE IT YOUR WAY,* 5.95. This is an overview of pregnancy, labor, and post-partum care which includes chapters on methods of childbirth preparation, choosing childbirth education classes, choosing health care, and choosing a hospital and a physician. There's also an in depth examination of labor and a number of case histories. The author has worked with the traditional system and she stresses the alternatives available in the hospital childbirth experience. The book has a nice tone and covers material not readily available elsewhere. Illustrations, glossary, index, 289pp. Php 76

WARD, CHARLOTTE and FRED. *THE HOME BIRTH BOOK,* 6.95. A beautifully illustrated book which explores the home birth alternative in all its dimensions: personal, medical, psychological, sociological, and historical. A sensitive essay by Ms. Ward accompanied by excellent photographs by her husband describes the actual home birth experience of the Ward family. Two doctors discuss the questions most frequently asked by couples considering home birth. Psychologists point out the advantages of home birth for the child and the child's family. There's also a sociological survey and interviews with typical home birth families. 7"x10", 149pp. INS 76

TANZER, DEBORAH and JEAN BLOCK. *WHY NATURAL CHILDBIRTH?* 3.95. To find out if natural childbirth is a better way to have children, Dr. Tanzer conducted a pioneering study of the psychological impact of childbirth. Through a series of tests and interviews, she studied two groups of women: one using conventional medication and a conventional approach, the other using the techniques of natural childbirth. She reports the results of her study here. The many cases cited overwhelmingly show the psychological benefits of the natural approach. Notes, index, 312pp. ScB 72

WEINER, JOAN and J. GLICK. *A MOTHERHOOD BOOK*, 1.95. A first person narrative of two young mothers and their experiences and thoughts about giving birth and the months afterward. Topics include: *Motherhood as a Possibility, Pregnancy, Giving Birth and Coming Down, Motherhood as a Physical Reality, Motherhood as a Psychic Reality.* The material is vividly written and should be illuminating and helpful to all mothers-to-be. Annotated bibliography, index, 131pp. McM 74

WHITE, GREGORY. *EMERGENCY CHILDBIRTH: A MANUAL,* 4.50. This is an excellent manual on emergency childbirth. All the essentials are succinctly covered under the following main topics: pregnancy and labor, delivery of the baby, unusual deliveries, hemorrhage, special care required by some babies, and pregnancy, labor, or delivery which is complicated by illness or accidental injuries. An especially useful section contains condensed instructions for emergency use, arranged for quick reference. This book is very well regarded and it has been very hard to get, so we are glad to make it more generally available. Spiral bound, 63pp. PTF 58

WRIGHT, ERNA. *THE NEW CHILDBIRTH,* 1.95. Ms. Wright is an authority on the Lamaze birth technique. Here she deals thoroughly with Lamaze preparation and birth. The explanations and diagrams

are complete, and the chapter on *The Necessary Father* is excellent.
Index, 205pp. S&S 67

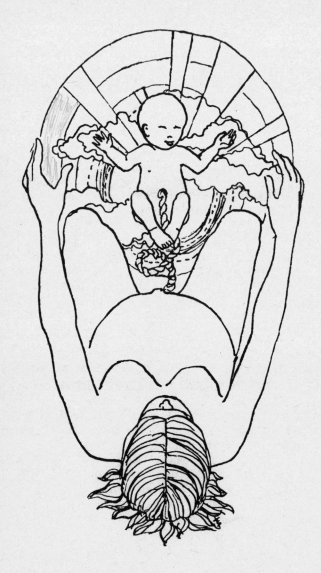

Nutrition

Nature, the transformation of energy from one form to another, universally expresses itself in three specific patterns. The first of such patterns swirls in *rotary* motion, evident in the movement of the atom, the human cell, the planets, our entire solar system, and all ordered movements of swirling spheres, evolving on the cosmic scale as a grand replica of the parent atom. The second of such patterns moves in *spirals,* evident in the mysterious helix of the chromosomes which stores the genetic blueprint for *each* cell in *each* cellular nucleus of the human body, evident in whirlpools swirling in great bodies of water, in the violent cone of a tornado sweeping across a midwestern plain, or in the fiery vortex that rises from a missile site at the moment of launching. Still a third pattern of energy thrusts itself *forward* to initiate some dramatic, evolutionary step in the universe: the passionate emission of sperm, the delicate growth of an embryo's spine, the rapid transportation of blood through the vascular system, or the overwhelming bolt of an electric current through an illumined skyscraper.

To give these patterns their free range of expression, nature takes the energy assembled in one form, disassembles it into the particles that supplied the form's energy, and reassembles them into a new form. When the new form follows closely upon the old, we readily recognize the transitory nature of the disassembling period. But when in some cases we cannot perceive any emerging new form, we specify the disassembling period as death. Death, for most investigators, declares an end to the old form—Period!

327

But as a footnote, it reflects proportionately our scientific incapacity to measure that further movement of the energy released from the old form.

Yet out of the myriad changes of energy patterns that *are* measurable in the universe, there is one grouping of transformations to which many of us lately are giving more thought and attention. In fact, people have currently become interested in their bodies as fields of energy transformations, discovering how to observe more intelligently the conditions that nature has imposed upon us for building and maintaining that constant flow of energy exchange within us.

In our bodies, the movements of energy which we spoke of—rotary, spiral, and forward—present the evidence of Nature at work disassembling the particles of one life form and reassembling them into another. The laws governing this transformation constitute the science of nutrition, a science that begins with food, a life form without, which becomes the cell, the life form within.

Nature's transformation of food into cells begins with the first stage of nutrient release, *ingestion*. Ingestion consists simply of thoroughly masticating and swallowing the food in order to trigger the second stage of release, *digestion*.

Digestion is the process whereby our body starts actually to transform the food energy by breaking down the protein, fat, and carbohydrate into micronutrient particles that become the building blocks of our body's mass and energy. The digestive processes reduce the protein foods to their *amino acids* and *nucleic acids*. They reduce the fat to *fatty acids*, and the carbohydrates to *glucose* or blood sugar. The forms of amino and nucleic acids, fatty acids, and glucose are simple enough to be carried through the body's elaborate transport system to the cell.

To feed the cell, to maintain its life and well-being, is the only reason we eat. To better understand the cell as a unit of life, we can compare it to one of its larger, more familiar analogues, the egg. The egg, we know, consists of a circular yolk engulfed in a clear liquid called albumen. Both the yolk and the albumen are encased by a brittle wall called the shell. Each cell in the human body is broadly similar to the parts of the egg. The yolk is the cell's nucleus; the albumen is the protoplasm; and the "shell" holding it all together is. . .the cell wall.

So much for the general similarities. Let's now look at some of the cell's specific differences. Our cell wall, of course, is not a brittle calcium composition like the egg shell. Imagine, rather, a network of interlacing strands, much like a seamless nylon stocking, but not quite. Instead of nylon, the netlike composition is a mixture of fat (lipid) and protein. Only through the pores of this lipoprotein membrane can the cell obtain its nutrition. The cell wall must therefore be kept permeable so that the amino and nucleic acids, the fatty acids, and the glucose (a bead of liquid sugar) can pass through. How these micronutrients are driven in their forward movement through the body's elaborate transport system to accomplish their osmotic passage into the rotating energy of the cell, and how the cell continues the transformation is called *metabolism*. Metabolism, the creation of mass and energy out of the simplest micronutrients, is what our physical preconscious life is all about.

Picture now, at the threshold of the cell wall, the arrival of the amino and nucleic acids from food protein, the fatty acids from food fat, and the glucose from food carbohydrate. The first task of these nutrients is to nourish the cell wall. This is the job of certain amino and fatty acids. They combine and form a new mass called lipoprotein. As lipoprotein they repair and strengthen, or if necessary, completely rebuild a cell wall. Next, the remainder of the fatty acids and the glucose pass osmotically through the pores of the cell wall to be oxidized, i.e., burned up, in the protoplasm for energy. This naturally requires oxygen which enters the cell in the same manner as the other nutrients, through the porous lipoprotein wall. This passage of oxygen is called *respiration*.

But how does the cell dispose of the waste produced by its oxidations? There appears in the protoplasm a group of inverted bubbles called vacuoles. Into these vacuoles, the cell deposits the waste materials resulting from the oxidation of glucose and fatty acids. Since the cell is in continual movement due to the property of latent heat characterizing the rotary movement of spheroid forms, the desultory movement of the vacuoles eventually brings them to the edge of the cell wall, and they pass through its pores into the bloodstream. This ejection of waste material is called *excretion*.

No cell can maintain its metabolic cycle of metabolism, respiration, oxidation, and excretion indefinitely. The cell must "die" so that other transformations of energy may continue on the broader, more inclusive planetary scale. The life cycle of a healthy cell is normally 120 days. After 120 days, the old cell decomposes and a duplicate cell takes its place. Its precise structure is due to the blueprint stored in the preceding nucleus and transmitted to the new nucleus so exact duplication can occur. Each nucleus, then, must be nourished with nucleic acid from food protein in order to sustain, by means of a genetic code, the plan for the structure of the entire body. The genetic code is an arrangement of permanent atoms transferred from cell lifetime to cell lifetime to maintain the unity and integrity of each cell. This is the process of cell *reproduction*.

And so we have the complete cycle of transformation: First, *ingestion*, whereby food nutrients, protein, fats, and carbohydrates are masticated and swallowed. Second, *digestion*, whereby these nutrients are broken down into amino and nucleic acids, fatty acids, and glucose. Third, *metabolism*, whereby the process of all cell nutrition begins with certain amino and fatty acids combining to make the cell wall. Fourth, *respiration*, the continuation of metabolism, whereby oxygen is brought into the cell so that fatty acids and glucose may undergo oxidation to make heat and energy. Fifth, *excretion,* the conclusion of metabolism, whereby the waste products of oxidation are dumped into vacuoles and floated out of the cell. Sixth, *reproduction,* whereby the nucleic acids which entered the nucleus in the metabolic cycle transmit the genetic blueprint from one cellular lifetime to another.

—from **Nutrition and Your Body** by Benjamin Colimore and Sarah Stewart Colimore

ADAMS, RUTH. *EATING IN EDEN,* 1.95. A survey of the dietary habits of a variety of so-called primitive societies combined with an examination of how the people kept so healthy. Ms. Adams is a good reporter and she writes in a lively manner. Bibliography, index, 196pp. Lar 76

ADAMS, RUTH and FRANK MURRAY. *BEVERAGES,* 1.95. The subtitle of this book—*All You Should Know for Your Health and Well Being*—sums up the contents as well as we can. The information seems to be solidly based on research and many tables and quotations are included. Index, 286pp. Lar 76

ADAMS, RUTH and FRANK MURRAY. *THE GOOD SEEDS, THE RICH GRAINS, THE HARDY NUTS,* 1.50. Written by a pair of prolific (and good) authors on nutritional subjects, this book first gives an up to date review of the evidence against refined carbohydrates that comprise half the average American diet, then goes on to discuss the many natural alternatives, their value and use. Tables, bibliography, index, 250pp. Lar 73

ADAMS, RUTH and FRANK MURRAY. *HEALTH FOODS,* **2.45. This is an excellent introductory book for those who are just getting into natural foods. Forty-eight of the most common foods and food products are discussed and their nutritional benefits analyzed. The information is clearly and succinctly presented. Index, 341pp. Lar 75**

AIROLA, PAAVO. *ARE YOU CONFUSED?* 3.95. Dr. Airola is our favorite naturopathic writer. Trained in Europe, he brings a wide background to all his books. In this one he examines the pros and cons of many issues still debated by nutritionists: high vs. low protein diets, whether to take supplements, the value of milk, how to fast, distilled vs. mineralized water, and much more. An excellent first reader on nutrition which will save you much confusion later. Index, 222pp. HPP 71

AIROLA, PAAVO. *REJUVENATION SECRETS FROM AROUND THE WORLD,* 3.25. *To make this book as short and concise as possible, I will not waste your time by describing various unproven theories, or controversial treatments and drugs. I will report to you only what is absolutely certain, solidly proven, and scientifically confirmed—or, as the title promises, I will reveal to you rejuvenation secrets from around the world THAT WORK.* —from the introduction. 128pp. HPP 74

AIROLA, PAAVO. *STOP HAIR LOSS,* 2.00. Airola reports on a Swedish discovery that purports to stop hair loss and aid new growth, even in advanced cases of baldness. 32pp. HPP 65

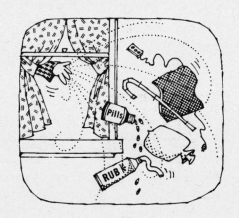

BIELER, HENRY. *DR. BIELER'S NATURAL WAY TO SEXUAL HEALTH,* 1.50. This book contains Dr. Bieler's views about health in general, with reference to sexual functions in particular. He believes that frigidity and impotence are frequently due to a high sugar, junk food diet and reflect high toxicity in the body. Maybe an interest in sex will lead people to read this book where they will probably learn more about general health and nutrition than they will about sex. 232pp. Ban 72

BIELER, HENRY. *FOOD IS YOUR BEST MEDICINE,* 1.95. In more than fifty years of practice, Dr. Bieler has had great experience with nutritional therapy. He believes disease is caused by toxemia which results in cellular impairment, that most use of drugs is harmful, and therefore that food is your best medicine. All readers might not go all the way with Dr. Bieler but there is a lot in here to learn about human physiology. The book has been very popular; unfortunately the print in the paperback edition is small and hard to read. Index, 236pp. RaH 65

BIRCHER-BENNER, M. *CHILDREN'S DIET,* 1.45. First published in 1935, this book sets out many of Dr. Bircher-Benner's ideas as applied to children. After discussing the deterioration of our civilized diet, he considers the relationship of diet and disease, discusses the particular problems of childhood, and then gives his recommendations as to what should and should not be given to children. He places great importance on raw foods but doesn't rely on these exclusively. These ideas have been more popular in Europe than here. We find much of value in them. 66pp. Dan 64

BIRCHER-BENNER, M. *EATING YOUR WAY TO HEALTH,* 1.95. This is primarily a cookbook with introductory material about the diet utilized over many years at the Bircher-Benner Clinic in Switzerland which avoids stimulants, meat or alcohol. To many, Dr. Bircher-Benner is best known as the inventor of *muesli,* that delicious cereal of grains, fruits and nuts. He believes that the high quality of food energy obtained from the freshest possible food as near as possible to its living state is of vital importance. Index, 341pp. Vik 61

BIRCHER-BENNER, M., et al. *SALT-FREE NUTRITION,* 2.75. Written by the staff of the Bircher-Benner Clinic, this is one of fifteen guides to diet for particular purposes. A fifteen-page discussion of salt metabolism and conditions requiring a salt free diet is followed by extensive diet suggestions and recipes. 132pp. Nas 67

CHEN, PHILIP. *SOYBEANS FOR HEALTH AND LONGER LIFE,* 1.50. This work goes beyond the usual books extolling the virtues of one food or another. Invaluable to any homesteader wishing to make the most of this remarkable food, it has directions for growing and storing soybeans, and making milk, curd and sauce, as well as many recipes. Bibliography, index, 178pp. Kea 73

CLARK, LINDA. *BE SLIM AND HEALTHY,* 1.50. Linda Clark is a prolific nutrition writer with a large following. This little book contains a wealth of good nutritional advice from the viewpoint of one who wants to reduce or stay slim. An important feature is her "Stop and Go Carbohydrate Computer," which simplifies low carbohydrate dieting. You merely look up each item, keep your intake to 60 grams, and favor the nutritional ones marked "go" and avoid those marked "stop." 161pp. Kea 72

CLARK, LINDA. *GO, STOP CARBOHYDRATE COMPUTER,* .95. A convenient pocket edition of the tables found in **Be Slim and Healthy.** 46pp. Kea 73

CLARK, LINDA. *KNOW YOUR NUTRITION,* 3.50. This is the most comprehensive of the recent Linda Clark books, adapted from the nutrition course that she ran in **Let's Live Magazine.** It deals primarily with the various vitamins and minerals, their effects, how and why to take them, and much else. Ms. Clark writes in a popular, easy to read manner and is generally well balanced. She does, however, frequently quote other popular writers such as Adelle Davis, rather than original sources. Index, 250pp. Kea 73

CLARK, LINDA. *LIGHT ON YOUR HEALTH PROBLEMS,* 1.50. Questions and answers, topically arranged, from Ms. Clark's column in **Let's Live Magazine.** 127pp. Kea 72

CLARK, LINDA. *STAY YOUNG LONGER,* 1.50. A well researched collection of nutritional suggestions for the aging, accompanied by a variety of related hints and guidelines. Notes, index, 396pp. Pyr 61

COLIMORE, BENJAMIN and SARAH. *NUTRITION AND YOUR BODY,* 4.95. Most nutrition books repeat the same information about what vitamins and minerals do and why they are important. That's all in here. But the refreshing thing about this book is that it gives a very good and clear presentation of the anatomy and physiology involved, so that if you are not technically trained you'll get a better understanding of what it's all about by reading this book than most others. Illustrated with photographs and line drawings that help explain the text. The book also contains various food tables, technical references, and a bibliography. Recommended. Index, 220pp. NAP 74

DAVIS, ADELLE. *LET'S EAT RIGHT TO KEEP FIT,* 2.25. The late Adelle Davis is so well known as to require no introduction here. This is her basic book which contains a great deal of useful information but is somewhat scattered and difficult to comprehend easily. It should not be read as a first book on nutrition—many people have unfortunately put off learning the basics of good nutrition after getting bogged down halfway through this book. Includes tables of food composition and an excellent index. 334pp. NAL 70

DAVIS, ADELLE. *LET'S HAVE HEALTHY CHILDREN,* 1.95. Extensively revised from the original edition, this was the last of the Davis books to come out in paperback. (It's a good practice to read the most recent editions of the Davis books, since she changed her views on a number of topics as new studies came to her attention.) This book should be read by all mothers-to-be and re-read as the children grow. It has advice on prenatal nutrition, how to have an easier delivery, and care and feeding of the child, as well as tables of food composition and an excellent index. 381pp. NAL 72

DAVIS, ADELLE. *YOU CAN GET WELL,* 2.25. This looks like a reprint of a pamphlet which Ms. Davis wrote years ago. There's no way to know the original date for sure. Half the book is devoted to short suggestions for treating a variety of ailments and the other half contains a table of food analysis which gives the calories, vitamins, and minerals of 287 foods. Index, 91pp. Lus 75

DOYLE, RODGER and JAMES REDDING. *THE COMPLETE FOOD HANDBOOK,* 5.95. This is an excellent reference book in which over 200 types of food are thoroughly evaluated in terms of nutritive value, processing effects, chemical additives, and environmental contaminants. Virtually all types of cereals, fruits, vegetables, dairy products, meats, poultry, fish, beverages, sweets, fats, and oils are discussed in detail. The authors also survey the role in health and disease of such controversial subjects as dietary fiber, fat, cholesterol, sugar, additives, vitamins, and organic food. The basic information is well organized and presented in a readable way. Glossary, bibliography, notes, index, 308pp. Grv 76

ELWOOD, CATHERINE. *FEEL LIKE A MILLION,* 1.95. We have long viewed this as one of the best beginning books on nutrition. The first section explains the various nutrients, the second section discusses health problems and their relation to nutrition, and the final section covers various foods and the fundamentals of good diet. There is an excellent chapter on the food value of sprouts and how to make them. Ms. Elwood is a trained nutritionist who also has the facility to write simply. Tables, bibliography, index, 366pp. S&S 56

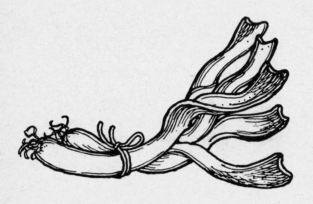

Food Pollution

First, the good news: The federal government, mainly the Food and Drug Administration of the Department of Health, Education and Welfare and to a lesser extent the U.S. Department of Agriculture, is empowered to keep your food safe for consumption and free of dangerous chemicals. Now the bad news: They do nothing of the kind. As a result our food supply is permeated with chemicals of dubious safety.

Such chemical foods are now quite familiar to you if you just glance at labels. You may have even become inured to the lists that run on like endless entries in a chemical dictionary. What can it matter? The food may taste good. It's convenient. And surely, you reason, your government would not permit you and 210 million others to eat it if it weren't safe.

But also—what about peanut butter and hot dogs and milk and bacon and potatoes and corn and eggs and beef? These are not mere food analogues concocted in a laboratory. These are real foods which you should be able to depend on not to be harmful. These are staples, basic foods, life-sustaining nutrients that you and your family eat every day.

These foods, too, are often not safe. Some knowledgeable scientists have given up eating hot dogs, bacon, ham, sausages, anything containing the chemical nitrite, after seeing how this chemical, interacting with others, has left laboratory animals grotesquely deformed with cancers. Peanuts, as well as peanut butter, corn, and other grains that go into bread and beer sometimes are contaminated with aflatoxin (a natural chemical produced by certain molds), one of the most potent cancer-causing agents ever discovered. Eggs and chickens may contains PCBs, industrial chemicals that have caused poisonings in Japan. Many foods, especially carbonated noncola beverages and gelatins, are infused with a red dye that in animals has caused birth defects and killed unborn fetuses. Monosodium glutamate (MSG) is still widely used in all kinds of processed foods, though it has been shown to cause brain damage in infant animals. Blighted potatoes have been implicated in birth defects such as spinal and head malformations. And ad infinitum—or, more appropriately, ad nauseam.

That things are this bad is not something your government is officially likely to tell you. There is not likely to be a press release from the FDA's public information office tomorrow saying: *Nothing's left that's fit to eat,* or *Whole population being slowly poisoned.* Nor is an official likely to suggest slapping a warning label on foods similar to that familiar to cigarette smokers: *Eating May Be Hazardous to Your Health.* After all, in most cases it was the government that allowed things to get into such a sorry state, and it does have a self-protective stake in the affair.

Yet, imagine how much easier it would be if the government would just out with the truth. It would end all that

337

intrigue, all the time-consuming hard work trying to cover up mistakes, juggling scientific data to make it come out right, always assuming a defensive posture, evading responsibility, playing footsie with the industry, assuring everyone that no matter what a few die-hard scientists say and do, there is no need for concern, that our food is the safest in the world and there's not a shred of evidence that anyone has ever been harmed by eating an additive.

Unfortunately, our food is not the safest in the world; at least, some other countries think it isn't. Sweden, for example, refused to import U.S. beef that had been raised on feed containing diethylstilbestrol (DES), a growth-promoting hormone known to cause cancer. Twenty-one nations, in fact, banned DES in livestock before this country got around to banning it in 1973 after much delay. Norway has outlawed the use of nitrites in certain food. Great Britain prohibited brominated vegetable oils in 1970 (they're still allowed here). In general the United States has a very relaxed attitude toward chemicals in foods compared with other countries, which follow a much more conservative policy. The Soviet Union is especially strict, allowing only a minimum of chemicals in food and quickly banning those found to be potentially harmful.

Notwithstanding the FDA's proclamations to the contrary, all is not right with our food supply and we had best do something about it. What your government is not telling you can hurt you, and unless there is public pressure the FDA and the USDA will not be swayed from a course they are now taking that in the future will expose us to even more potential danger—without our knowledge or consent.—from **Eating May Be Hazardous to Your Health** by Jacqueline Verrett and Jean Carper

BANIK, ALLEN. *YOUR WATER AND YOUR HEALTH,* 1.25. Dr. Banik is the foremost advocate of distilled water for health. He reviews the arguments that soft water is associated with heart disease, suggesting the problem is not lack of minerals but other pollutants that soft water dissolves out of the pipes. If you want to get a home still, this is the book for you. Bibliography, 126pp. Kea 74

CALDWELL, GLADYS and PHILIP ZANFAGNA. *FLUORIDA-TION AND TRUTH DECAY,* 3.50. *Fifteen years of total involvement in viewing the American fluoridation scene has convinced me that fluoridation is the most disastrous and costly consumer fraud of this polluted century. . . .The purpose of this book is to tell you the truth about fluoridation, and in doing so we take you behind the scenes to show you that the fertilizer factories are unable to control or dispose of their deadly fluoride, to show you the tank truck labeled "Danger Corrosive Acid" unloading its fluoride garbage into the nation's drinking water under the guise of a public health program, and to reveal how dangerous fluoridation is to your health.*—from the introduction. This is a very well documented study. 301pp. Top 74

CLARK, LINDA. *ARE YOU RADIOACTIVE?* 1.25. Ms. Clark discusses radioactivity from x-rays, luminous dials, food irradiation, microwave ovens, fluorescent lights, color television, microwave towers, and nuclear plants, its effects on our bodies, and what foods or remedies can be taken to mitigate these effects. Bibliography, 128pp. Pyr 74

GARRISON, OMAR. *THE DICTOCRAT'S ATTACK ON HEALTH FOODS AND VITAMINS,* .95. Don't read this book if you don't want to be outraged or if you wish to preserve your faith in the goodness and disinterest of the federal officials who protect us from "nutritional nonsense." It documents the fact that many official acts have been motivated by economic, political, and personal considerations rather than by concern for consumer protection, discusses the vendettas against Carlton Fredericks, Adelle Davis, Rachel Carson and others, and shows the connections between the U.S. agencies, big food business, and large universities. 340pp. Arc 70

GRANT, DORIS. *RECIPE FOR SURVIVAL,* 3.95. Doris Grant is a popular English writer on health topics. By exploring subjects

339

such as environmental contaminants of air, water and food, Ms. Grant demonstrates how modern man's mode of life is related to modern diseases, and how we can help ourselves to reduce the damage. Particularly interesting data on bread. While written for an English audience, most of the information translates well to our society. 224pp. Kea 73

HALL, ROSS. *FOOD FOR NOUGHT—THE DECLINE IN NUTRI-TION,* 3.95. A biochemist attacks the increased use of chemicals to produce larger crops, fatter livestock, and better textured, tenderer flavor—not because the chemicals are dangerous in themselves (although they often are) but because they destroy basic nutritional values. A well documented technical survey, geared toward awakening the general public. Glossary, notes, index, 324pp. RaH 76

HIGHTOWER, JIM. *EAT YOUR HEART OUT,* 1.95. This is an important book which reveals how the food we buy in the supermarkets is controlled in price and quality by huge conglomerates who bleed the helpless consumer dry while reaping exorbitant profits for themselves. This book documents just how high the costs are, and why they are getting higher. It is subtitled *How Food Profiteers Victimize the Consumer* and Hightower presents a good case backing up his claims. It's a technical study, but one that is well worth reading. Extensive notes, index, 294pp. RaH 75

HUNTER, BEATRICE. *CONSUMER BEWARE,* 3.95. Fifteen years ago, Beatrice Trum Hunter received an award from the Friends of Nature for her work in educating the public to the dangers of pesticides. She is the Rachel Carson of today. This book says it all and as well as anybody has said it. With a wealth of detail about the machinations of industry and the FDA, this book tells you just what you can expect to find in your supermarket foods. If this doesn't drive you to your local natural foods store, we don't know what will. Well documented with fifty pages of notes. Recommended. Index, 431pp. S&S 71

HUNTER, BEATRICE. *FOOD ADDITIVES AND YOUR HEALTH,* 1.25. Which food additives are dangerous, which are not? This slim book (not as comprehensive as Jacobson's) provides some of the answers. Slip it in your purse when you go to the supermarket and start reading labels. Bibliography, index, 116pp. Kea 72

HUNTER, BEATRICE. *THE MIRAGE OF SAFETY,* c9.95. Subtitled *Food Additives and Federal Policy,* Ms. Hunter's latest book describes how safety tests for food additives are conducted and why present methods are inadequate. Physicians are reporting adverse effects of specific additives on their patients and new startling information about the hazards of additives is being revealed in various basic research projects. All these are documented by Ms. Hunter along with suggestions about what can be done at both the policy level and the personal level. Bibliography, index, 192pp. Scr 75

JACOBSON, MICHAEL. *EATER'S DIGEST,* 2.50. This is the best collection of data on food additives we have seen. Reasoned, balanced, and scientifically based, Dr. Jacobson tells us what to beware of and what is all right. Over a hundred additives, good and bad, are carefully discussed in terms of usage, history, and relevant experimental data. Another very useful section gives many of the FDA's food standards which state what foods may or must contain which do not have to be listed on labels. Read the standards for bread and ice cream and you'll never feel the same about them again. Appendices include a list of additives that have been banned, much of the GRAS (generally recognized as safe) list, chemical formulas and an excellent glossary of terms. Bibliography, index, 260pp. Dou 72

LAPPE, FRANCES MOORE and JOSEPH COLLINS. *FOOD FIRST: BEYOND THE MYTH OF SCARCITY,* c12.95. The authors direct the Institute on Food and Development Policy in San Francisco and Ms. Lappe is the author of **Diet for a Small Planet.** This book is written in a question and answer format. The authors tackle certain long held assumptions and demonstrate how these have actually impeded efforts to end starvation. The questions center around the following themes: Are there truly too many mouths to feed? Why can mechanized farming be both inefficient and harmful? Have pesticides actually created scarcities? Who has really profited from the "green revolution"—and how has it been responsible for famine in India and Africa? This is an important new book. Bibliography, notes, index, 448pp. HMC 77

LERZA, CATHERINE and MICHAEL JACOBSON, eds. *FOOD FOR PEOPLE, NOT FOR PROFIT,* 1.95. Prepared for Food Day, 1975, this is a complete, up to date fact book including everything you want to know about the food crisis and then some. Contains fifty-four articles, organized around food production, costs, nutrition, world food, food and the poor, the government and the food industry. If you have to write a speech or an article, or simply want to be a well informed citizen about the food problem from all angles, this is your book. Also contains a chapter on action ideas for the activists, and a number of useful appendices including excellent notes and other sources of further information and action. 466pp. RaH 75

MARINE, GENE and JUDITH VAN ALLEN. *FOOD POLLUTION: THE VIOLATION OF OUR INNER ECOLOGY,* 2.95. Written by two reporters who claim not to be food freaks, this book runs through all the usual information about what the greedy manufacturers are doing to our food and what the government isn't doing about it. An interesting, well documented narrative. As they say in the preface: *If you know what this book tells you, and choose white bread and poison-riddled food, you are an adult making a free choice. If you eat it because you don't know any better, or cannot afford better, you are a victim.* Index, 385pp. HRW 72

NICHOLS, JOE and JAMES PRESLEY. *PLEASE DOCTOR, DO SOMETHING!* c6.95. Dr. Nichols, longtime president of the Natural Foods Associates, tells how he became involved in the natural foods movement and how he discovered the importance of a fertile, living soil. He discusses how a farmer can restore and maintain the fertility of his soil without using cancer causing chemicals and also gives the backyard gardener many hints. In the process Dr. Nichols relates many case histories and discusses natural foods and the importance of specific nutrients for healthful living. Bibliography, index, 197pp. DAC 72

NULL, GARY. *BODY POLLUTION,* c5.95. Another book on the additives and other substances we put into our bodies—polluting our vital systems and destroying our health. Includes an alternative program of natural nutrition. Gary Null is a young health food store owner, health food magazine publisher, and, with his staff of research assistants, a prolific writer. His books are readable compilations of material in the general literature, sometimes, however, showing evidence of hasty putting together without a consistent point of view. Index, 214pp. Arc 73

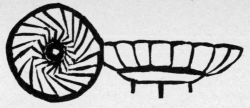

ROBBINS, WILLIAM. *AMERICAN FOOD SCANDAL,* 3.50. *William Robbins carefully documents and forcefully presents the facts about agribusiness giants and huge food companies—they are not more efficient at farming and processing; they're more efficient at farming us, the taxpayers and consumers.*—Former Sen. Fred Harris. Index, 280pp. Mor 74

SCHROEDER, HENRY. *THE POISONS AROUND US,* c10.00. Mankind has, throughout time, seen fit to dig up metals from deposits in the earth and scatter them over the face of the globe. That some of them are toxic has worried him little in the past. But now he is slowly becoming concerned. In this book one of the world's foremost authorities on the relations of metals to human health discusses metals and other elements as pollutants and as substances beneficial to life. He places the industrial metals and elements to which man is exposed today in their proper perspective, and explains which are toxic, which are necessary, and which are inert. His findings are based on experimental evidence amassed in studies and the book is written in nontechnical language. Bibliography, notes, index, 146pp. IUP 74

SULLIVAN, GEORGE. *ADDITIVES IN YOUR FOOD,* 1.95. A dictionary of the most common food additives, with a full description of each. Sullivan is a journalist and he has consulted a wide variety of sources. This is the most simplified of the books on additives. 128pp. S&S 76

TAUB, HAROLD. *KEEPING HEALTHY IN A POLLUTED WORLD,* 2.95. Taub is former executive editor of **Prevention.** In this book he not only tells us about all the dangers of our polluted environment, but goes on to prescribe practical measures by which we can defend ourselves. These include nutritional programs, intelligent use of vitamin supplements, special exercises, and other simple modifications of our way of life that can increase our chances of survival. Bibliography, index, 246pp. Vik 74

VERRETT, JACQUELINE and JEAN CARPER. *EATING MAY BE HAZARDOUS TO YOUR HEALTH,* 2.95. *This is a soberly gripping book by a courageous Food and Drug Administration scientist and a lucid consumer writer. The story they tell about the silent violence in your food—how it got there and the FDA's abysmal lack of courage to make the food companies obey the law—makes you want to do something about it. As* **Eating May Be Hazardous to Your Health** *points out, you can help do it as a tough and active citizen. The choice is clear: if consumers don't control their government, the food industry will.*—Ralph Nader. Dr. Verrett is the scientist who first blew the whistle on cyclamates. Since she has been a biochemical researcher within the FDA for over fifteen years, this book is more of an inside expose than most of this genre. Notes, index, 256pp. Dou 74

WERTHEIM, ALFRED. *NATURAL POISONS IN NATURAL FOODS,* c7.95. This book reviews a lot of the ingredients in common natural foods which can be toxic in excessive amounts or under special conditions. A well researched study which is easy to understand. Tables, bibliography, index, 210pp. Stu 74

WESTLAKE, AUBREY. *LIFE THREATENED,* c5.80. Dr. Westlake is a well known British physician who has intensively studied alternative methods of healing and alternative methods of thinking. The concepts in this volume are derived from the work of Rudolf Steiner. *In Part I I have endeavoured to establish that a grave menace confronts us in the indiscriminate. . .use of all these chemical poisons. . . .In Part II I discuss what can be done about it. . . .This resolves itself into two aspects. The first is how to restore the balance between matter and spirit. . . .The second,. . .whether there is any way in which the long-term effects of paratoxic environment can be detected, and can be rectified before irreversible damage has been done, both in the world of nature and in man himself.* Index, 193pp. Wat 67

WINTER, RUTH. *A CONSUMER'S DICTIONARY OF FOOD ADDITIVES,* 3.95. An extremely complete presentation, in dictionary form, which defines, in simple language, all the mysterious ingredients listed on food labels. Ms. Winter is a reliable reporter. Introduction, notes, 235pp. Crn 72

FREDERICKS, CARLTON and HERBERT BAILEY. *FOOD FACTS AND FALLACIES,* 1.75. Carlton Fredericks has a PhD in Public Health Education, and has taught nutrition at NYU and several other universities in addition to teaching over the radio for many years. We find his views eminently sound, anti-establishment of course, but also critical of the health food stores where criticism is needed (and it often is). This book covers a wide range of subjects: supplements, fluoridation, various diseases, aging, mental illness, sex and diet, weight, the FDA and AMA, and much else. Tables, index, 380pp. Arc 65

FREDERICKS, CARLTON. *LOOK YOUNGER, FEEL HEALTHIER,* 2.95. This is Dr. Fredericks' most comprehensive book. He covers gynecological problems, low blood sugar, diabetes, weight control (including sample diets), nutrition for pregnant women, megavitamin therapy, aging, additives, supplements, nutrition for babies, and much more. There is a good chapter on how to shop in a health food store. Individual vitamins and minerals are discussed. A hypoglycemic diet is provided. All in all, a very readable, sometimes mind-boggling book which should increase your alienation from the system but at the same time give you a plethora of good scientific facts with which to defend yourself and your health. Recommended. Formerly entitled *Eating Right For You.* Index, 310pp. G&D 72

FRIEDLANDER, BARBARA. *THE VEGETABLE, FRUIT AND NUT BOOK,* 4.95. A beautifully illustrated encyclopedic compendium of almost every vegetable, fruit, and nut in North America and Europe. Includes facts, myths, charts, and recipes. 300pp. G&D 74

FRYER, LEE and ANNETTE DICKINSON. *DICTIONARY OF FOOD SUPPLEMENTS,* 5.95. This dictionary defines vitamins, minerals, whole foods, dietary foods, oils, proteins, and cosmetics, plus words and phrases commonly used to describe these various food supplements. It also has information about the origin and use of a variety of foods. It is cross-referenced and illustrated and contains a sampling of other information about general nutrition. Index, 119pp. MCh 75

GREGORY, DICK. *DICK GREGORY'S NATURAL DIET FOR FOLKS WHO EAT: COOKIN' WITH MOTHER NATURE,* 1.75. "An introduction to natural foods written with an eye to good health and an ear for the witty line. Even for those not ready to replace sirloin with soy bean (economic considerations notwithstanding), Gregory's discourse on the typical mistreatment of the digestive tract should be informative—it certainly is amusing. There are sections on Gregory's various fasts (with how to hints for the interested), suggested diets for putting on and taking off weight, and even a discussion of natural food substitutes (fruit and vegetable juices) for your favorite alcoholic concoction. Good fun and a good guide for those who feel they are what they eat."—*New York Times*. A popular book. Bibliography, index, 171pp. H&R 73

HALSELL, GRACE. *LOS VIEJOS*, c6.95. Ms. Halsell spent some time in a small, isolated mountain village in Ecuador. She lived with the villagers and acted as interpreter and assistant for a team of American health experts who came to study the people and evaluate the reasons for their unusual longevity (many live to 132). In this book Ms. Halsell examines these doctors' observations and discusses the lifestyle of *los viejos* and their philosophy of life. Index, 186pp. Rod 76

HARRIS, BEN CHARLES. *KITCHEN MEDICINES*, .95. *The more one studies the therapeutic values of our everyday Nature-all foods, the more will he understand that these foods become the healing agent of most, if not all, organic ailments. Proper selection and balance of organically grown vegetables and fruits, plus proper eating and hygienic habits, become the required fraction of prevention of such disorders.* From allspice to wheat, this book collects a wealth of data, both scientific and traditional, about the medicinal value of the common foods we eat. Interesting reading as well as a useful reference work. Bibliography, indices of diseases and symptoms, 174pp. S&S 61

HAUSCHKA, RUDOLF. *NUTRITION,* 10.50. Dr. Hauschka, a follower of Rudolf Steiner, based this book on many years of research at the Clinical-Therapeutic Institute in Arlsheim, Switzerland. It is a serious, important, and difficult book, of interest to those who wish to explore the effects of cosmic forces on nutrition. It represents a scientific study of the proposition that matter is merely a solidification of a spiritual process and that, where life is involved, the mechanical and chemical laws covering the mineral kingdom are insufficient to explain what happens. Not recommended for general readers but if you are into bio-dynamic gardening or anthroposophy, you will find a great deal to ponder here, going far beyond other nutritional texts. Bibliography, index, 212pp. Wat 51

HAUSER, GAYLORD. *DICTIONARY OF FOODS,* 1.95. Brief descriptions of nutritional values and uses of common (and some uncommon) foods. Lists of acid and alkaline forming foods, table of how long various foods stay in the stomach, index, 135pp. Lus 70

HAWKSEY, H. *GET WELL WITH FOOD,* 1.35. Explains the close association between illness and dietary deficiencies and includes information on overcoming a variety of ailments with a balanced diet. 64pp. TPL 76

HITTLEMAN, RICHARD. *YOGA FOR HEALTH, BOOK 3: PRINCIPLES OF NUTRITION,* 2.35. See the Yoga subsection of Body Work.

HUNTER, BEATRICE. *FACT BOOK ON FERMENTED FOODS AND BEVERAGES,* 1.25. This is another uniquely valuable little book for the homesteader's or do it yourselfer's library. Fermentation is an effective method of preserving many foods—it increases digestibility and adds zest to the diet. Ms. Hunter has looked far and wide to tell us about a great variety of fermented foods from many corners of the world and, better yet, how to make many of them ourselves. Bibliography, index, 116pp. Kea 73

HUNTER, BEATRICE. *FACT BOOK ON YOGURT, KEFIR, AND OTHER MILK CULTURES,* 1.50. Notes, index, 117pp. Kea 73

HUNTER, BEATRICE. *THE NATURAL FOODS PRIMER,* 2.50. Subtitled *Help for the Bewildered Beginner,* this might be a good book to slip to anyone whom you are trying to turn on to good food. It tells what to look for, how to shop, how to prepare natural foods, what equipment you need, and how to adjust your favorite recipes. Includes a long glossary and a description of the basic natural foods. Index, 156pp. S&S 72

JACOBSON, MICHAEL. *NUTRITION SCOREBOARD,* 2.50. Michael Jacobson, a PhD in microbiology, is Co-Director of the Center for Science in the Public Interest in Washington, D.C. He has been an indefatigable campaigner for a greater sense of responsibility on the part of the big food industry in avoiding dangerous additives and providing more nutritious food. The book discusses all the important nutrients and then provides a unique rating of many common foods. The rating formula gives positive credit to protein, unsaturated fat, starch, and naturally-occurring sugars, five vitamins, two minerals, trace elements, and fiber. A food loses points for saturated fat, a fat content above twenty percent, and added sugar and corn syrup. Orange juice ranks 62, soda pop is -92, granola and milk are 45, chuckles candy is -98. A very useful compendium. 102pp. Avo 73

JENSEN, BERNARD. *HEALTH MAGIC THROUGH CHLORO-PHYLL,* 4.45. Bernard Jensen has been a well known naturopath and nutritionist for some forty-five years. This book, though somewhat scattered, contains a wealth of material about the use of chlorophyll and greens in the diet for health and healing. He also gives useful tips on food in relation to survival should our society seriously break down. Index, 154pp. Jen 73

JENSEN, BERNARD. *SURVIVE. . .THIS DAY,* 6.65. *This is a book about survival, not only facts of survival and nutrition, but a philosophy for survival and nutrition that should underlie your choice of direction in the coming days. . . .Survive This Day looks closely at the. . .basic survival foods, the seed family, berries, and sprouts, and rounds out your survival program with many hints and survival directions.*—from the preface. Index, 265pp. Jen 76

KADANS, JOSEPH. *ENCYCLOPEDIA OF FRUITS, VEGE-TABLES, NUTS, AND SEEDS FOR HEALTHFUL LIVING,* 2.95. Kadans, a PhD and naturopath, is President of Bernadean University, an organization which gives correspondence courses in naturopathy. This book is in three parts: I, a brief discussion of various nutrients and metabolic factors; II, a detailed listing of the various foods giving nutritive values, reported health benefits, and preparation and use; and III, a useful "Symptomatic Locator Index," which lists all the foods under symptom headings. Lots of good information but marred by poor printing—page 41 is from another book by the same publisher! 215pp. PrH 73

KEYES, KEN. *LOVING YOUR BODY,* 3.50. Ken Keyes is known to many as the author of the **Handbook to Higher Consciousness.** This book, originally published as **How to Live Longer-Stronger-Slimmer,** combines Keyes' easy way of writing with the usual good advice on how to eat an optimal diet, plus two special features: an excellent food table which includes Keyes' own "Vitamin-Mineral Index," giving a rating of food value per 100 calories for hundreds of foods, and a nutrition analysis form that you can fill out for yourself. 238pp. LLC 74

KINDERLEHRER, JANE. *HOW TO FEEL YOUNGER LONGER,* c8.95. The author is senior editor of **Prevention Magazine**. This book is the best thing we've seen for older people, discussing the nutritional aspects of the ailments and diseases of aging. Chapters on feet, teeth, digestion, menopause, arthritis, heart, back, sleep, sex, how to handle hospital visits, and much more. Written in a sprightly, upbeat style. We particularly enjoyed the chapter on digestion, which points out the evils of antacids and the virtues of HCL, another case where most people do exactly the wrong thing to solve their problem. Index, 220pp. Rod 74

KUGLER, HANS. *SLOWING DOWN THE AGING PROCESS,* 1.50. This is one of the best books on this subject. Dr. Kugler, a chemist by training, teaches and does research on gerontology at Roosevelt University. This is a careful distillation of the literature, including much recent research, written in a clear, nontechnical fashion. Advice: cut down on carbohydrates and fats, increase proteins, drink raw vegetable juice, take vitamins B,C, and E, avoid quick weight loss diets, exercise, and learn to cope with stress. Beyond this is a review of promising leads in nucleic acid therapy and other cell therapies, antioxidant therapies, blood cleaning, and various drugs such as procaine. A final chapter quotes the theories and advice of a number of leading gerontologists. Notes, 236pp. Pyr 75

MAGAZINES: There are a number of magazines devoted to nutrition and healing. The best known ones are the following monthlies: **Bestways Magazine, Inc.** (466 Foothill Blvd., La Canada, CA 91011, single issue, 50 cents, year's subscription, $5.00), **Prevention Magazine** (Rodale Press, Inc., 33 East Minor St., Emmaus, PA 18049, single issue, 75 cents, year's subscription, $7.85), and **Let's Live** (444 N. Larchmont Blvd., Los Angeles, CA 90004, single issue, 75 cents, year's subscription, $7.50).

MCGRATH, WILLIAM. *BIO-NUTRONICS,* 1.50. Good general advice on health and nutrition by a naturopathic doctor. His "Ten Commandments" of bio-nutronics include: *Feast on the Bread of Life,* i.e., by loving, *Avoid Eating the Bread of Affliction,* i.e., stress, *Eat Fresh, Organic Foods as Close to the Original State as Possible, Avoid Highly Processed, Chemicalized, De-Vitalized*

Foods, Eat 75% Live Carbohydrates, 20% Protein and 5% Saturated Fat, Eat More Light-Filled Foods, etc. Index, 216pp. NAL 72

MCCAMY, JOHN and JAMES PRESLEY. *HUMAN LIFE STYLING*, 2.95. Subtitled *Keeping Whole in the Twentieth Century*, this book presents a synergistic program designed to help the body and mind work together better, thereby creating a healthier, more disease resistant human being. Dr. McCamy's plan focuses on four areas: nutrition, ecological living, exercise, and stress reduction. Many specific suggestions are offered and the authors have documented their assertions well. Bibliography, notes, 191pp. H&R 75

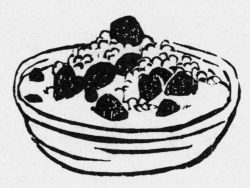

MILTON, R.F. *BASIC NUTRITION AND CELL NUTRITION*, 1.50. This slim volume goes into more details about cells, how they operate and their needs, enzymes, etc., than most. It simplifies with the aid of diagrams and should be quite helpful to someone who wants to go beyond knowing what to eat and understand better why. 70pp. Prv 70

MORELLA, JOSEPH. *NUTRITION AND THE ATHLETE*, 3.95. A general explanation of the basics of nutrition accompanied by advice on how to relate this knowledge to a variety of specific sports. There are also charts on the nutritional content of foods and diet regimes for both gaining and losing weight. Index, 264pp. MCh 76

MOYLE, ALAN. *MOLASSES AND NUTRITION*, 1.50. This book explains the nutritional significance of molasses and its value in treating many disorders, including constipation, intestinal troubles, and rheumatism. Recipes are also included. Index, 64pp. TPL 76

Natural Beauty

Ever since woman's reflection was caught in still water or the polished surface of the first mirror in ancient China, her vanity and her desire to improve and keep her beauty have caused her to experiment with all the growing things around her in search of good and lasting beauty products. This pursuit of beauty is as old as the love of beauty.

Few things have been overlooked in the relentless search for maintaining and creating loveliness. The herbs of the field and the very soil itself have been put to use as sources of life so necessary to beauty.

Until recent generations, women had to rely on their own ingenuity in producing cosmetics, for preparation in commercial quantity is a modern innovation. For a time, the novelty and excitement of purchasing creams, lotions and pomades which promised incredible rewards of restored youth turned women away from their homemade cosmetics. But interest has been aroused once again in simple preparations which feed, nourish and soothe the complexion.

A young woman has only to look at her mother's troubled skin and her own and compare them with her grandmother's smooth complexion to realize that grandmother's simple applications must have been better.

There is no reason to suppose that numerical years should unduly decimate one's youthful appearance. With proper care given to all parts of the body, one can remain vitally alive and attractive throughout life. We begin proper care with a nutritionally wise diet that eliminates all non-foods. A non-food is any food that in any way has been processed, refined, preserved chemically or devitalized.

In addition, exercises must be performed in order to keep muscles flexible, ligaments supple, skin tissue elastic and the bloodstream clean. With these attentions given to the body, the discipline of serenity for mental health becomes easier to practice, and life then becomes the joy that reflects itself in beauty.

While these rules are being practiced, one can turn to nature for external applications that will further beautify the body. Only by following this complete program can youth, beauty and health be achieved and maintained.

Fading and weakness accompany abuse of the body, whereas careful nurturing will prolong the years of beauty and comfort. And even if the body has been mistreated and subjected to the strains and indulgences of today's feverish pace, it is still rarely too late to reverse the ravages of the years. Such a transformation is not only highly possible, but highly probable when the simple laws of nature are used to pave the path to beauty.—from **The Handbook of Natural Beauty** by Virginia Castleton

BUCHMAN, DIAN. *COMPLETE HERBAL GUIDE TO NATURAL HEALTH AND BEAUTY,* **2.95. A herbal guide to natural beauty and health. Many of the recipes in this book are unusual and it is a great deal more comprehensive than most of the natural beauty books. It also has a nice feeling to it. We like it better than any of the other books. Many of the recipes came from Ms. Buchman's grandmother and she includes folklore in her discussion. In addition to the face, the recipes are for hair, hands, feet, and sleep. Index, 146pp. Dou 73**

CASTLETON, VIRGINIA. *THE HANDBOOK OF NATURAL BEAUTY,* c9.95. A comprehensive volume, featuring hundreds of ways to make homemade cosmetic preparations and explaining which type of individual needs each preparation. Ms. Castleton also offers a variety of tips and suggestions and explains exercise routines. An appendix contains a table of *Basic Beauty Foods and What They Do For You.* Index, 305pp. Rod 75

CLARK, LINDA. *FACE IMPROVEMENT THROUGH EXERCISE AND NUTRITION,* 1.75. Illustrated with full page drawings, Ms. Clark presents a systematic approach to eye area problems, double chins, foreheads, etc. Includes cosmetics, diet, exercises, and even the art of serenity. 124pp. Kea 73

CRENSHAW, MARY ANN. *THE NATURAL WAY TO SUPER BEAUTY,* 1.95. Ms. Crenshaw is not a nutritionist but a **New York Times** fashion and beauty reporter. The book is based on her own personal experiences plus a lot of research. It is the book that launched the lecithin-cider vinegar-B-6-kelp craze that helped to fatten the vitamin manufacturers, whatever it did for the consumers. (A number of our nutritional buffs have read this book and reported that it does have a lot of valuable information in it.) Very extensive food nutrition tables, but in very small type. Index, 432pp. Del 75

MESSEGUE, MAURICE. *WAY TO NATURAL HEALTH AND BEAUTY,* c6.95. Described as the world's most famous natural healer, M. Messegue here describes how, using only vegetables, fruits and herbs, one can prepare many treatments for ailments, health, and beauty. Lots of good practical advice and a few recipes as well. Index, 254pp. McM 74

NULL, GARY. *THE NATURAL ORGANIC BEAUTY BOOK,* 1.25. Nutritional advice on hair, skin, yoga, etc. Bibliography, index, 220pp. Del 72

NULL, GARY and STEVE. *HANDBOOK OF SKIN AND HAIR,* 1.75. This concise volume covers a wide area and does so in fairly good depth. The Nulls discuss skin and hair care, cosmetics, allergies, dandruff, and a variety of related problems. Regimens are also suggested. Index, 176pp. Pyr 76

PREVENTION MAGAZINE, ed. *NATURAL WAY TO HEALTHY SKIN,* 2.95. Based on articles in **Prevention** over the years, this book discusses a wide variety of skin conditions (burns, shingles, acne, athlete's foot, warts, etc.) as well as the functions of skin, how to maintain it in a healthy condition, and cosmetic advice. Index, 202pp. Rod 72

ROSE, JEANNE. *JEANNE ROSE'S HERBAL BODY BOOK,* 4.95. See the Herbs section.

ROSE, JEANNE. *KITCHEN COSMETICS: USING PLANTS AND HERBS IN COSMETICS,* 3.95. See the Herbs section.

STEINHART, LAURENCE. *EDGAR CAYCE'S SECRETS OF BEAUTY THROUGH HEALTH,* 1.50. Because of Edgar Cayce's excellent track record in diagnosis and prescription, whatever he said about health and beauty is well worth listening to. This book collects all the relevant readings: care of the skin, eyes, teeth, hair, food and exercise, physiotherapy, elimination. The last part of the book goes beyond most health and beauty books, delving into reincarnation, recycling the mental body, vibratory influences, dreams, and rejuvenation. Steinhart has done a good job of integrating the readings with other relevant information and putting it all together in easily readable fashion. 216pp. Ber 74

THOMAS, VIRGINIA. *MY SECRETS OF NATURAL BEAUTY,* 2.95. Organic beauty treatments, facial and figure exercises, and formulas for money-saving lotions and cosmetics you can make yourself at home from the beauty editor of **Prevention Magazine.** 148pp. Kea 72

TRAVEN, BEATRICE. *THE COMPLETE BOOK OF NATURAL COSMETICS,* 1.95. This book gives recipes for a wide variety of natural cosmetics. It appears to be as good as the other books of type and the instructions are clear and easy to follow. An added feature is a thirty-five page glossary which describes the origins and uses of over a hundred widely used ingredients. The book has been reviewed in places like **Vogue** and **Mademoiselle,** and its orientation is toward those who wear make-up. 205pp. S&S 74

WINTER, RUTH. *A CONSUMER'S DICTIONARY OF COSMETIC INGREDIENTS,* 4.95. Recently promulgated regulations will soon require that all of the ingredients of cosmetics be listed in descending order of amount contained. This can be of great help to persons who have found themselves allergic to various cosmetics without knowing what it was in them that caused the problem. To most of us, a list of ingredients will be fairly meaningless for—far more than food ingredients—they are chemicals we have never heard of. Hence the need for this dictionary with hundreds of definitions and indications of possible toxicity. 236pp. Crn 76

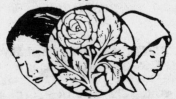

NITTLER, ALAN. *A NEW BREED OF DOCTOR,* 1.50. Dr. Nittler was an ordinary doctor who got interested in nutritional rather than drug therapy, and was expelled from the medical societies as a result. This book tells his personal story and gives sound advice. It is directed, in part, to other doctors, in the hope that it will encourage them to take part in the medical revolution that is now beginning. Some parts of the book are therefore quite technical, though most can be read by the layman. If you are interested in going to a nutritional doctor, this book is good advance preparation. Index, 202pp. Pyr 74

NULL, GARY. *FOOD COMBINING HANDBOOK,* 1.25. This says more about food combining than any other book we know of. It explains in great detail the digestive system, the function of enzymes, analyzes the various foods and the effects of different combinations on digestion, has a chapter on ulcers, and one on fasting. If digestion is your problem, you should find a great deal in here which will be of help. Bibliography, 140pp. Pyr 73

NULL, GARY and STEVE. *THE COMPLETE HANDBOOK OF NUTRITION,* 1.75. This is probably the most useful, and certainly the most comprehensive of the Gary Null books. It is one of the better general nutrition texts including, in addition to the usual information on vitamins, minerals, etc., food combining, acid-alkaline balance, fruit and juices, fasting, herbs, beauty hints, poison in foods, and much else. Good value. Bibliography, index, 413pp. Del 72

NUTRITION SEARCH, INC. *NUTRITION ALMANAC,* 5.95. This is not a book to sit down and read. It is, however, the best single sourcebook on nutrition available, the product of team research over several years. It can be used to help the reader work out a total plan for personal nutrition, or it can answer questions about food, nutrition and health. The first and largest section discusses over forty vitamins and minerals in terms of description, absorption and storage, dosage and toxicity, deficiency effects and symptoms, beneficial effect on ailments, and human and animal tests. This is followed by a section on synergistic effects, providing an easy to follow guide for understanding which nutrients are compatible or antagonistic. Next is a brief section on available forms of nutritive supplements and their relative effectiveness. Then a long discussion of various diseases and ailments, in layman's language, accompanied by a list of nutrients (and quantities) that have been found to be beneficial. Next a discussion of various foods and their values, including a list of rich sources of nutrients. A table of food composition gives the complete nutrient analysis of over 600 foods. Other tables include essential amino acid contents of foods and a nutrient allowance chart. There is an extensive bibliography, a good glossary, and an index. Highly recommended. 8"x10", 263pp. MGH 75

PAGE, MELVIN. *YOUR BODY IS YOUR BEST DOCTOR,* 1.25. Dr. Page, a dentist, has been one of the pioneers in nutritional studies for more than forty years. This book, co-authored by an anthropologist, reports many of his findings. The theme is that our bodies contain a built in blueprint for good health but most of us spend our lives trying to tear it up. Page shows how to cooperate with it, in terms of what to eat and not to eat. Good discussion of body chemistry, functions of glands, etc. Extensive discussion of degenerative diseases and effects of sugar, milk, and coffee. Good bibliography, 236pp. Kea 72

PASSWATER, RICHARD. *SUPERNUTRITION,* 1.95. Relying on extensive research in medical and scientific literature, the author, a biochemist, demonstrates that nutritional deficiencies exist in almost everyone's diet and that these deficiencies maintain the current high incidence rates of heart disease, cancer, and mental and emotional disturbances. He presents the evidence showing that low cholesterol diets have not decreased heart disease and he states that such diets are, in fact, detrimental to health. In the concluding chapter he presents a program of megavitamin therapy easily tailored to anyone's specific needs and makes the challenge that such a program can reduce the incidence of heart disease by sixty percent, cancer by thirty percent, cure most cases of schizophrenia, and save over a million lives a year. All in all an excellent book. Charts, tables, 256pp. S&S 75

PELSTRING, LINDA and JO ANN HAUCK. *FOOD TO IMPROVE YOUR HEALTH,* 1.50. This is a reference book in two parts: One, an alphabetical listing indicating the vitamin and mineral content of hundreds of foods from abalone to zucchini, along with a discussion of how these elements work for or against your body; Two, a listing of common health problems with information about nutritional deficiencies that cause them and what to eat to help make up those deficiencies. Bibliography, 221pp. Pin 74

PFEIFFER, CARL. *MENTAL AND ELEMENTAL NUTRIENTS,* c9.95. Subtitled *A Physician's Guide to Nutrition and Health Care,* this book will appeal not only to physicians but to educated lay-persons who want a more in depth discussion of nutritional treatment of disease. Part I, *Nutritional Background,* contains a lot of material familiar to health food types, written at a fairly simple level (perhaps on the assumption that many physicians are abysmally ignorant in such matters). There is a good discussion of cholesterol and the widespread misunderstandings about it within the profession. Parts II and III deal with the vitamins and trace elements in depth, discussing effects on various conditions, dosages, overdosages, etc. Niacin and megavitamin therapy gets first billing since Dr. Pfeiffer is Director of the Brain Bio Center in Princeton, N.J., a research-educational organization for the diagnosis and treatment of biochemical imbalances, with emphasis on mental illness. Part IV, *Clinical Problems,* goes into milk, alcoholism, hypoglycemia, schizophrenia (good detailed treatment), insomnia, headache, aging and senility, arthritis, skin problems, nutrients for a better sex life, and much else. This section is primarily for doctors but any reader wishing to expand their repertory of drugless healing methods would doubtless find much of value here. This book should be regarded as a useful reference work, rather than one to curl up with and attempt to read through. Bibliography, name and subject indices, 519pp. Kea 75

POPOV, IVAN. *STAY YOUNG,* 3.95. Dr. Popov is the medical director of the Renaissance Revitalization Center. His career has been devoted to preventing premature aging and he has pioneered many techniques, including the controversial embryotherapy and cell therapy. In the former, a chick embryo, incubated under special conditions, is ingested and helps maintain youth; in the latter, the cells of a specific organ are extracted from animal embryos, cut into tiny pieces, mixed into a saline solution, and injected into the muscular tissues of a patient in cases where this organ contains degenerated or deficient cells. Dr. Popov cites case studies from his practice and research and includes a variety of practical treatments—many of which can be done at home. Bibliography, notes, 286pp. G&D 75

PRICE, WESTON. *NUTRITION AND PHYSICAL DEGENERATION: A COMPARISON OF PRIMITIVE AND MODERN DIETS AND THEIR EFFECTS,* c20.50. This is a landmark study of the effects of "civilized" food, showing how the food we eat today is a

357

primary cause of disease and physical degeneration. Dr. Price was a dentist who spent much of his adult life researching the diets and nutritional practices of so-called primitive people all over the world. The study is extensively documented and very carefully prepared. There's a wealth of information for all who are seriously interested in nutrition and physical degeneration—though the book could stand a great deal of editing. 560pp. PPF 70

Raw Foods

Raw foods contain nutrients and enzymes vital to our health, many of which are lost when the same foods are cooked. This has been proven by a number of experiments. More than thirty years ago, Francis Pottenger, M.D., carried out a ten year experiment using 900 cats who were placed on controlled diets. The cats that ate only raw food produced healthy kittens from generation to generation. Those on a similar diet, but with all the food cooked, developed our modern ailments: heart, kidney, and thyroid disease, pneumonia, paralysis, loss of teeth, difficulty in labor, diminished or perverted sexual interest, diarrhea, irritability. Liver impairment on cooked protein was progressive, the bile in the stool becoming so toxic that even weeds refused to grow in soil fertilized by the cats' excrement. The first generation of kittens was sickly, the second generation were often born dead or diseased. The experiment could not continue past the third generation because by this time all the females were sterile.

There have also been a number of experiments with humans. Dr. Koratsune, a Japanese researcher, reported in 1951 that as long as he ate uncooked whole rice and raw radishes, spinach, kale and grated raw potatoes, he found he had excellent quality blood, even though his diet was poor in protein and calories. However, as soon as he ate the same quantity of vegetarian food in a cooked form, he began to notice symptoms of edema and anemia.

Some people advocate eating nothing but raw food. This is an extreme position. Nonetheless, it is generally agreed that at least a third of our total daily intake should be raw if we wish to maintain optimum health.

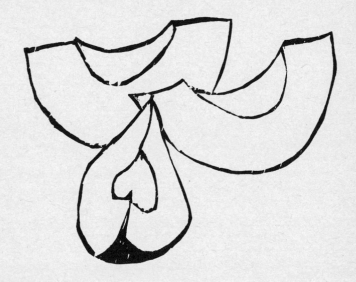

ANDREWS, SHEILA. *NO-COOKING FRUITARIAN RECIPE BOOK,* 4.55. A collection of imaginative recipes utilizing only raw foods. No sweeteners are included in any of them. A bit of fruitarian philosophy is also included. Index, 96pp. TPL 75

BIRCHER-BENNER. *NUTRITION PLAN FOR RAW FOOD AND JUICES,* 2.75. A discussion of the benefits of a raw food diet along with menus and recipes. 63pp. Nas 72

ABRAMOWSKI, O.L.M. *FRUITARIAN HEALING SYSTEM,* 7.10. This is the most complete discussion available for the benefits of a fruitarian diet for healing and regeneration. Unfortunately it's far from well written, but there's not much else on the subject. Index, 187pp. EsH 76

KROK, MORRIS. *FORMULA FOR LONG LIFE,* 5.80. Krok, a

South African, favors a diet primarily of raw fruits and vegetables. In addition to reading what others have said, he has experimented on himself, eating one food at a time to determine its effects. There is a lot of interesting information in this book about the effects of different foods, cooking, fasts, about cleansing and disease and acid/alkaline reactions. He has an interesting chapter on pregnancy, asserting that a woman with a clean body will not suffer from morning sickness and other symptoms usual in most pregnancies. 138pp. EsH 62

KROK, MORRIS. *FRUIT THE FOOD AND MEDICINE FOR MAN,* 5.80. A scattered discussion of the benefits of a raw food diet. Both philosophy and specific diets are included. 88pp. EsH 61

KULVINSKAS, VIKTORAS. *LOVE YOUR BODY–LIVE FOOD RECIPES,* 2.50. Kulvinskas is Co-Director of Ann Wigmore's Hippocrates Health Institute, where people are cured by eating live (raw) foods and fasting on wheat grass juice. This book gives a few pages of theory; the rest is recipes—ways to make live food interesting, even delicious. We once spent a week with Kulvinskas sampling many of these recipes and can testify that he has done as much to elevate raw food cuisine as any man alive. 90pp. Oma 74

SEMPLE, DUGALD. *THE SUNFOOD WAY TO HEALTH,* 4.65. A terribly written argument for a raw food diet which includes information not available elsewhere. Index, 138pp. EsH 76

SZEKELY, EDMUND. *TREASURY OF RAW FOODS,* 1.75. Szekely recommends a diet of twenty-five percent cereals and seventy-five percent raw foods. We found him a little rigid in this book, but there are a lot of interesting points in here about good foods and diet. He introduces us to the word *trophology* to describe the science of food combining. In addition to discussing body needs and the contribution of various foods, this book includes suggested menus and a number of raw food recipes. 42pp. Aca 73

WALKER, N.W. *DIET AND SALAD SUGGESTIONS,* 3.35. A comprehensive discussion of the nutritional benefits of a wide variety of raw fruits and vegetables. Walker also includes a miscellany of nutritional information, especially in reference to the digestive system and many raw food menus. Illustrations, charts, 156pp. NoP 40

READ, ANNE, CAROL ILSTRUP, and MARGARET GAMMON.
EDGAR CAYCE ON DIET AND HEALTH, 1.50. Selections from
the Cayce readings containing his most practical suggestions for
practical diet. He emphasized eating the right foods in the right
combinations at the right time. The books also include a series of
questions and answers on vitamins, minerals, cooking methods, sleep
and rest, the correct psychological attitude to eating, and much
else. Index, 191pp. War 69

RODALE, J.I. and STAFF. *ENCYCLOPEDIA FOR HEALTHFUL
LIVING,* c13.95. A topically and alphabetically arranged discussion
of over 1300 topics. Each of the listings is an essay in itself and reviews the research up to the date of publication. A vast and somewhat outdated but still highly useful volume. 1055pp. Rod 60

RODALE, J.I. and STAFF. *THE HEALTH SEEKER,* c10.95. Like
the previous book, this one reprints material on a variety of diseases
and health problems ranging from accidents and acne to water soft-
eners and x-rays. Lots of good material here but it must be kept in
mind that the original articles represented particular points of view
and were not written in an encyclopedic fashion. Good index,
928pp. Rod 62

RODALE PRESS, eds. *NUTS AND SEEDS–THE NATURAL
SNACKS,* 2.95. Following an introductory discussion of the value
of seeds as food, this book reprints a number of articles on different seeds and their health value, follows with a section on growing
nuts and seeds (comprehensive as to varieties but not sufficiently
detailed to be a good farmer's guide), and finally presents a few
snack recipes. Index, 173pp. Rod 73

SHEARS, C. CURTIS. *NUTRITIONAL SCIENCE AND HEALTH
EDUCATION,* 7.95. Shears is a former successful lawyer who cured
himself nutritionally and, since 1959, has been studying and teaching nutrition full time. He is currently Professor of Nutrition at the
British College of Naturopathy and Osteopathy. This carefully researched and documented book is not recommended for beginners
but should be stimulating to persons who already have some knowledge of nutrition. Shears is very eclectic in his research and in addition to the standard sources he draws heavily on Rudolf Steiner
and metaphysical concepts. Major topics covered include: *The Sickness Crisis, Essential Minerals, Unsaturated Fatty Acids, Acid-Alka-*

line Balance, Essential Vitamins, Metabolism, Problems of Reforms, The Creative Approach, Beneficial and Harmful Foods, and *Diet and Health Around the World.* Bibliography, index, 189pp. NuS 74

SHELTON, HERBERT. *FOOD COMBINING MADE EASY,* 1.50. Dr. Shelton is one of the leading lights of the American Natural Hygiene Society, composed of people who favor eating the right food (mostly raw), fasting, and generally avoiding or eliminating toxicity in the body. This small book summarizes his views on food combining, explains the digestive process and shows how wrong combinations can play hob with that process. There's a lot to this, though we admit our own weaknesses keep us from following these principles very often. Includes suggested menus. 71pp. Shl 51

SHELTON, HERBERT. *HEALTH FOR THE MILLIONS,* 1.60. This is a good introduction to the whole natural hygiene story: how our bodies utilize food, what to eat and what not to eat, cooking, food combining, how to eat, physical activity, keeping the body clean, and much else. The hygienic way involves moderation and self discipline—something that few of us are very good at. But it holds up for us a standard against which to measure our shortcomings. 314pp. NHP 68

SHELTON, HERBERT. *THE HYGIENIC CARE OF CHILDREN,* 1.95. This is one of the few books entirely devoted to an exposition of sound nutritional practices for infants and children. Over half the book covers prenatal care and the care and feeding of infants. The second half discusses what to feed children and gives some common diseases of infants and children. The approach—as with all of Shelton's other books—is somewhat stringent, but many excellent suggestions are advanced. Index, 473pp. NHP 70

SOBEL, DAVID and **FAITH HORNBACHER.** *TO YOUR HEALTH,* 4.95. "The initial idea for this book came from a headache. The headache said, in its own insufferable way, 'There are many simple, practical things you could do to take care of yourself, why don't you do them?' " The text is handwritten and illustrated and includes a wide variety of practical techniques and exercises on the following topics: eyes and seeing, feet, hair and skin, tooth care, good eating, breathing, relaxation, body movement, the great laughter cure, body rhythms, creating healthy environments, body mind and inner work. Also includes a good, topically arranged annotated bibliography, 8½"x11", 191pp. Vik 74

STEINER, RUDOLF. *PROBLEMS OF NUTRITION,* .95. A brief lecture on the spiritual effects of consuming meat, alcohol, coffee, milk. *If by eating meat a person is relieved of too large a portion of his inner activities, then activities will develop inwardly that would otherwise be expressed externally. His soul will become more externally oriented, more susceptible to, and bound up with, the external world. When a person takes his nourishment from the realm of plants, however, he becomes more independent and more inclined to develop inwardly. He will become master of his whole being. The more he is inclined to vegetarianism, the more he accepts a vegetarian diet, the more he will be able also to let his inner forces predominate.* 22pp. API 69

TILDEN, J.H. *FOOD: ITS INFLUENCE AS A FACTOR IN DISEASE AND HEALTH,* 3.50. Dr. Tilden was one of the founders of the Natural Hygiene movement. This book was written in the early twentieth century and it is one of his most important statements. He believed in proper food combinations and in the consumption of unrefined, pure foods. The language is archaic at times—but the ideas are modern and still important today. Index, 250pp. Kea 76

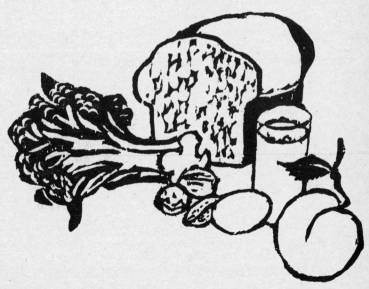

Vegetarianism

The cause of vegetarianism has always had its champions, and their arguments have always been enthusiastic and impressive, if not always accepted by the general public. Perhaps the vegetarian ethos was summed up best by George Bernard Shaw, when he added this postscript to his letters: *Be kind to animals; don't eat them!*

Nevertheless, in spite of the often splendid health of its crusading adherents, and in spite of the testimonies to a meatless diet in the writings of all the major religions, we feel very strongly that the ethical side of vegetarianism should remain a personal question. To kill an animal for the purpose of eating its flesh will cause one person to feel guilty and another to feel hungry. It is against the principles of democracy to impose morality on others; if they do not come from a deep-felt personal conviction, they are useless morals anyway.

However, there is another side of vegetarianism which exists, not in the dark light of faith, but in the bright light of the scientist's laboratory. It is plain, scientific fact that the two greatest dangers in our food consumption today, from the standpoint of the world's greatest killer, heart disease, are animal fats and refined carbohydrates. A vegetarian diet, followed scientifically (that is, to include all the basic requirements of proteins, vitamins, minerals, enzymes, and the right kind of fats and carbohydrates), will inevitably prolong life, strengthen vitality and increase resistance to disease. Disease cannot exist in a normal metabolism, and a normal metabolism can be achieved and maintained by following the principles of scientific vegetarianism. It is as simple as that.—from the preface to **Scientific Vegetarianism** by Edmund Szekely

ALTMAN, NATHANIEL. *EATING FOR LIFE*, 2.45. This is the best single book on vegetarianism that we have seen. It draws on material from many sources, particularly those that are objective and scientific and have no vested interest in vegetarianism. Altman looks at the subject from the standpoint of morality, anatomy and physiology, health and nutrition, the world food shortage, and ecology. He includes a good summary of the main principles of nutrition, recipes and food value charts. Well documented. Bibliography, index, 142pp. TPH 73

BARKAS, JANET. *THE VEGETABLE PASSION,* c8.95. Only incidentally a nutrition book, this is primarily a social history of vegetarianism, full of anecdotes and gossip about famous vegetarians, for example, what Hitler had for breakfast. Well researched and full of details, fascinating and otherwise. Illustrations, bibliography, index, 224pp. Scr 75

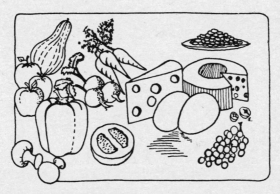

HUR, ROBIN. *FOOD REFORM: OUR DESPERATE NEED,* c10.95. This is a far out and controversial book. It is also a very thoroughly researched book. The author spent three years doing nutritional research for this book and he has 600 footnotes and many more references. Where does he come out? He advocates the SGA diet: sprouts, greens and algae—up to two pounds per day of greens, a similar amount of sprouts, and a very small amount of seaweed. Mr. Hur's arguments for this diet are both nutritional and ecological. This is not an easy book to read and is not suggested for someone just getting into the subject. But if you are ready to go deep and test your ideas against a lot of relevant research, you'll find a great deal in this book to mull over. 264pp. Hei 75

LAPPE, FRANCES. *DIET FOR A SMALL PLANET,* 5.95/1.95. See the Cookbooks section.

NULL, GARY. *PROTEIN FOR VEGETARIANS,* 1.50. Goes beyond the title to deal generally with how vegetarians (and others, for that matter) can be assured of an adequate diet. Includes extensive food value tables, including a table of the contents of many foods in terms of the twelve principal amino acids. Bibliography, 189pp. Pyr 75

SZEKELY, EDMUND. *SCIENTIFIC VEGETARIANISM,* 1.75. A good summary of the basic argument for vegetarianism which combines a scientific rationale with a spiritual focus. Szekely deals with theory, types of food to eat and not to eat, ecological considerations, and effects of thoughts on the body. 47pp. Aca 74

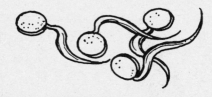

Vitamins & Minerals

The two greatest discoveries in 20th century medicine are the importance and the multiple role of minerals and vitamins in the human body, as well as their pronounced influence on the basic biological functions of the human organism in health and disease. I am very often asked the question, *How is it that we didn't know about this vital role of vitamins and minerals before the 20th century?* There are two reasons. First, only in the 20th century did the science of biochemistry reach its full development and become the most important branch of medical science. Second, 90 percent of the discoveries concerning vitamins and minerals were made during the last forty years. And it is not accidental that these vital biochemical discoveries were not made before. *Necessity is the mother of invention* and wherever the urgency for solution of a problem appears, the discovery of the means for the solution will always follow.

In the good old days there was no need for knowledge concerning the minerals and vitamins simply because we didn't have mineral or vitamin deficiencies. The mineral and vitamin deficiency diseases are natural, direct conseuqences of the appearance and development of our present economical and technical system of production, transportation and distribution.

The most disastrous condition in our basic biological functions is a deficiency of the most important minerals and vitamins. In the ultimate analysis, they determine and direct the assimilation and distribution of all food substances ingested by the organism. Minerals and vitamins represent the general staff of the army of the organism while the other food substances—starches, sugar, etc.—represent only the mass of soldiers. Our organism, lacking the important minerals and vitamins, is nothing but a defeated, disorganized army deserted by its general staff. During the past few decades, the various deficiency diseases have deteriorated the public health to such an enormous scale in the Western world, that the study of mineral and vitamin deficiencies, their influence on the basic biological functions of the organism and the practical application of the conclusions of these studies became imperative.—from the preface to **The Book of Vitamins** by Edmund Szekely

ADAMS, RUTH. *THE COMPLETE HOME GUIDE TO ALL THE VITAMINS,* 1.95. This is a basic book about vitamins and what they are—with a brief rundown of each of the major ones. Tables, index, 253pp. Lar 72

ADAMS, RUTH and FRANK MURRAY.*MINERALS,* 1.65. A very interesting, detailed account of the minerals and trace elements—both those important to health and those which pose a threat. A great deal of attention is paid to the problems of pollution. A good account of the fluoridation controversy with many detailed studies for those looking for "ammunition" is included. Bibliography, index, 290pp. Lar 74

ADAMS, RUTH and FRANK MURRAY. *VITAMIN C: THE*

POWERHOUSE VITAMIN, CONQUERS MORE THAN JUST COLDS, 1.65. A comprehensive journalistic review of the potential benefits of vitamin C for a wide variety of ailments. All the relevant research is cited and case histories are interspersed. Index, 191pp. Lar 72

ADAMS, RUTH and FRANK MURRAY. *VITAMIN E: WONDER WORKER OF THE SEVENTIES?* 1.25. A readable survey of what vitamin E can and cannot do. Introduction by Dr. Evan Shute. Bibliography, index, 128pp. Lar 71

BAILEY, HERBERT. *VITAMIN E,* 1.65. This was one of the first books to awaken the public to the importance of vitamin E, in face of the suppressions and distortions of the medical establishment. Written by a veteran medical writer, it provides extensive research details and references. 203pp. Arc 64

BAILEY, HERBERT. *THE VITAMIN PIONEERS,* .95. This is a fascinating account of the key discoveries of various vitamins and their importance to our health. It details the great resistances of the FDA and much of the medical profession to many usages which are generally accepted today and some which still are not, thus giving us a good background from which to judge many of the criticisms we still hear from the establishment. For many, this will prove an easier way to begin learning about vitamins than books packed with technical details. 239pp. Pyr 70

BOCK, RAYMOND. *VITAMIN E: KEY TO YOUTHFUL LONGEVITY,* 1.95. Based on his many years of experience and observation as a practicing gynecologist, Dr. Bock presents a detailed case for the many benefits of vitamin E on general health and as a sort of miracle worker in specific diseases. Dr. Bock is primarily concerned with the applications of vitamin E in gynecology. 62pp. Arc 77

CYAN, ERWIN DI. *VITAMIN E AND AGING,* 1.25. Among the various theories on aging, two—the oxidation and free radical theories—suggest an important role for vitamin E. Free radicals are portions of chemical compounds in the body which break off, are highly reactive, and enter into connections with unsaturated fatty acids, causing them to oxidize rapidly. Vitamin E is an anti-oxidant and it helps to neutralize the effects of free radicals. This book, conservatively written, includes material from the International Conference on Vitamin E and Its Role in Cellular Metabolism, held in 1971. Glossary, bibliography, index, 176pp. Pyr 72

CYAN, ERWIN DI. *VITAMINS IN YOUR LIFE,* 2.95. This is an excellent survey of vitamins and minerals and their importance to our health. The author, who has been a drug consultant for over thirty years, writes essentially from the health establishment point of view, but he is not unsympathetic to the "heretical" views of Pauling on vitamin E, Hoffer and Osmond on niacin, and others. Each vitamin is discussed with respect to use, deficiency effects, and sources. Toxicity levels and use of supplements are also covered. The treatment of trace elements is quite thorough. Recommended. Bibliography, index, 223pp. S&S 74

PAULING, LINUS. *VITAMIN C, THE COMMON COLD, AND THE FLU,* 3.45. Since the publication of Pauling's original work over six years ago countless additional studies have been carried out to determine the value of vitamin C in relation not only to the common cold but also to influenza and other diseases. In this book Dr. Pauling surveys these studies and reports on his own findings. He also discusses a variety of related material. 241pp. Fre 76

PREVENTION MAGAZINE EDITORS. *VITAMIN A,* 2.95. Recent studies have shed new light on the many ways vitamin A is important to our health. At the same time, deficiencies seem to be more widespread than with virtually any other vitamin among North Americans of all income groups. This reflects both bad nutritional habits and the effects of pesticides and pollutants. This book tells the story in a clear and readable way. Index, 130pp. Rod 72

ROSENBERG, HAROLD and A.N. FELDZAMEN. *THE DOCTOR'S BOOK OF VITAMIN THERAPY,* 2.45. This is our favorite of the vitamin books. Dr. Rosenberg is one of that rare breed of nutritionally well educated MDs and is past president of the International Academy of Preventive Medicine. Dr. Feldzamen (a PhD) is former editorial director of the Encyclopaedia Britannica Educational Corporation. This up to date book covers all the vitamin issues as well as providing basic information. It makes a strong case for vitamin supplementation in our society. Its most useful feature is a series of tables by age, sex and weight, giving recommendations for optimum levels of vitamin intake: on the order of 1,000-1,500 mg of vitamin C, 200-600 IU of vitamin E, and 200-1,000 mg of vitamin B3. There is also an excellent critique of the Government's Recommended Daily Allowances of vitamins. Unfortunately the book lacks footnotes and an index. Highly recommended. 350pp. Ber 74

SCHROEDER, HENRY. *THE TRACE ELEMENTS OF MAN,* c7.95. This is not a popular nutrition book but a serious, heavy (and fascinating) book by a distinguished scientist who is Professor Emeritus of Physiology, Dartmouth Medical School. Dr. Schroeder believes that when animals—including man—became terrestrial, they brought with them a need for those trace elements that occur naturally in sea water. Other elements locked into the earth's crust are poisonous to man and have recently been released into the environment by industrial man. Good reading for those who ask *why?* Index, 171pp. DAC 73

SHUTE, WILFRED. *VITAMIN E BOOK,* c8.95. This is Dr. Shute's latest update on the use of vitamin E for heart patients, and also its use in the treatment of burns, diabetes, skin ailments, and circulatory diseases. He reviews various methods of treatment (proposed, widely used, and rejected), discusses the ineffectiveness of many current drugs, and demonstrates why many treatments now in common use are not only valueless but essentially dangerous. Bibliography, notes, index, 225pp. Kea 75

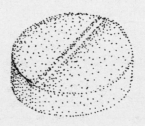

RODALE, J.I. and STAFF. *THE COMPLETE BOOK OF MINERALS FOR HEALTH,* c13.95. Another of the Rodale Press' encyclopedic compilations of articles about various subjects. It is divided into six books: I. *The Macronutrients,* II. *Trace Minerals,* III. *Harmful Elements,* IV. *Mineral Deficiency Diseases,* V. *Foods and their Minerals,* and VI. *Vitamin and Mineral Interactions.* Not a book to read through, but good to dip into or look up a wider variety of information about various minerals than you are likely to find anyplace else. Index, 786pp. Rod 72

RODALE, J.I. and STAFF. *THE COMPLETE BOOK OF VITA-MINS,* c14.95. This classic has a great deal of interesting material but it is overpriced and outdated. Much of it is reprinted from **Prevention Magazine** without re-editing and all the references are at least ten years old. Nevertheless it provides a lot of general information, including useful documentation for supporters of natural vitamins and large doses. Good index, 688pp. Rod 66

STONE, IRWIN. *THE HEALING FACTOR: VITAMIN C AGAINST DISEASE,* 1.95. This is the definitive book on vitamin C. Stone, a noted biochemist, has been researching ascorbic acid for some forty years—it was he who turned Linus Pauling on to its virtues in large doses. Man is virtually alone among animals in not producing his own vitamin C. If s/he did in similar amounts to other animals relative to body size, s/he would utilize two to four grams a day, rising to fifteen grams under stress. By treating ascorbic acid as a "minimum daily requirement" instead of the crucial enzyme it really is, we are living in a state of sub-clinical scurvy, symptoms of which have been attributed to other ailments. Glossary, extensive notes, 258pp. G&D 72

SZEKELY, EDMUND. *THE BOOK OF MINERALS,* 1.50. Similar to his vitamin book, this is a brief guide to the role of each mineral in our basic biological functions, our requirements for each, mineral deficiency symptoms, best natural sources in order of importance, and a list of symptoms with minerals to take for each. For quick reference it's hard to beat. 38pp. Aca 71

SZEKELY, EDMUND. *THE BOOK OF VITAMINS,* 1.95. This is a neat little summary, in outline form, of a lot of useful information. It begins with lists of vitamin deficiency symptoms in the various systems of the human body, then goes on to deal with each vitamin, listing role, positive biological functions, deficiency symptoms, and best natural sources. An easy to use quick reference. 38pp. Aca 71

VITA CHART. *VITAMINS AND MINERALS CHART,* 3.00. This 11"x14" plastic chart is the neatest summary of vitamin and mineral information we've seen. Printed in color on both sides, it is not a substitute for a book about the vitamins but is an excellent memory jogger for those of us who've read many of the books and still can't keep all the details in mind. We particularly like the information on dosage—both the government's RDA and suggested supplementary ranges, complemented by specific information on the amounts contained in standard qualities of principal sources. Highly recommended. VCh 76

WADE, CARLSON. *MAGIC MINERALS,* 1.95. Following a review of the minerals, Wade devotes chapters to their relationship to various aspects of health. Useful information, though we don't care for his vivid writing: *How to Make Your Blood Stream A River of Eternal Youth, How Three Magic Mineral Sources Can Give You Added Mineral Power,* etc. 229pp. Arc 72

WADE, CARLSON. *VITAMINS AND OTHER FOOD SUPPLE-MENTS,* 1.25. A useful, brief guide for the newcomer to the shelves of a health food store. Explains the use of vitamins, minerals, and items such as lecithin, wheat germ, and yoghurt. 119pp. Kea 72

WEBSTER, JAMES. *VITAMIN C,* 1.25. A good, straightforward review of the research, expressed in terms comprehensible to the layman. 158pp. ASC 71

WADE, CARLSON. *FACT BOOK ON FATS, OILS AND CHO-LESTEROL,* 1.50. *This book will offer you the vital facts about fats and cholesterol and how a slight adjustment can add years to your lifeline of health. You will learn the difference between saturated and unsaturated fats and what they mean for your heart and artery health. You will learn how to plan a low fat diet that has all the delicious taste of a high fat diet. You will also be given the latest doctor-approved fat-controlled diet plans to help you cooperate with your own doctor for your individual case. You will discover how you can use natural foods to help control and even "wash" the cholesterol in your system.*—from the introduction. 125pp. Kea 73

WADE, CARLSON. *HELPING YOUR HEALTH WITH ENZYMES,* 1.95. Discusses how enzymes help build resistance against disease, help us recover from illness and tiredness, help relieve aches and pains, subdue skin irritations, affect weight, and much else. Also deals with fasting, food combining, raw foods, proper breathing, and acid-alkaline balance. Index, 224pp. Arc 66

WADE, CARLSON. *MIRACLE PROTEIN: SECRET OF NATURAL CELL-TISSUE REJUVENATION,* c8.95. Wade points out ways in which protein can nourish cells and tissues and help them to regain vitality. Many specific case studies and treatment suggestions are offered. Index, 231pp. PrH 75

WADE, CARLSON. *NATURAL HORMONES,* 2.45. The idea of this book is to eat foods and to take mineral baths, fast, and exercise in ways which stimulate the glands that produce hormones. The foods include grapes, beans and peas, rose hips, herbs, seeds, sprouts, apple cider vinegar, carob meal, honey, millet and fresh juices. Wade also discusses the various glands, what they do and how they may be helped. Index, 236pp. PrH 72

WATT, BERNICE K. *HANDBOOK OF THE NUTRITIONAL CONTENTS OF FOOD,* 4.00. This is a reprint of a survey of food nutrition prepared by the U.S. Department of Agriculture. The material is in the form of two tables, one measuring nutrients in 100 grams of edible food and the other measuring nutrients in the edible portion of one pound of food. Both tables give values for calories, fat, carbohydrate, vitamins, and minerals. 9"x12", 192pp. Dov 63

WIGMORE, ANN. *BE YOUR OWN DOCTOR,* 2.25. Ann Wigmore, D.D., N.D., is head of the Hippocrates Health Institute in Boston where she specializes in treating many difficult cases with spiritual concern and a raw food diet, making particular use of wheat grass juice—a rich source of potent chlorophyll. This book explains these health principles, how to sprout wheat and make wheat grass juice, and gives many recipes for delicious raw food. We've had some exposure to her ideas and methods and while we're not prepared to go all the way with raw food, we have great respect for what can be accomplished by those who will go the whole way. One added advantage of her "live food" diet is that it is very cheap. 192pp. Hem nd

WIGMORE, ANN. *WHY SUFFER,* 3.25. Ms. Wigmore's personal testament including her statements about why she got involved in the natural foods movement, what it has done for her, and what she hopes it will do for everyone. Many case studies are included along with a great deal of Dr. Ann's personal philosophy. 219pp.

Hem 64

WILLIAMS, ROGER. *NUTRITION AGAINST DISEASE,* 1.95. Dr. Williams is perhaps responsible for more original work in the field of vitamin research than any living scientist. He was the first man to identify pantothenic acid, he also did pioneer work on folic acid and gave it its name. He is past president of the American Chemical Society and has received many awards and honorary degrees. His basic thesis is that the nutritional microenvironment of our body cells is crucially important to our health and that deficiencies in this environment constitute a major cause of disease. He has found that our inherited needs for various nutritive factors vary tremendously. This book discusses his general theory, then applies it to birth defects, heart disease, obesity, dental disease, arthritis, old age, mental disease, alcoholism and cancer. The work is supported by some 1100 medical and scientific citations. Recommended. Index, 370pp. Ban 71

WILLIAMS, ROGER. *NUTRITION IN A NUTSHELL,* 1.95. In this small book, Dr. Williams undertakes to set forth in simple language some of the basic facts of nutrition, such as what nourishing food contains, where nutrition starts, and what a vitamin is, and what it does. It is written from a biochemical point of view, is scientifically sound, and can be helpful in giving us the kind of information that will permit us to sort out sound nutritional ideas from those that proceed from an excess of zeal and a lack of hard evidence. Index, 171pp. Dou 62

WILLIAMS, ROGER. *PHYSICIAN'S HANDBOOK OF NUTRITIONAL SCIENCE,* c13.10. This is a book which should be read by physicians. It is generally too heavy for the lay reader, however it contains a great deal of information which is needed to turn physicians on to good food. Dr. Williams is a prominent biochemist and former president of the American Chemical Society. He discovered a couple of vitamins and is most noted for his work on biochemical individuality. Notes, index, 127pp. Tho 75

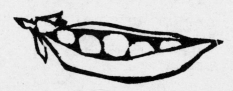

Organic Gardening

T wo distinctively different economic principles apply to our relation to the world. They cannot be mixed up without causing harm to each other. One embraces our relation to goods and commodities, if you like: the world of inanimate things. The other concerns our relation to living organisms. In the first we are the recipients of things; in the second, the administrators of processes.

A close look at food substances will show that these belong to the first area while agriculture itself belongs to the second. . . .At the moment they are severed from the living organism, one could say, food substances are born. They immediately, like all goods, become subject to different principles and laws than before, economic laws that apply to all material things. These goods generate, serve and sustain our socio-economic life. In doing so, however, they are subject to a process of diminution and destruction.

The second principle applicable to living organisms is quite different. All living organisms—plants, animals, men— are dependent on laws which, contrary to the above laws of economics, lie outside man's jurisdiction and control, such as day and night, seasons, weather, etc. All life roots in these rhythmic processes. The earth with its most sensitive part, the soil, is part of this living organization and subject to the same processes. Therefore a garden, and particularly a farm, is a living organism. Our individual life as man depends on this living organism.

Because of increasing demands, the land has been invaded by a principle valid only for goods. The use of spare land

375

(as long as available), cheap labor, artificial fertilizers, forced breeding of plants and animals, mechanization—all these have, because of their seeming success, prevented our recognition of the fact that they are largely compromises, obscuring the effect of inappropriate economic principles on the land.

The now apparent global limits of capital resources, including soil fertility, may make us ask, how can we reverse this trend? A community of people would have to recognize that the land is our host, and that we are indebted to it. This recognition would allow the farmer, gardener or forester to be placed in a different position than is customary today. He would become a mediator between the land and a community of people. From composting to sowing to harvesting, he should be given full freedom to administer the land according to its needs, according to methods and principles which are in harmony with the living organism of the farm. He would then be assured of his true position, that of a mediator between a community of men on the one hand and divine forces working in the organism of the land on the other.—adapted from **Bio Dynamics**, Spring 1975 by Hartmut von Jeetze

ABRAHAM, GEORGE and DOC. *RAISE VEGETABLES, FRUITS, AND HERBS WITHOUT A GARDEN,* 2.95. This is the best book of type that we have ever seen. All the crops you would want to grow are clearly covered and problems which may come up are also discussed. There's also plenty of background information. Illustrated throughout with excellent line drawings and color photographs. Index, 8¼"x10½", 86pp. H&R 74

CAMPBELL, STU. *LET IT ROT: THE HOME GARDENER'S GUIDE TO COMPOSTING,* 3.95. A complete discussion of composting, beginning with instructions on constructing a compost pile and containing an exhaustive guide to materials which can be composted. Campbell also talks about the many uses of compost and simplifies the technical terminology. There's really no need to buy a whole book on composting—most of the larger organic gardening books contain chapters on it—but if you are interested in getting one, this is your best bet. Bibliography, index, 152pp. Gar 75

CAMPBELL, STU. *THE MULCH BOOK,* 3.95. A comprehensive, illustrated guide to mulching your garden. Notes, index, 147pp. Gar 73

FELL, DEREK. *HOW TO PLANT A VEGETABLE GARDEN,* 3.95. This is an excellent handbook for the beginning gardener. It includes over 100 of the nicest line drawings we have ever seen. All the basic vegetables are covered as well as a number of fruits, nuts, and berries. There's also information on soil preparation, seed starting and transplanting, composting, and canning, freezing and dry storage. 8¼"x10½", 96pp. H&R 75

FOSTER, CATHARINE. *THE ORGANIC GARDENER,* 2.95. This is an excellent book for the beginning gardener. Ms. Foster speaks from almost forty years of working with the soil and she has a wealth of experience to draw on. She also writes wonderfully; unlike many of the dry gardening books, this one is a joy to read. Virtually everything of interest to the gardener is covered, and many neat tips are offered. Vivid line drawings abound throughout. We recommend this book highly. Bibliography and directory of resources, index, 250pp. RaH 72

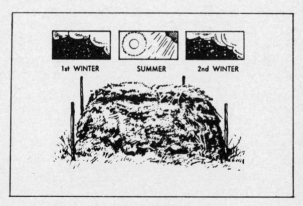

Compost Pile

GRIFFITH, ROGER. *VEGETABLE GARDEN HANDBOOK,* 3.95. A spiral bound planning and planting record book which also includes complete planting data on fifty-seven vegetables, graph pages to plot garden plans, and much else. Index, 126pp. Gar 74

HECKEL, ALICE, ed. *THE PFEIFFER GARDEN BOOK: BIO-DYNAMICS IN THE HOME GARDEN,* 5.50. The bio-dynamic system of farming and gardening developed out of advice and instructions given to farmers by Rudolf Steiner. *Working with living plants on a soil that has life in it, we endeavor to work with the ultimate processes that shape and maintain life rather than just with a few of its material bricks.* The bio-dynamic gardeners differ from organic gardeners in their emphasis on a high humus content in the soil, their desire for balanced nutrients, and especially in their consideration of cosmic factors as they affect plant life. This book provides an adequate overview of the subject—although it is not a comprehensive discussion. The book begins with information on starting a bio-dynamic garden and goes on to a discussion of specific crops. Index, 230pp. BID 67

HOWARD, ALBERT. *AN AGRICULTURAL TESTAMENT,* c7.95. Since this book first appeared, it has been regarded as one of the most important contributions to the solution of soil rehabilitation problems ever published. It has also been regarded as the keystone of the organic movement. Howard's object was to draw attention to the loss of soil fertility, brought about by the vast increase in crop and animal production, that has led to such disastrous consequences as a general unbalancing of farming practices, an increase in plant and animal diseases, and the loss of soil by erosion. He stresses that such losses can only be repaired by maintaining soil fertility through the manufacture of humus by composting. Tables, illustrations, index, 253pp. Rod 40

HOWARD, ALBERT. *THE SOIL AND HEALTH,* 4.95. A fascinating study of the relationship of organic cultivation of the soil to health in plants, animals, and humans. Every page of the book is filled with practical knowledge and stimulating ideas and speculation. Index, 307pp. ScB 47

JEAVONS, JOHN. *HOW TO GROW MORE VEGETABLES THAN YOU EVER THOUGHT POSSIBLE ON LESS LAND THAN YOU CAN IMAGINE,* 4.00. One of the modern day heroes of the organic gardening movement is Alan Chadwick who introduced this subject into the curriculum of the University of California at Santa Cruz using a method which combined bio-dynamic principles with the intensive practices developed by French market gardeners a century ago. The essence is using small raised beds, dug very deeply, with the soil carefully enriched, so that plants can be spaced very close together with their leaves acting as a kind of mulch. This 8½"x11", typewritten, saddle stitched book is the first distillation of Chadwick's teaching by a group of his students. We're using this method in our own garden and recommend this little book as the best presentation of it to date. Bibliography, 82pp. Eco 74

KOEPF, HERBERT. *BIO-DYNAMIC AGRICULTURE: AN INTRODUCTION,* c12.00. This is the most comprehensive discussion imaginable. Every aspect of agriculture is discussed from a bio-dynamic viewpoint and it's often very heavy material. We had problems getting into the book and so will most people. If you are seriously interested in the bio-dynamic methods, then this is the book for you. But beware, it takes a deep study. Many case histories and practical examples are offered. Bibliography, index, 439pp. API 76

MCKILLIP, BARBARA, ed. *GETTING THE BUGS OUT OF ORGANIC GARDENING,* 2.95. A discussion of organic pest control by the editors of **Organic Gardening Magazine.** The book includes a discussion of the constituents of healthy soil, natural soil guardians, companion planting, organic sprays, and much else. Suppliers of various products are also given. Index, 124pp. Rod 73

OLKOWSKI, HELGA and WILLIAM. *THE CITY PEOPLE'S BOOK OF RAISING FOOD,* 4.95. A fine book for city dwellers which shows how they can become more food self-sufficient, despite space limitations, poor city soil, and other problems inherent in living in a city. They cover all the basics as they relate to city food production. Index, 239pp. Rod 75

ORGANIC GARDENING AND FARMING MAGAZINE (Rodale Press, Inc., 33 East Minor Street, Emmaus, PA 18049). This is *the* magazine for those who are interested in organic gardening. It's a monthly and is packed with useful articles and case histories from readers. The Rodale organization has been at the forefront of the organic movement and they conduct an extensive research program which is reported on in their magazine. Single issue, 75 cents, year's subscription, $7.85.

ORGANIC GARDENING AND FARMING STAFF, eds. *ORGANIC FERTILIZERS: WHICH ONES AND HOW TO USE THEM,* 2.95. A readable discussion which covers virtually all kinds of organic fertilizers. Index, 129pp. Rod 73

PETRICH, PATRICIA and ROSEMARY DALTON. *THE KIDS GARDEN BOOK,* 3.95. Kids love the magic of seeing things grow and almost no child is too small to enjoy having her own garden. This profusely illustrated book is filled with gardening ideas for kids. Many, if not all, of the illustrations appear to have been drawn by kids and almost half of them are in color. The book reads easily and is suitable for pre-schoolers. 8¼"x5¼", 188pp. Nit 74

PFEIFFER, EHRENFRIED. *THE ART AND SCIENCE OF COMPOSTING,* 1.50. A technical paper outlining Pfeiffer's observations and his testing methods. 20pp. BID 59

PFEIFFER, EHRENFRIED. *WEEDS AND WHAT THEY TELL,* 3.25. A bio-dynamic analysis, discussing how weeds grow, what they reveal about their surroundings, and how their powers may be harnessed for the benefit of the human beings who appreciate and use them. Illustrations, index, 96pp. BID nd

PHILBRICK, HELEN and RICHARD GREGG. *COMPANION PLANTS AND HOW TO USE THEM,* 3.95. This was the pioneering book on companion planting, and it is the source for all later works. We find Louise Riotte's book more useful, but there are some things in here that have not been duplicated in Ms. Riotte's book. Alphabetically arranged. Bibliography, index, 128pp. DAC 66

PHILBRICK, JOHN and HELEN. *THE BUG BOOK: HARMLESS INSECT CONTROL,* 3.95. A bio-dynamic exploration of ways to identify and control the pests that are damaging your crops. 126pp. DAC 72

RAYMOND, DICK. *DOWN-TO-EARTH VEGETABLE GARDENING KNOW-HOW,* 5.95. This is a neat collection of hints from an experienced gardener—full of photographs, charts, and tables. Covers choosing the right site for your particular needs, soil conditioning, planting techniques, weeding methods, diseases, pest control, harvesting, weeding methods, fertilizing, and much else. We have found many neat ideas here that we haven't seen elsewhere. And, as the title says, it's all down to earth! Index, 8½"x11", 160pp. Gar 75

RIOTTE, LOUISE. *THE COMPLETE GUIDE TO GROWING BERRIES AND GRAPES,* 3.50. A clearly written study, covering

380

virtually every aspect of the subject. Illustrations, index, 144pp. Gar 74

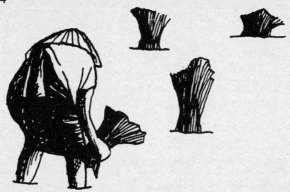

RIOTTE, LOUISE. *NUTS FOR THE FOOD GARDENER,* 4.50. A complete how to grower's guide to raising, storing, and using thirteen kinds of nut crops. Each chapter covers the full range of cultivation, care, harvesting, and pest control information for each kind of nut. Illustrations, index, 179pp. Gar 75

RIOTTE, LOUISE. *PLANETARY PLANTING: A GUIDE TO ORGANIC GARDENING BY THE SIGNS OF THE ZODIAC,* 4.95. Ms. Riotte discusses the centuries old method of planting and harvesting according to the signs of the zodiac and the phases of the moon, in harmony with the natural rhythms of life. She shows how these techniques can be adapted to small home gardens. The book contains information on growing trees, berries, flowers, vines, lawns, herbs, and house plants. There's also material on organic methods of pest control. An unusual, neat book. Illustrations, bibliography, index, 352pp. S&S 75

RIOTTE, LOUISE. *SECRETS OF COMPANION PLANTING FOR SUCCESSFUL GARDENING,* 4.95. Companion planting takes advantage of th fact that vegetables and fruits have natural friends that they prefer to be with. This book is far and away the most complete book on the subject and it should be in the library of everyone who is seriously interested in gardening. Ms. Riotte has incorporated information from a number of disciplines, including bio-dynamics. The book is alphabetically arranged and very clearly written. Recommended. Illustrations, bibliography, index, 226pp. Gar 75

RIOTTE, LOUISE. *SUCCESS WITH SMALL FOOD GARDENS USING SPECIAL INTENSIVE METHODS,* 4.95. An excellent, practical survey of all types of intensive gardens for fruits, vegetables, and berries. Ms. Riotte supplements her text with a variety of lot plans and illustrations. Index, 192pp. Gar 77

RODALE, J.I. and **STAFF.** *THE COMPLETE BOOK OF COMPOSTING,* c11.95. Everything you could possibly want to know—and more—about the science of composting. Illustrations, bibliography, index, 1007pp. Rod 75

RODALE, J.I. and **STAFF.** *ENCYCLOPEDIA OF ORGANIC GARDENING,* 12.95. For over seventeen years, this has been the organic gardener's bible. Its 1145 pages cover over 1500 topics (alphabetized for quick reference), and provide information on just about every fruit, vegetable, flower, shrub, nut, herb, tree, organic technique and principle that you could possibly think of. Hundreds of related topics are also covered. If you are seriously involved in organic gardening, this book is a must. Illustrated throughout. Rod 59

RODALE, J.I. and **STAFF.** *HOW TO GROW VEGETABLES AND FRUITS BY THE ORGANIC METHOD,* c13.95. This book differs from the *Encyclopedia* in that it covers fruits, vegetables, nuts, and herbs only—and it discusses these in far greater detail than the latter book. Seventy-five kinds of vegetables and sixty-three kinds of fruit are covered at length and information is included on range and soil, seed and planting, maintenance, culture, enemies, and harvesting. The book is packed with charts, diagrams, and testimonials from organic gardeners. There are also detailed chapters on the mechanics of planning and planting vegetable gardens and orchards, improving soil structure, mulching, composting, pruning, natural pest control, and much else. This is the book we use the most, and we recommend it highly. Illustrations, index, 926pp. Rod 61

RODALE, ROBERT, ed. *THE BASIC BOOK OF ORGANIC GARDENING,* 1.95. A compilation written by the editors of **Organic Gardening Magazine.** As the title suggests, this book covers all the basics and is full of information and suggestions. An excellent book for the beginner who wants to know where to start. Glossary, index, 377pp. RaH 71

STEINER, RUDOLF. *AGRICULTURE,* 6.50. A new edition of

these long out-of-print lectures. Fascinating material for all gardeners, including color illustrations and practical advice. 175pp. Bio 74

STOUT, RUTH. *HOW TO HAVE A GREEN THUMB WITHOUT AN ACHING BACK,* 1.95. This is a delightful book, filled with hints for gardening the easy way. The easy way for Ms. Stout involves building up a thick layer of mulch on your garden and planting in the mulch. It's not as easy as it sounds, but the technique does yield often amazing results. 160pp. S&S 73

STOUT, RUTH and RICHARD CLEMENCE. *THE RUTH STOUT NO WORK GARDEN BOOK,* 1.50. A collection of the articles that the authors wrote for **Organic Gardening Magazine** between 1953 and 1971. The later ones at times contradict the earlier ones, so the reader can learn as the authors did. Index, 161pp. Ban 71

WOLF, RAY, ed. *MANAGING YOUR PERSONAL FOOD SUP-PLY,* c11.95. This book is a hard one to categorize. It is a cookbook, a manual on basic nutrition, and a discussion of the basic principles of organic gardening. We have put it in the organic gardening section because that's where it seems to most belong. The emphasis throughout is on home management of resources—on spotting where problems lie and forestalling them before they crop up. The authors suggest ways of planning and means of record keeping. Every conceivable topic is covered at some length. Bibliography, index, 476pp. Rod 77

YEPSEN, ROGER, ed. *ORGANIC PLANT PROTECTION,* c12.95. A comprehensive study of basic preventive measures, including extensive information on how to identify and combat thousands of common pests. Written by the editors of **Organic Gardening Magazine.** 688pp. Rod 76

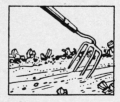 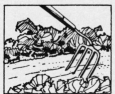 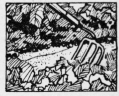

Oriental Medicine

The life of the universe and the life of an individual are essentially the same and are made from the same elements. According to the ancient Oriental philosophers, each life, everything in the universe, even the universe itself, follows the same life cycle. Yin and yang are the opposing forces of the universe which must be maintained in balance if Oneness is to be attained. Yin is a negative or minus force. Yang is positive. The moon is considered yin—the sun, yang. Night is yin—day is yang; water is yin—fire, yang. Within the concept of yin and yang there are no absolutes, and it is thought that although the forces are opposing they are also in harmony. For instance, man is yang to woman, yin. Since neither yin nor yang is an absolute, each contains the other, and everything is made of both yin and yang. Men and women both have male and female hormones.

It is also thought that yin and yang forces are not static; that they are changing constantly, and an excess of yin becomes yang and too much yang becomes yin. When water (yin) is frozen (yin), it becomes ice (yang).

Since its beginnings, Oriental medicine has been closely related to the philosophy of Oneness and the idea of yin and yang forces of the environment and the body. The belief was that diminished health occurred only when the equilibrium between yin and yang was broken. The approach to healing was preventive, to keep the body in harmony. If, however, the harmony was lost, it had to be restored. This attitude of prevention has been carried down through the years to shiatzu, for it is first and foremost a method to maintain health and keep the body in harmony.

The ancient Chinese healers and philosophers made intensive studies of human ailments. The system which grew out of these studies was quite different from that developed by modern Western medicine thousands of years later. The Oriental approach is empirical: practices are based on experience and observation. The Chinese sages observed that certain ailments affected certain points on the surface of the body: various points became hot, cold, numb, hard, painful, oily, dry, discolored or stained. They located 657 such points on the body and observed that some of these points appeared to be related to one another. Acting like medical map makers, they charted the lines between these related points and determined that there are twelve pathways or meridians connecting the points on each half of the body. In addition to these twelve pairs of body meridians, they traced out two coordinating meridians which bisect the body. One, known as the meridian of conception, runs up from the base of the trunk, up the center of the abdomen, the center of the chest, and ends at a point in the front center of the lower jaw. The second, the governor meridian, begins in the center of the upper gum, traces up and over the center of the skull, down the spine, and ends at the base of the tailbone. The meridian of conception was so named because the sexual organs are located along this line. It acts mainly on yin energy. The governor meridian received its name because of the extreme significance of the spine as the main pillar of the body. It acts mainly on yang energy. These two bisecting meridians control the energy which flows constantly through the twelve pairs of body meridians. Interconnected, the twelve pairs of body meridians or pathways form the single energy system which maintains the health of the body.

The accuracy of the sages' observation is attested to by the fact that their ideas of the functions of these meridians correspond in many cases to the functions of the various networks discovered so many centuries later by Western medicine, i.e., the circulatory and nervous systems, the endocrine system, the reproductive system, etc.

The early sages believed that the meridians were pathways through which the energy of the universe circulated throughout the body organs and kept the universe and the body in harmony. They conceived that illness or pain occurred when the pathways became blocked, disrupting the energy flow and breaking the body's harmony. By inserting extremely fine needles into the body at the affected points on the pathways and into related points, they believed that the pathways' blockage was broken and the flow of energy was restored. They also believed that periodic treatment of a healthy person helped to preserve the flow of energy and to prevent illness. This grew into the science of acupuncture.

Over the years acupuncture has become a sophisticated and medical discipline still based upon its early concept—that it is necessary to maintain balance between all areas of the body within itself as well as within the external environment.—from **Shiatzu: Japanese Finger Pressure for Energy, Sexual Vitality and Relief from Tension and Pain** by Yukiko Irwin with James Wagenvoord.

Many of the books in this section specifically discuss the practice of acupuncture. Others survey the whole realm of oriental medicine, ancient and modern. Books on oriental herbalism are described in the Herbs section and the Healing section contains a number of books on Tibetan and Indian medicine.

ACADEMY OF TRADITIONAL CHINESE MEDICINE. *AN OUTLINE OF CHINESE ACUPUNCTURE,* c12.50. *The aim of compiling this book is to provide source material for study by medical personnel in China and other countries, and to popularize the science of acupuncture and moxibustion. After studying this book one should have a preliminary understanding of the development of acupuncture and moxibustion in China, together with their basic theory and application in clinical treatment. . . .In the selec-*

tion of material for this book, every effort has been made that it be concise, practical, and easily understood. The book was published in mainland China and is an extremely detailed study which should be of great interest to all practitioners. 133 plates, many in color, including two 20"x13" full views of the human body. Index, 10½"x7½", 319pp. FLP 75

ACUPUNCTURE RESEARCH INSTITUTE. *ACUPUNCTURE MADE EASY,* **6.95.** "This is a little classic produced by experienced teachers of this modernized ancient art, intended as a textbook for use by the up to one million bare-foot doctors. I warmly recommend it even for any western beginning student. . . ."—Wong Kwan-Pak, the Hong Kong acupuncturist who gave the translators the original book. Includes a good general introduction, a section detailing the most commonly used acupuncture points (including the Chinese characters for the point, transliteration, location, indocation, and technique—along with a detailed drawing), and a subdivided section on ailments treatable with acupuncture. Indices to points and ailments, 97pp. ChB 75

AUSTIN, MARY. *TEXTBOOK OF ACUPUNCTURE THERAPY,* c15.00. Dr. Austin is a physician who has practiced and taught acupuncture at the Albert Einstein Medical School in New York City. In this excellent textbook she explains the bipolar energy of the body and the ways in which it can be balanced, gives anatomical descriptions, and illustrates the exact location of acupuncture points, discusses the nature of the five elements, and much else. She also gives practical advice on how the needle can be used correctly, the techniques of massage and moxa therapy, and the daily and seasonal effects upon acupuncture therapy. A comprehensive study which should prove extremely useful to both practitioners and students. Notes, 276pp. ASI 72

CADRE. *ACUPUNCTURE MANIKIN,* 90.00. The official teaching model used in China today. Soft, plastic body, hand painted meridians, and varnished mahogany stand. Twenty inches tall. Available either with English numbering system or Chinese calligraphy (specify which you want). Includes an explanatory booklet of acupuncture points. (A 10" tall display model is available for $30—Chinese calligraphy, no booklet.) Cad

CADRE. *ACUPUNCTURE WALL CHART,* 5.00. Includes meridian points, extra points, points used for anesthesia, three full length views of the body, plus seven detailed inserts including one showing ear points. 23"x35". Cad

CADRE. *ATLAS OF THE EAR,* 16.00. A spiral bound atlas containing four illustrations, 12"x12", three in color, on heavy card stock. Shows the front and back of the ear with individual views of acupuncture points, nerves, veins, and arteries, and the paths of the six ear meridians. Cad

CADRE. *FOUR CHARTS,* 7.00. A comprehensive package of four full color anatomy charts, each 14"x30", English reference atlas, and pamphlet on acupuncture anesthesia—drawn in the old Chinese style and suitable for framing. Includes explanatory material. Cad

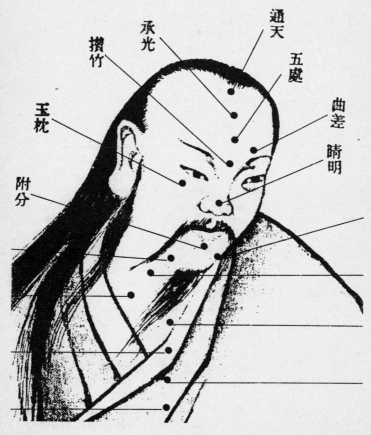

CADRE. *LIFE SIZED EAR MODELS,* 13.00/pair. Plastic, showing the ear points and stylized morphology. Cad

CADRE. *TEXOPRINT CHARTS,* 25.00. A set of three 24"x37½" wall charts on cleanable, wrinkle resistant texoprint. The numbering system has been especially prepared by the AJCM committee on nomenclature. Cad

CHAITOW, LEON. *THE ACUPUNCTURE TREATMENT OF PAIN,* 12.95. A very well illustrated, specific discussion of the role acupuncture can play in relieving pain. Precise details of anatomical location are given adjacent to each detailed diagram. Both body and auricular points are given for each cause of pain. Dr. Chaitow is an osteopath who has studied acupuncture under Dr. J. Lavier. He emphasizes the treatment of pain in his professional practice and this book is geared to practitioners. Index, 8½"x11", 160pp. TPL 76

CHAN, PEDRO. *ACUPUNCTURE, ELECTRO-ACUPUNCTURE, ANAESTHESIA,* 1.95. What is acupuncture and what are the new discoveries? Chan offers information from his experience and research. Copiously illustrated with pictures from China. 44pp. ChB 72

CHAN, PEDRO. *ANIMAL CHART,* 8.50. Shows pertinent acupuncture points in anatomically correct locations for the horse, cow, pig, chicken, and duck. Also illustrates several types of needles used for animal acupuncture. Full colors, 20"x29". ChB

CHAN, PEDRO. *BODY CHART,* 12.00, flat/6.50, folded. Bilingual, Chinese and English (Dr. Mann's number code). Originally designed by the Chinese Medical College of Peking. Shows the positions of acupuncture meridians and points in relation to the human body and internal organs. The courses of the meridians are indicated with different colors or patterns. Three views: anterior, posterior, and lateral. ChB

CHAN, PEDRO. *EAR ACUPUNCTURE CHART,* 8.50. Shows ear points and prescriptions on eighty-three diseases where ear acupuncture has proved to be beneficial. Also describes all points and combinations used in acupuncture anesthesia. In addition it shows ideographic diagrams (front and back) of the auricle for ear acupuncture.

Translated from a number of authoritative Chinese sources. Three colors, 20"x29". ChB

CHAN, PEDRO. *EAR POINT CHART,* 10.00, flat/5.00, folded. Bilingual, Chinese and English. Two main views: one full anterior showing over 100 auricular points; another shows thirty-eight points on the back of the ear. Also includes a preliminary presentation of therapeutic functions of some major ear points, compiled by the Zoological Research Institute of the Chinese Academy of Sciences. Full colors, 20"x29". ChB

CHAN, PEDRO. *ELECTRO-ACUPUNCTURE,* 8.50. *Electro-acupuncture therapy is a new concept in the healing sciences integrating conventional acupuncture with modern technology. Its uniqueness is a therapeutic apparatus which transmits electrical currents of different characteristics through acupuncture needles to human subjects, in order to give symptomatic relief and therapeutic results.* Subtitled *Its Clinical Applications in Therapy,* this is a compilation of Chinese translations and references, well organized and including introductory and instructional material as well as detailed chapters on the treatment of various ailments. Extensive illustrations of the points and of the equipment. Notes, 103pp. ChB 74

CHAN, PEDRO. *HAND ACUPUNCTURE CHART,* 8.50. Shows all new points of the hand in relation to the surface and anatomical location. Each point is clearly defined and indicated for many specific symptoms. Also includes a series of diagrams showing needling techniques in hand acupuncture. Three colors, 20"x29". ChB

CHAN, PEDRO. *WONDERS OF CHINESE ACUPUNCTURE,* 4.50. *This monograph by Pedro Chan has encompassed traditional Chinese medicine for those who desire a short but concise explanation and correlation of Chinese and Western medicine. . . .There is a good correlation between the two types of medical practice and the application of an integrated medical approach to patient treatment.* —Howard Morse, M.D., Chairman, Department of Anesthesia, White Memorial Medical Center. Many illustrations, 133pp. ChB 73

CHANG, STEPHEN. *THE COMPLETE BOOK OF ACUPUNCTURE,* 6.95. Dr. Chang is a direct descendant of a long line of Chinese physicians and his great grandfather was physician to an Empress of China. He is a practicing acupuncturist and his goal in this book is to give the Western reader as understandable a picture as possible of the rationale and practice of acupuncture. The drawings that illustrate the text are adequate, but little more, however, the text itself is well above the average. The chapter on energy is especially fine. The second half of the book is devoted to a specific discussion of regional acupuncture points throughout the body—material which is of little practical value to the nonpractitioner. And there's a final section of treatment for specific ailments. 263pp. CeA 76

CLAUSEN, TORBEN, ed. *PRACTICAL ACUPUNCTURE,* 7.95. "The main purpose of translating this book has been to provide some insight into fundamental aspects of acupuncture as practiced today by millions of health workers in China. Therefore, a short popular and contemporary handbook was selected (more than 2.5 million copies sold in China up to 1970). As stated in the preface to the Chinese edition, the present text is written with the intention of making basic techniques of acupunture available to people with a minimum of medical training." This is by no means an easy introduction. It is designed for practical use and is fully illustrated. Includes two introductory sections: "How to Locate Acupuncture Points" and "The Techniques of Acupuncture and Moxibustion" along with a detailed analysis of the position of the individual points. The terminology used corresponds to the classification system proposed by Felix Mann on the basis of Soulier de Morant's now classical system. This is considered the best overall work available for the beginning practitioner. Notes, 160pp. Cad 73

DA LIU. *TAOIST HEALTH EXERCISE BOOK,* 3.95. This is more than a mere illustration of exercises. Da Liu has attempted to explain the philosophy behind the exercises and how this philosophy relates to Western wo/man. Included are tai chi chuan movements, breathing exercises, explanations of the acupuncture meridians, and material on curative herbs. Nicely illustrated. 135pp. QFx 74

DIMOND, E. GREY. *MORE THAN HERBS AND ACUPUNCTURE,* c8.95. In 1971 Dr. Dimond, a cardiologist, made the first of three trips to the People's Republic, playing a key role in developing the original medical exchanges between the U.S. and China. He was specifically interested in learning about the medical education, acupuncture anesthesia, herbal medicine, and medical care. This is a very readable account of his experiences in China and of his observations of the Chinese medical system. 223pp. Nor 75

DUKE, MARC. *ACUPUNCTURE,* 1.50. A detailed introduction for the layman as well as the serious student which surveys the current work being done all over the world plus the technique and philosophy of acupuncture. Well illustrated, bibliography, index, 201pp. Pyr 72

EWART, CHARLES. *THE HEALING NEEDLES,* 1.25. Charles Ewart was a patient of Dr. Louis Moss, one of England's pioneering acupuncturists. Here he tells us the story of Moss' battle to gain recognition for acupuncture in England and includes many detailed case histories of patients with widely varying ailments. 137pp. Kea 73

FITZGERALD, WILLIAM and EDWIN BOWERS. *ZONE THERAPY,* 5.50. This is actually three books in one, including George S. White's **Zone Therapy.** Fitzgerald was the pioneer in the field and this is the basic source book—not as readable as some of the later manuals, but important, nonetheless. HeR 72

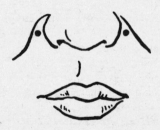

GEOGRAPHIC HEALTH STUDIES PROGRAM. *A BAREFOOT DOCTOR'S MANUAL,* 5.95. This is an amazing book which was originally put together in 1970 by the Institute of Traditional Chinese Medicine. The manual lists and describes 197 common and prevalent diseases, some 522 herbs (with 338 illustrations), and offers several hundred tried and tested remedies based on effectiveness, popular use, ease of preparation, and economy. The manual was prepared for use by the rural "barefoot doctors" and has been translated under the auspices of the U.S. Department of Health, Edcation, and Welfare. We recommend the manual highly to all who are interested in healing and particularly in Chinese medicine. Oversize, 974pp. RuP 74

HALL, MANLY P. *THE MEDICINE OF THE SUN AND MOON,* 1.50. A well written philosophical treatise on the principles behind the Chinese concept of healing. 32pp. PRS 72

HASHIMOTO, M. *JAPANESE ACUPUNCTURE,* 1.75. Dr. Hashimoto runs a successful acupuncture clinic in Tokyo. This book embodies her system of pulse diagnosis and her philosophy of healing. Glossary, 80pp. Liu 68

HUANG, HELENA. *EAR ACUPUNCTURE,* c14.50. This is a translation of a medical book written and published in the People's Republic of China. It was compiled and edited after more than ten years of experience in the development and practice of the technique by a team of acupuncturists. Ear acupuncture involves the treatment of disease through the application of acupuncture techniques to the external ear. The technique seems to be effective in treating a large variety of common diseases. This work also describes the interrelationship between the ear and internal organs of the body in the theory of traditional Chinese medicine, and includes much related material. Twelve full page plates and numerous charts detailing the points used in treating common diseases are included. An excellent reference work for the practitioner and serious researcher. Index, 149pp. Rod 72

HUARD, PIERRE and MING WONG. *CHINESE MEDICINE,* 2.45. A historical text by two French doctors, both of whom are leading authorities on oriental medicine. Contents include the evolution of Chinese medicine, Western medicine in modern China, and traditional medicine in modern China. Extensively illustrated, 237pp. MGH 68

JAIN, K.K. *AMAZING STORY OF HEALTH CARE IN NEW CHINA,* c7.95. Dr. Jain is a Canadian neurosurgeon who visited China in 1971. He recorded what he saw and learned and here he presents an overview of all aspects of medical care in China today. Acupuncture is just one of the many methods of Chinese medicine that he evaluates. Other topics include herbs, folk medicine, and China's medical traditions. Observations and impressions of the Chinese lifestyle and the future of Chinese medicine are also included along with many photographs. Index, 184pp. Rod 73

KUSHI, MICHIO. *AN INTRODUCTION TO ORIENTAL DIAG-*

NOSIS FROM LECTURES BY MICHIO KUSHI, 4.95. *The art of diagnosis is based upon the understanding of what man is, within the order of the universe. The immortal law of endless change of all phenomena, yin and yang, which governs all physical, mental and spiritual phenomena as well as visible and invisible worlds in this universe is a way to approach the art of diagnosis. . . .Accordingly, those who observe people through the art of diagnosis are able to eventually understand the meaning of life.*—from the foreword by Michio Kushi. The book is illustrated throughout and each area of the body is discussed in turn. Bibliography, 92pp. RMP 76

LANGRE, JACQUES DE. *ACUPUNCTURE, DO-IN AND SHIATSU ATLAS,* 4.25. All acupuncture meridians are shown in relation to surface anatomy and skeletal configuration. Thirty-six of the major treatment points are specifically indicated. Printed in three colors, 23"x35". Hap

LAVIER, J. *POINTS OF CHINESE ACUPUNCTURE,* c5.00. A detailed technical text translated, indexed, and edited by Dr. Philip Chancellor. It is divided into four parts: *General Topography of the Meridians, Regional Topography of the Points of Acupuncture, Bioenergy,* and *Synthesis of Symptomatic Treatment.* Each of the numbered points is illustrated and named. 115pp. HSP 74

LAWSON-WOOD, DENIS and JOYCE. *ACUPUNCTURE HANDBOOK,* c7.00. A textbook for students and practitioners which presents a westernized form of the science. Correspondences are indicated which link the therapeutic effect of each acupuncture point to a specific homoeopathic remedy. A preface describes the discoveries of Professor Kim Bong Han of North Korea. Includes photographs of the meridian points. 141pp. HSP 64

LAWSON-WOOD, DENIS and JOYCE. *FIVE ELEMENTS OF ACUPUNCTURE AND CHINESE MASSAGE,* c4.80. The authors present an approach which stresses foreseeing and preventing disease rather than suppressing symptoms. The terms used are readily understandable to the layman. 96pp. HSP 65

LAWSON-WOOD, DENIS and JOYCE. *THE INCREDIBLE HEALING NEEDLES,* 1.25. This is a good general layman's introduction to acupuncture, with material on the individual meridians, yin and yang, diagnosis, and oriental theories on health. A well written exposition, with many clear diagrams. 63pp. Wei 74

LAWSON-WOOD, DENIS and JOYCE. *MULTILINGUAL ATLAS OF ACUPUNCTURE,* c20.30. Seventeen color plates (19¼"x18") of anatomical drawings of the major acupuncture points as they are located on the body. Explanatory text in English, French, German, Russian, Spanish, and Swedish. The drawings are large and the points clearly illustrated. HSP 67

LEONG, LUCILLE. *ACUPUNCTURE, A LAYMAN'S VIEW,* 1.50. This is an overview of acupuncture by a woman who has academically studied the literature and has had a close relationship with a number of acupuncturists. Includes chapters on the philosophy of acupuncture, acupuncture in practice, why it works, and case studies of acupuncture treatments. There are also many illustrations, photographs and a glossary. Bibliography, 139pp. NAL 74

LIU ZHAOYUAN. *ACUPUNCTURE CHARTS,* c22.75. This is the finest set of charts that we know of. All the information is drawn from and all the drawings are based upon Chinese medical books and charts published by the People's Republic. Four color charts are included: three showing all 361 points of the fourteen principal meridians, the 117 "strange" points, and 110 newly discovered points, and one chart showing ear and hand acupuncture points and head acupuncture areas. Each point is referenced by the abbreviations and numbers commonly adopted in the West, and the Chinese name of each point is given along with its transliteration, as is the equivalent point number. The charts fold out of a bound book and measure 26"x14". They are also available in a larger size as wall charts for $25.00. CCC 75

MCGAREY, WILLIAM. *ACUPUNCTURE AND BODY ENERGIES,* c6.95. Dr. McGarey has been Director of the Medical Research Division of the Edgar Cayce Foundation since 1965 and has been instrumental in activating research programs designed to evaluate concepts in the Cayce readings as they pertain to physiology and therapy. Since 1970 he has been the Director of the A.R.E. Clinic in Arizona, a medical group actively engaged in various research projects designed to explore the material in the Cayce readings at a clinical and laboratory level. *This book. . .will deal with my ideas of how acupuncture fits into the Western scheme of things; how these various laws and concepts of acupuncture appear to the Western doctor who is philosophically inclined; and. . .what might be expected as one learns about this ancient art of healing the body* *and puts it to the test.* McGarey spent over two years studying and practicing acupuncture before beginning this book. Illustrations, notes, index, 146pp. Gab 74

MANAKA, YOSHIO and IAN URQUHART. *THE LAYMAN'S GUIDE TO ACUPUNCTURE,* c7.95/3.95. In addition to presenting a concise but thorough introduction to the concepts underlying acupuncture, the authors discuss diagnosis, uses of different kinds of needles, treatment procedures, treatment of children, moxibustion and pressure massage, and some empirical experiments now going on. The text is amplified by a wealth of illustrations, including both traditional woodcuts and up to date photographs and drawings. This is the best work on acupuncture for the layman that we have seen. 143pp. Wea 72

MANN, FELIX. *ACUPUNCTURE–THE ANCIENT CHINESE ART OF HEALING,* 1.95. Mann, a leading British acupuncturist, here describes the basic principles and laws, according to the theories of traditional Chinese medicine. There are chapters on yin and yang, the five elements, theories of pulse diagnosis, the laws of acupuncture, Ki–the energy of life. This second edition contains about fifty percent new material and has been almost entirely rewritten. Sixty-eight drawings, bibliography, 253pp. RaH 71

MANN, FELIX. *ACUPUNCTURE: CURE OF MANY DISEASES,* 1.95. This is Mann's least technical book. It briefly surveys many aspects of the theory and practice of acupuncture and is illustrated throughout. 121pp. HeG 71

MANN, FELIX. *ATLAS OF ACUPUNCTURE,* c15.00. This is considered the definitive acupuncture atlas. Includes front, rear, and side views, giving the points and meridians in relation to surface anatomy. Done in book form on heavy paper with the illustration continuing from page to page without a break. 7½"x14". HeG 66

MANN, FELIX. *THE MERIDIANS OF ACUPUNCTURE,* c9.00. The course, function and symptomatology of the fifty-nine meridians which constitute the basis of classical Chinese acupuncture are portrayed in detail. In addition, the traditional Chinese physiology and pathology of the twelve main groups of internal organs are described and correlated with Western scientific medicine wherever possible. Fifty-three full page drawings, index, 174pp. HeG 64

MANN, FELIX. *THE TREATMENT OF DISEASE BY ACU-PUNCTURE,* c12.00. In Part I, *Function of Acupuncture Points,* each point is listed separately and a full account of the symptoms and diseases that may be influenced by stimulating a specific point is given, following the classical Chinese pattern. In Part II, *The Treatment of Disease,* the majority of diseases amenable to acupuncture are tabulated with the corresponding acupuncture points used for treatment. The first part of this section is based entirely on Chinese sources, while the second describes the experiences of Mann and other European doctors. Bibliography, 222pp. HeG 63

MATSUMOTO, TERUO. *ACUPUNCTURE FOR PHYSICIANS,* c19.60. This is a very technical survey with extensive illustrations and photographs of the clinical practice of acupuncture. Also includes many case studies and a description of research going on now as well as proposed research. The language and approach make this book suitable only for practitioners. Extensive bibliography, notes, index, 203pp. Tho 74

MEDICINE AND HEALTH PUBLISHING COMPANY. *AN EX-PLANATORY BOOK OF THE NEWEST ILLUSTRATIONS OF ACUPUNCTURE POINTS,* 5.50. A detailed study which analyzes the points illustrated in Cadre's **Newest Illustrations of Acupuncture Points.** Includes the transliteral name, location, main treatment, and needling methods for the meridian points in each of the parts of the body discussed. Over 640 new points are covered in all. Fully indexed by the parts of the body and the transliterated name and Chinese characters. 11½"x8½", 113pp. Cad 73

MEDICINE AND HEALTH PUBLISHING COMPANY. *NEWEST ILLUSTRATIONS OF ACUPUNCTURE POINTS,* 6.95. A set of three charts, each 15½"x34", showing many new acupuncture points and giving detailed views of the hands, throat, neck, and ear. Available in English translation. Cad

NAKATANI, YOSHIO. *A GUIDE FOR APPLICATION OF RYO-DORAKU AUTONOMOUS NERVE REGULATORY THERAPY,* 5.00. A technical study, fully illustrated with photographs, drawings, and tables. 25pp. ChB 72

NOGIER. *TREATISE OF AURICULAR THERAPY,* c44.50. A classic of the French school. Cad 72

PALOS, STEPHAN. *THE CHINESE ART OF HEALING,* 1.50. This is a well written, comprehensive discussion which begins with a history of the Chinese healing arts and a treatise on man and nature and the human body in ancient Chinese thought. The second half of the book is devoted to a discussion of traditional methods of treatment and the orientation here, as elsewhere in the book, is toward practical information, simply stated. Illustrations throughout. Bibliography and extensive notes, index, 251pp. Ban 71

PORKERT, MANFRED. *THE THEORETICAL FOUNDATIONS OF CHINESE MEDICINE,* c20.00. A systematic account of the system of correspondences that underlies all of Chinese medicine. The book is based directly and exclusively on Chinese sources, including recent Chinese secondary literature. Illustrations, bibliography, index, 384pp. MIT 74

Reflexology

Reflexology is a process of zone therapy that involves deep massage of the soles of the feet. Pressure is applied to the nerve endings in the soles. Each of the pressure points corresponds to specific organs and functions. The idea behind reflexology is that the application of pressure relaxes nerve tension, increases circulation in the blood and lymphatic systems, and helps the body throw off accumulated poisons.

BERGSON, ANIKA and VLADIMER TUCHACK. *ZONE THERAPY,* 1.25. A fully illustrated step-by-step guide to applied pressure therapy, arranged according to ailments. Each of the discussions is brief, but the directions are clear. While this is by no means a definitive volume, it serves as an adequate introduction. 149pp. Pin 74

CARTER, MILDRED. *HAND REFLEXOLOGY: KEY TO PERFECT HEALTH,* c8.95. Ms. Carter is a well known professional reflexologist, whose book on foot reflexology is the most popular one on the subject. This is the only book on hand reflexology and it is as well organized and clearly illustrated as the author's previous text. She begins with general techniques and then goes on to detail techniques for specific ailments. Index, 257pp. PrH 75

CARTER, MILDRED. *HELPING YOURSELF WITH FOOT RE-FLEXOLOGY,* 2.95. The various organs, nerves, and glands in your body are connected with certain reflex areas on the bottoms of your feet, such as the soles and toes. This book shows how it is possible, through massaging those reflex areas in certain simple ways known as reflexology, to bring relief from pains and diseases. Illustrated with many pictures and charts. Mildred Carter is a professional reflexologist who has been in practice over fourteen years. She studied under Eunice Ingham. 190pp. PrH 75

GRAZIANO, JOSEPH. *FOOTSTEPS TO BETTER HEALTH,* 4.00. This is an overpriced book for the amount of material it contains. However it is the only book on pressure point therapy that is illustrated with large photographs of the feet with the appropriate point for each ailment marked. 32pp. Grz 73

INGHAM, EUNICE. *STORIES THE FEET CAN TELL,* 4.45. Ms. Ingham was the first important reflexologist. She worked with patients and physicians for many years and her work is the basis of all that is done today. This is her first book. Many case studies are cited and there is extensive instructional material. Introductory chapters explain the method and the rest of the text deals with specific ailments. Includes a reflexology chart. 109+pp. Ing 38

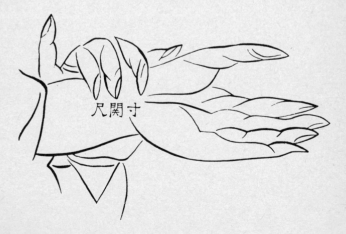

INGHAM, EUNICE. *STORIES THE FEET HAVE TOLD,* 4.45.
This second book presents a detailed account of the Ingham Reflex
Method of Compression Massage. The material is along the same
lines as the earlier work, but this book incorporates more advanced
techniques and later findings. Includes a reflexology chart. 110pp.
Ing 51

NATIONAL INSTITUTE OF REFLEXOLOGY. *FOOT CHART,*
9.00. A 22"x31" color wall chart which shows the anatomical relationship of the body to the foot's reflexology points. Ing

Shiatsu & Acupressure

Shiatzu developed during the eighteenth century in Japan
as a combination of acupuncture and the traditional amma
form of Oriental massage. Am (press) ma (stroke) was a
simple pressing and rubbing of painful spots on the body
by the fingers and palms of the hands. It was determined
that instead of needles, direct thumb and finger pressure
on the acupuncture meridian points would gain similar
results. The points are, in effect, the floodgates which
when stimulated with steady direct pressure keep the
energy systems in motion. This innovation is regarded as
the beginnings of shiatzu as we know it, although it was
nearly two hundred years later, in the 1920's, that the
name shiatzu became part of the Japanese language. Today there are over 20,000 licensed shiatzu therapists in
Japan, and the art itself is a part of nearly every Japanese
life.

Although shiatzu is closely allied to acupuncture and shares
its effects on the body, I strongly favor shiatzu as an individual discipline for a normally healthy person. Acupuncture is primarily a way to treat ailments, while
shiatzu's main function is to maintain health and well-
being—although it does overcome many ailments and

aches. Shiatzu is free of the risks of infection or rupture that are inherent in needle therapy. While it is not possible for a layman to give acupuncture, virtually anyone can learn the basic shiatzu techniques. And you can apply shiatzu to yourself easily.

We often take our hands and fingers for granted, but they serve us as a means of communication and a way to ease pain. When in love, people hold hands or touch each other. When one is in pain, one's hands reach directly to the area of the pain. Being at one with your hands is the essence of shiatzu. Whether you are giving to another or practicing self-shiatzu, energy is transmitted from your hands.

Specifically, shiatzu is given with the thumbs, fingers and palms, but these serve only as the outlet for your energy. In fact, you give shiatzu with your entire body, focusing your weight and consciousness at your fingers.

Whether you are a man or a woman, shiatzu can enhance your life. When it is used intelligently and consistently, in concert with proper diet and exercise, its purposes become its results. Muscles relax, pains are alleviated, nervous tensions diminish. Take advantage of it. You'll find that as an ancient sage once said, *Healthy thoughts and vitality spring from the healthy body.*—from **Shiatzu: Japanese Finger Pressure for Energy, Sexual Vitality and Relief from Tension and Pain** by Yukiko Irwin with James Wagenvoord

BEAN, ROY. *HELPING YOUR HEALTH WITH POINTED PRESSURE THERAPY,* c8.95. Dr. Bean is a naturopath who has used the techniques he outlines here for twenty years in his private practice. The book is organized according to specific ailments and the methods for relieving the discomfort are fully discussed. Unfortunately, the discussion is not accompanied by illustrations; however, general instructions on Dr. Bean's technique are offered at the beginning of the book. Index, 204pp. PrH 75

BERGSON, ANIKA. *SHIATZU: JAPANESE PRESSURE POINT*

MASSAGE, 1.50. An extremely simplified discussion of shiatsu. The illustrations are profuse but are little more than adequate and the text is in summary form. The bulk of the book is devoted to suggestions for the use of shiatsu in a variety of ailments. 144+pp. Pin 76

BLATE, MICHAEL. *THE G-JO HANDBOOK*, 6.95. *G-Jo. . .is roughly translated from the Chinese as meaning "first aid." However, the techniques described in the following pages are substantially different from the splinting, bandaging, and such, one often considers when thinking of Western-style first aid. The G-Jo techniques primarily rely upon fingertip stimulation of tiny pressure points. . . .This handbook details a number of ancient, oriental techniques that may. . .supplement and add to the effectiveness of standard, Western first aid methods. This traditional, Eastern way of first aid is not limited to emergency situations. The same techniques may be effective in relieving pain or various symptomatic disorders.*—from the introduction. The material is organized by ailments which are cross referenced to the appropriate point and illustrated. There's also some instructional material. Bibliography, 223pp. Flk 76

BRESSLER, HARRY. *ZONE THERAPY*, 4.50. Zone therapy relieves pain and distress in the body by giving pressure on certain parts of the body to bring relief, by reflex action, to other parts of the body. This is a discussion of the history of the therapy and extensive instructions for treatment of various ailments. Spiral bound, 73pp. HeR 55

CHAN, PEDRO. *FINGER ACUPRESSURE*, 2.95/1.75. Chan, using his own experience as well as that of other professionals, has picked out the most effective acupuncture points to treat certain common disorders by utilizing the finger technique known generally as shiatsu. Here he presents the treatment for about thirty common disorders. Following each is the name of the point and a description of the location as well as a drawing of the anatomical location with relation to the skeletal structure, and a photograph illustrating the treatment. With simple instructions. 67pp. ChB 75

CERNEY, J.V. *ACUPRESSURE: ACUPUNCTURE WITHOUT NEEDLES*, 2.95. A text on acupressure geared toward its use in the cure of various common ailments. Includes a general explanatory section as well as detailed chapters on home treatment of ailments in the head, neck, chest, back and spine, sex organs, legs and feet, and gastro-intestinal and abdominal tract. Fully illustrated and geared toward the layman. Index, 299pp. S&S 74

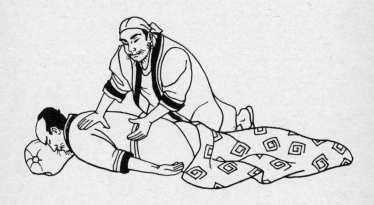

HOUSTON, F.M. *THE HEALING BENEFITS OF ACUPRESSURE,* 4.95. This is a very clearly illustrated guide to the practice of acupressure. Each of the acupoints is shown in a large drawing of the part of the body in which it is found along with an analysis of the parts of the body the point affects. There's also a detailed analysis of how to manipulate the point. The material is arranged according to the parts of the body in which the points are found. In addition, there's introductory instructional material, a long glossary, and an extensive index. 8½"x11", 96pp. Kea 74

IRWIN, YUKIKO and JAMES WAGENVOORD. *SHIATZU,* 5.95. Ms. Irwin has practiced shiatsu for over twenty-five years and was trained in Japan. Her book is one of the few pressure point manuals which is written by a Western practitioner and her discussion is geared to the Westerner and to Western ailments. She begins with a discussion of shiatsu techniques and goes from there to a survey of shiatsu as a remedy for the following disorders: insomnia, headaches, stiff neck and sore shoulders, lower back pain, constipation and diarrhea, and tennis elbow. The book is illustrated throughout with line drawings and the step-by-step instructions are exceedingly clear. Recommended. 6"x9", 239pp. Lip 76

LANGRE, JACQUES DE. *FIRST BOOK OF DO-IN,* 1.50. Presents a therapeutic and restorative technique of self-massage written in both French and English and containing over sixty photographs which show every step of the technique. A glossary contains all common health problems and internal-external natural remedies. The material is not very well organized and is often hard to follow. 8½"x11", 30pp. Hap 71

LANGRE, JACQUES DE. *SECOND BOOK OF DO-IN,* 7.50. The material that de Langre introduced in the first book has been greatly expanded here. The emphasis is on practical exercises and techniques, all of which are well explained and illustrated with photographs and line drawings. The techniques range from yogic-type exercises to various forms of self massage utilizing acupressure points. A great deal of background philosophy is also presented incorporating Oriental ideas with Western ones. A very popular, self learning instructional manual. 8½"x8½", 150pp. Hap 74

LAWSON-WOOD, DENIS and JOYCE. *ACUPUNCTURE VITALITY AND REVIVAL POINTS,* c4.80. An illustrated discussion of the points which, when massaged in a certain manner for a very short period, stimulate organs and glands to overcome fear, fatigue, mental and physical lethargy, fainting, congestive conditions, and much else. 63pp. HSP 75

MANAKA, YOSHIO. *QUICK AND EASY CHINESE MASSAGE,* 2.50. This pocket sized book is the clearest presentation of the material we've seen. The first four chapters cover the basic principles, the next eight demonstrate specific practices, and the other sixteen discuss treatments for various physical problems. Clear photographs illustrate each remedy. Spiral bound, 62pp. Jap 73

NAMIKOSHI, TOKUJIRO. *SHIATSU: JAPANESE FINGER PRESSURE THERAPY,* 3.95. When a part of the human body is in pain, the instinct is to touch it. When the eyes are tired, the instinct is to rub them. The word "shiatsu," composed of the element *shi* (fingers) and *atsu* (pressure) means a method of treating illness with digital compression. Pressure points are well illustrated and easy to follow. One of the important features of shiatsu treatment is that you can do it anywhere and by yourself. Three minutes of proper shiatsu massage when you are tired will have you feeling like a new person. Namikoshi is a leading Japanese shiatsu practitioner. 7¼"x 10¼", 82pp. Jap 69

NAMIKOSHI, TOKUJIRO. *SHIATSU THERAPY,* 5.50. A companion volume to Namikoshi's earlier work, *Shiatsu,* this book is divided into two parts: "The Theory of Shiatsu Therapy" and "Shiatsu Techniques." The section on techniques is the major part of the book. First Namikoshi gives instructions on general techniques and then he goes from there to details on giving a shiatsu treatment to each part of the body. All of the instructions are illustrated and the material is well organized and clearly presented. An excellent, practical work. Recommended. 7¼"x10¼", 89pp. Jap 74

OHASHI, WATARU. *DO-IT-YOURSELF SHIATSU,* 5.95. This is a self-help acupunture manual directed at Westerners by a man who has been teaching and practicing shiatsu in the U.S. for a number of years. The book is well illustrated with photographs and line drawings of the points and of actual shiatsu practice and all the instructional material is clear and easy to follow. Each part of the body is discussed in its own chapter and the book begins with introductory explanations of Ohashi's techniques. There's also a section on treatments for common ailments. Recommended. 8½"x11", 144pp. Dut 76

SERIZAWA, KATSUSUKE. *MASSAGE: THE ORIENTAL METHOD,* 4.50. With the help of photographs and diagrams, the author explains how to get relief from headaches, body pain and stiffness through the use of Japanese massage, a unique method which combines Western massage, shiatsu, and Chinese amma (which stimulates nerves). Lots of photographs and drawings explain exactly where and how to rub, tickle, punch, kick, and bat the body into divine bliss! 7¼"x10¼", 78pp. Jap 72

SERIZAWA, KATSUSUKE. *TSUBO: VITAL POINTS FOR ORIENTAL THERAPY,* c18.00. According to the medical philosophy of the East, the human body is operated and controlled by means of two groups of organs. As long as these organs operate harmoniously, the body remains healthy. Disturbances in any of them mean illness. A system of energy circulation provides the power by means of which the organs can operate in harmony. This larger system is broken down into fourteen smaller systems, called meridians, extending throughout the whole body. Along them are points where the flow of energy to the organs tends to stagnate. These points, called the *tsubo,* are the basic subject of this book. At the *tsubo,* actual physiological changes occur, revealing internal disorders and malfunctions in one or more of the organs. The *tsubo* are more than indicators of trouble; they are the places where therapy can be expected to produce maximum effects. Serizawa, the leading authority on *tsubo* research, explains how to locate the *tsubo* and how to apply acupuncture, massage, shiatsu, and moxa therapy to them. His text is clear and straightforward enough for the layman while being detailed and informative enough for the professional. Hundreds of excellent charts and diagrams make the locations of the *tsubo* and the practical aspects of treatment easy to understand. Index, 7"x10", 256pp. Jap 76

SILVERSTEIN, M.E. and I LOK CHANG and NATHANIEL MA-CON, trs. *ACUPUNCTURE AND MOXIBUSTION,* 2.95. This is the actual handbook used by the barefoot doctors in the People's Republic of China. This includes all the basics the Chinese practitioners need to know. It lists dozens of common illnesses and tells precisely how to treat them, illustrating the acupuncture points with clear diagrams and discussing the theory behind the practices. 118pp. ScB 75

TAN, LEON, MARGARET YOU-CHING TAN and ILLSA VEITH. *ACUPUNCTURE THERAPY: CURRENT CHINESE PRACTICE,* c19.00. A definitive explanation of acupuncture as it is currently practiced in the People's Republic of China. Includes sections on needles, techniques for insertion, moxibustion, and electric acupuncture. The essential acupuncture points, their locations, and treatment of specific diseases are all carefully described. A final chapter surveys acupuncture anesthesia. Many illustrations and tables, notes, index, 159pp. ChB 72

TOGUCHI, MASARU. *THE COMPLETE GUIDE TO ACUPUNC-TURE,* c6.50. A comprehensive handbook which begins with a discussion of the specific values of acupuncture and follows with a detailed survey of a number of diagnostic techniques. The next section outlines some methods of treatment and the rest of the book is devoted to an in depth presentation and analysis of acupuncture treatments for a wide variety of specific ailments. The directions are explicit and line drawings (fairly inadequate ones) accompany the text throughout. The text itself is geared to the general reader who wants to become a practitioner—though it takes a good deal more than book knowledge to practice acupuncture successfully and safely. Nonetheless, this volume does present a great deal of useful information in an easy to understand form. 267pp. TPL 74

VEITH, ILZA. *THE YELLOW EMPEROR'S CLASSIC OF INTERNAL MEDICINE,* c10.50/3.95. Written in the form of a dialogue in which the emperor seeks information from his minister on all questions of health and the art of healing, **The Yellow Emperor's Classic** has become a landmark in the history of Chinese civilization. It is the oldest known document of Chinese medicine. In her translation and introductory study, Dr. Veith has succeeded in giving an excellent picture of early Chinese medicine. Many illustrations and notes. An essential work for anyone studying oriental medicine. Index, 253pp. UCP 49

WADE, CARLSON. *HEALTH SECRETS FROM THE ORIENT,* 1.75. This is a survey of healing techniques from China, Japan, India, Tibet, Korea, Polynesia, and Hawaii. Wade has written countless books on healing and nutrition and, while his writing style tends toward hyperbole, his books contain a great deal of information and they are easy to read and understand. Many case histories and specific techniques are offered. Index, 239pp. NAL 73

WALLNOFER, HEINRICH and A. VON ROTTAUSCHER. *CHINESE FOLK MEDICINE AND ACUPUNCTURE,* 1.25. Deals less with acupuncture and more with traditional Chinese folk medicine than most books in this area. The ingredients, recipes, and remedies are printed just as they have been handed down from one generation to another. Contains sections on fundamentals of Chinese medicine, its evolution, Chinese anatomy and physiology, Chinese pathology and treatment methods, as well as medicinal herbs, drugs, and love potions. Well illustrated, index, 186pp. NAL 75

WARREN, FRANK and THEODORE BERLAND. *THE ACUPUNCTURE DIET,* c7.95. It has recently been found that acupuncture, in coordination with a special diet, can have a dramatic effect on body weight. By using a medically inserted ear staple or needle, you can influence the activity of the vagus nerve on stomach action, and therefore influence the perception of hunger and appetite. This book is written by a physician who has successfully used this technique with his patients and Dr. Warren includes case studies along with an analysis of the physiological reasons for this phenomena. He also gives three diets especially formulated to coordinate with an acupuncture program. 136pp. STM 76

WEXU, MARIO. *THE EAR, GATEWAY TO BALANCING THE BODY: A MODERN GUIDE TO EAR ACUPUNCTURE,* c24.50. A comprehensive textbook of ear acupuncture, the first written by a Western acupuncturist. Dr. Wexu combines his extensive personal clinical experience with traditional and modern Chinese and Western sources. Anatomical descriptions and detailed charts clearly illustrate how to locate and work with over 300 ear points, both alone and in combination with body points. Case histories illustrate the applications for specific ailments. 191pp. ASI 75

WORSLEY, J.R. *IS ACUPUNCTURE FOR YOU?* 2.95. A good introduction, presented in question and answer format. Beginning with *What is Acupuncture?* and *How does it work?* Dr. Worsley then discusses the techniques with needles and moxa, treatable illnesses, consultation and diagnosis, and duration and effects of treatment. 81pp. H&R 73

WU WEI-PING. *CHINESE ACUPUNCTURE,* c7.50. This is essentially a textbook for practitioners who wish to follow the classical Chinese tradition. Dr. Wu is the sixteenth generation in his family of acupuncturists. He is the President of the Chinese Acupuncture Society and head of the School of Acupuncture in Tai-Pei, Taiwan. This book was written to serve as a text for his students. 181pp. HSP 62

YAU, P.S., tr. *SCALP-NEEDLING THERAPY,* c7.50. Acupuncture on the scalp is a new technique worked out by a young Chinese physician. It has proved effective in a variety of cases. This is a translation of a text on the technique and it includes general instructions as well as specific applications. Illustrations, 65pp. M&H 75

Afterword

We hope you have found reading this guide both useful and enjoyable. We'd like to hear from you with any comments you have, pro or con. We'd also like to see you if you come to Washington.

Yes! is more than just a bookshop. We provide food for spirit, mind and body, as we also have a natural food store and a lovely self-service vegetarian restaurant. We occupy three old buildings in Georgetown with a delightful patio in the middle with a fountain and plants and birds.

The bookshop is very open, with carpeting, lots of seats, plants and classical music. You can browse and read and when you get hungry, step into the garden for a meal or a snack.

Yes! is a business which exists to provide goods and services to the public, honestly, efficiently and profitably. Yes! is also a spiritual place. The extent to which this is true is a function of the collective input of the forty-five people who work here and the people who come here, as well as the aspirations of the principal owners, managers, and long-time staff. A two-way flow is involved: we put our energy into Yes!'s development, and being at Yes! has a strong impact on our development.

Why do we call ourselves Yes!? We say Yes! to life. If we have any unifying concept, it is that of living in harmony with nature, our own as well as that around us. Along with this is the belief that our purpose in this world is to work on our own development and evolution, and through that the development and evolution of humankind in general. We recognize that there are many paths, and if they are trod by committed seekers they all ultimately lead to the same place. Some people on the Yes! staff are followers of particular spiritual disciplines. Others are not. We get along by not trying to convert others to our own path, but by remaining open to others, whatever path they are on, and wherever on it they are. We try to create at Yes! a warm, loving atmosphere which will welcome people of all ages, races, and cultures.

We hope we will have the opportunity one day to welcome you to Yes!

Appendices

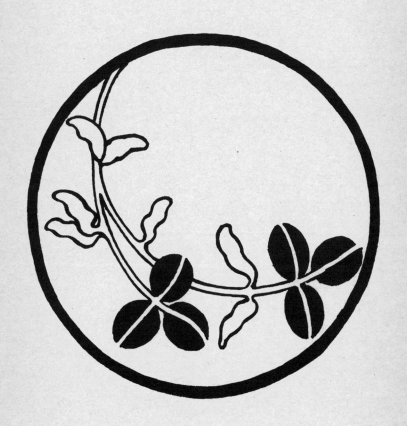

How To Obtain These Books

If you wish to read any of these books and they are not in your local library, show the reviews to your librarian and ask him to order them for you. In this way you will help to awaken your librarian to the importance of these books and help to make them more widely available to others.

The same thing goes for bookstores. Try to get the books at the store where you bought **Wellness.** If they don't have them in stock, ask if they will special order them for you. We have provided the publishers' addresses for the benefit of other bookstores who wish to order these books. Or check your yellow pages for a local store that might stock these kinds of books.

BUYING BY MAIL

If you cannot obtain these books locally, you can buy them from us. That's the business we are in, and we normally have all these books in stock. We do a large mail order business all over the world and we get the books out the same day the order comes in. So if you wish to get the books from us, read the following ordering information carefully:

All sales are final. We can accept no returns unless the book is defective in some way. We have tried to say enough in the reviews to give you good guidance on the books. However, if you would like some additional information about a book before you buy it, write and ask us.

413

Our prices are net. We sell at retail only. If you are interested in buying at wholesale, contact the publishers of the books. We offer a five percent discount on orders over $50.00 and ten percent for ten or more copies of the same book.

Book prices are continuing to rise as books are reprinted. If an increase is substantial, we'll notify you before filling the order. If it's slight, we'll send you the book and let you pay the balance later. If the price has dropped or we can substitute a paperback, we'll do so, and send you a credit slip. We will automatically supply the paperback edition whenever possible, unless you specifically request hardcovers. If you wish hardcovers on books not so shown in **Wellness,** query us and we'll tell you if we can special order them for you.

If we are temporarily out of stock on a title, we will back order it and send it to you as soon as it is available. If the book is out of print we will let you know and send you a credit slip.

Domestic orders, please send us a check or money order payable to Yes! Inc.; D.C. residents please add 5% sales tax. We do not take credit cards or sell on credit; however, we can keep money on account for you which you can draw on as you order. Overseas orders, please send us a bank check or money order, payable in U.S. dollars. We cannot accept personal checks from foreign banks (including Canada). We send our books by surface mail. If you wish your order sent airmail, send us an amount for postage equal to the cost of the book. We will refund any unused money or bill you for the balance.

POSTAGE AND HANDLING CHARGES

Domestic

Our charge for domestic postage and handling is $.60 for the first book and $.30 for each additional book. Alternatively, if it will save you money, you may figure 8% of

414

the total order with a minimum of $1.25. Books and records are sent special fourth class mail or UPS. We automatically insure, at our expense, all orders over $30.00.

International

Our charge for international postage and handling is $.65 for the first book and $.35 for each additional book. Alternatively, if it will save you money, you may figure 9% of the total order with a minimum of $1.50. Registration fees are additional.
We cannot insure international parcels and we cannot take responsibility for their safe arrival. We recommend that they be sent registered. Registration costs $2.10 for each $22.00 worth of books, except to Canada where up to $140 worth of books can be registered for $2.10.

Supplements

We plan to issue periodic supplements to **Wellness**, which will provide reviews of new books and indicate new paperback editions. They will be arranged according to the same subject headings used in **Wellness**.

These supplements will be sent free automatically to our mail order customers.

Others, such as libraries or bookstores, who wish to obtain this information may do so at a cost of $2.00 per year (a minimum of three supplements). If you wish to subscribe to this service, please send us a check for $2.00.

yes! BOOKSHOP
1035 31st Street, NW
Washington, DC 20007

Enclosed is ___ $2.00 for one year, ___ $4.00 for two years, of ___ issues of **Wellness** supplements.

_____
Name

_____
Address

_____
City/State/Zip

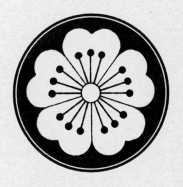

Publishers' Codes & Addresses

A&U   Allen & Unwin, 198 Ashe St., Reading, MA 01867
A&W   A&W Promotional Book Corp., 95 Madison Ave., New York, NY 10016
Aca   Academy Books, 3085 Reynard Way, San Diego, CA 92103
ADE   Assn. for Documentation and Enlightenment, P.O. Box 180, Virginia Beach, VA 23458
AmM   American Media, P.O. Box 4646, Westlake Village, CA 91359
Amo   AMORC, Rosicrucian Park, San Jose, CA 95114
AMP   Ananda Marga Pub., % Golden Lotus, Inc., 847 E. Colfax Ave., Suite 210, Denver, CO 80218
AnP   Ananda Publications, Allegheny Star Route, Nevada City, CA 95959
AOP   And/Or Press, 3431 Rincon Annex, San Francisco, CA 94119
API   Anthroposophic Press, Inc., 258 Hungry Hollow Rd., Spring Valley, NY 10977
APM   Acad. of Parapsychology & Medicine, P.O. Box 18541, Denver, CO 80218
Arc   Arco, 219 Park Avenue South, New York, NY 10003
ARE   ARE Press, P.O. Box 595, Virginia Beach, VA 23451
AsA   Astro-Analytics Pub., 16440 Haynes St., Van Nuys, CA 91406
ASC   Award Sales Corp., P.O. Box 800, Bergenfield, NJ 07621
ASI   ASI Publishers Inc., 127 Madison Ave., New York, NY 10016
Asl   Aslan Enterprises, P.O. Box 1858, Boulder, CO 80306
AUM   Assoc. for the Understanding of Man, P.O. Drawer 5310, Austin, TX 78763
Aut   Autumn Press, P.O. Box 469, Kanagawa, CA 95073
Avo   Avon Books, 250 West 55th Street, New York, NY 10019

B&J   Barrie & Jenkins, 24 Highbury Crescent, London N5 1RX England
Bak   Douglas Baker, *Little Elephant,* High Road, Essendon, Herts., England
Ban   Bantam Books, 666 Fifth Avenue, New York, NY 10019
BaP   Barre Publishers, South St., Barre, MA 01005
Bea   Beacon Press, 25 Beacon St., Boston, MA 02108
Ber   Berkley Books, 390 Murray Hill Pkwy., E. Rutherford, NJ 07073
Bha   M. Bhattacharyya & Co., Ltd., 73, Netaji Subhas Rd., Calcutta, India
BID   Bio-Dynamic Literature, P.O. Box 253, Wyoming, RI 02898
BoM   Bobbs Merrill, 4300 West 62nd St., Indianapolis, IN 46208
BPC   Book Publishing Co., Route 1, Box 197A, Summertown, TN 38784
BrH   British Homoeopathic Assn., 27a Devonshire St., London W1N 1RJ England
BSR   Borderland Sciences Research Fdn., P.O. Box 548, Vista, CA 92083

Cad   Cadre, 124 28th Ave., San Mateo, CA 94403
Can   Cancer Book House, 2043 N. Berendo St., Los Angeles, CA 90027
CCC   China Cultural Corp., P.O. Box 3724, Hong Kong
CCP   Christian Community Press, 34 Glenilla Rd., London NW3 England
CeA   Celestial Arts, 231 Adrian Road, Millbrae, CA 94030
CFS   Center for Science in the Public Interest, 1779 Church St., N.W., Washington, D.C. 20036
ChB   Chan's Books, 2930 W. Valley Blvd., Alhambra, CA 91803
ChP   Diana's Nutrition Center, 505 S. Glendora Ave., Glendora, CA 91740
CiP   Citadel Press, 120 Enterprise Ave., Secaucus, NJ 07094
Cla   James Clarke & Co., Ltd., 7 All Saints Passage, Cambridge CB2 3LS England
CMG   Coward, McCann & Geoghegan, Inc., 200 Madison Ave., NY, NY 10016
CMP   Century Medical Pub., P.O. Box 706, La Porte, IN 46350
CPT   Chinmaya Publications Trust, 175, Rasappa Chetty St., Madras 3, India
CRC   CRCS Pubs., Prof. Mall Bldg., 231 E St., Suite 8, Davis, CA 95616

419

Crn	Crown Publishers, One Park Avenue South, New York, NY 10016
Cro	T. Crowell Co., Conklin Book Center, Inc., Baker Dr., Conklin, NY 13748
Crs	Dr. John Christopher, P.O. Box 352, Provo, UT 84601
Css	Crossing Press, Trumansburg, NY 14886

DAC	Devin-Adair Co., Inc., 143 Sound Beach Ave., Old Greenwich, CT 06870
DaH	Dance Horizons, 1801 East 26th St., Brooklyn, NY 11229
Dan	C.W. Daniel, 60 Muswell Road, London NW10 England
Del	Dell, One Dag Hammarskjold Plaza, New York, NY 10017
DeV	DeVorss & Co., P.O. Box 550, Marina Del Rey, CA 90291
DHP	Dawn Horse Press, 1530 Custer Ave., San Francisco, CA 94124
Dia	Dial/Delacourte, One Dag Hammarskjold Plaza, New York, NY 10017
Dou	Doubleday & Co., 501 Franklin Ave., Garden City, NY 11530
Dov	Dover Publications, 180 Varick St., New York, NY 10014
DTP	Doubletree Press, Inc., P.O. Box 1321, Walla Walla, WA 99362
Dut	E.P. Dutton & Co., 201 Park Avenue South, New York, NY 10003

ECa	El Cariso Publishers, P.O. Box 176, Elsinore, CA 92330
Eco	Ecology Action of the Midpeninsula, 2225 El Camino Real, Palo Alto, CA 94306
Ehr	Ehret Publishing Co., Beaumont, CA
EsH	Essence of Health Publishing Co., P.O. Box 2821, Durban, S. Africa
EsP	Esoteric Publications, P.O. Box 1529, Sedona, AZ 86336
Esp	Espiritu, 124 Miramar, Houston, TX 77006
EvC	M. Evans & Co., 216 East 49th St., New York, NY 10017
EWF	East West Foundation, 359 Boylston St., Boston, MA 02116
ExP	Exposition Press, 900 South Oyster Bay Road, Hicksville, NY 11801

Fab	Faber Books, 3 Queen Square, London WCiN 3AU England
Faw	Fawcett Publishing, Fawcett Building, Greenwich, CT 06830
Flk	Falkynor Books, P.O. Box 8060, Pembroke Pines, FL 33023
FLP	Foreign Language Press, Peking, China
FoI	Formur, Inc., 4200 LaClede Ave., St. Louis, MO 63108
Fou	W. Foulsham & Co., Yeovil Road, Slough SL1 4JH England
Fow	L.N. Fowler & Co., 1201/1203 High Rd., Chadwell Heath, Romford, Essex, England
FPC	Freestone Publishing Co., P.O. Box 357, Albion, CA 95410
Fre	W.H. Freeman & Co., 660 Market St., San Francisco, CA 94104
FSG	Farrar, Straus & Giroux, 19 Union Square West, NY, NY 10003

G&B	Gordon & Breach Science Pubs., Inc., One Park Ave., NY, NY 10016
G&D	Grosset & Dunlap, Inc., 51 Madison Ave., NY, NY 10010
Gab	Gabriel Press, 4018 North 40th St., Phoenix, AZ 85018
Gar	Garden Way Publishing Co., Charlotte, VT 05445
Geo	Mrs. Karl George, 1405 Valley Dr., Laurel, MT 59044
GEP	Georgetown Press, 483 Francisco St., San Francisco, CA 94133
GeP	Genesis Press, Cupertino, CA
GPO	U.S. Gov't Printing Office, Asst. Public Printer, Superintendent of Documents, Washington, DC 20402.
GrP	Stephen Greene Press, Box 1000, Brattleboro, VT 05301
Grv	Grove Press, Inc., 53 East 11th St., New York, NY 10003
Grz	Joseph Graziano, 2207 West Clarendon Ave., Phoenix, AZ 85015

H&R	Harper & Row, 10 East 53rd St., New York, NY 10022
Ham	Hamlyn Publishing Group Ltd., Hamlyn House, The Centre, Feltham, Middlesex, England
Hap	Happiness Press, 160 Wycliff Way, Magalia, CA 95954
Har	Hart Publishing Co., Inc., 15 West 4th St., New York, NY 10012
Haw	Hawthorne Books, Inc., 260 Madison Ave., New York, NY 10016

HBJ	Harcourt Brace Jovanovich, 757 Third Ave., New York, NY 10017
HDI	Human Dimensions Institute, 4380 Main St., Buffalo, NY 14226
HeG	Heineman Group—Windmill Press, Kingswood, Tadworth, Surrey, KT 206 TG England
Hei	Heidelberg Publishers, 1003 Brown Bldg., 708 Colorado, Austin, TX 78731
Hem	Hemisphere Press, 263 Ninth Ave., New York, NY
HeP	Hemkunt Press, One—E/15 Patel Rd., New Delhi, 8, India
HeR	Health Research, 70 Lafayette St., Mokelume Hill, CA 95245
Her	Heritage Store, P.O. Box 444-B, Virginia Beach, VA 23458
HeS	Health Science, Box 15000, Santa Ana, CA 92705
HeY	Healing Yourself, P.O. Box 752, Vashon, WA 98070
HFA	Health for All Publishing Co., Gateway House, Bedford Park, Croydon, CR9 2AT Surrey, England
HHI	Hippocrates Health Institute, 25 Exeter St., Boston, MA 02116
Him	Himalayan Institute, 1505 Greenwood Rd., Glenview, IL 60025
HMC	Houghton Mifflin Co., Wayside Rd., Burlington, MA 01803
HME	Home Oriented Maternity Experience, 511 New York Ave., Takoma Park, MD 20012
Hod	Hodder & Stoughton, Mill Rd., Dunton Green, Sevenoaks, Kent TN 13 2XX England
HPG	Hutchinson Publishing Group, 3 Fitzboy Sq., London W1P 6JD England
HPP	Health Plus Publishers, P.O. Box 22001, Phoenix, AZ 85028
HRA	Huna Research Associates, 126 Camellia Dr., Cape Giradeau, MO 63701
Hrm	Hermes Press, Box 4642, Boulder, CO 80306
HRW	Holt, Rinehart & Winston, 383 Madison Ave., New York, NY 10017
HSD	H.S. Dakin, 3456 Jackson St., San Francisco, CA 94118
HSP	Health Science Press, Rustington, Sussex, England
Hum	Humata Publishing, Bos 56, CH-3000, Bern 6, Switzerland
HUP	Harvard University Press, 79 Garden St., Cambridge, MA 02138
Hur	Dr. and Mrs. Frank Hurd, Box 86A, Route 1, Chisholm, MN 55719

IHC	International Health Council, 15328 Edolyn Ave., Cleveland, OH 44111
III	Inter-American Indian Institute, Ninos Heroes 139, Mexico 7, D.F.
Ing	Eunice D. Ingham, P.O. Box 948, Rochester, NY 14603
INS	InScape Corp., Publishers, P.O. Box 978, Edison, NJ 08817
Int	International University Press, 315 Fifth Ave., New York, NY 10016
IUP	Indiana University Press, 10th & Morton Sts., Bloomington, IN 47401
IWP	Illuminated Way Press, P.O. Box 2449, Menlo Park, CA 94025

Jap	Japan Publications Trading Co. (USA) Inc., 200 Clearbrook Road, Elmsford, NY 10523
Jen	Jensen's Nutritional & Health Products, P.O. Box 8, Solana Beach, CA 92075
JHU	Johns Hopkins University Press, Baltimore, MD 21218
JPC	B. Jain Publishers, XV/2793, Raj Guru Rd., Chuna Mandi, Pahar Ganj New Delhi 55, India

Kau	William Kaufmann, Inc., One First Street, Los Altos, CA 94022
Kea	Keats Publishing Co., 36 Grove St., (P.O. Box 876), New Canaan, CT 06840
Kod	Kodansha International/USA, Ltd., 10 E. 53rd St., NY, NY 10022

Lar	Larchmont Books, 25 West 45th St., New York, NY 10036
LBC	Little Brown & Co., 34 Beacon St., Boston, MA 02106
LEP	Life Energy Products, Inc., P.O. Box 75 GPO, Brooklyn, NY 11202
LFP	Life Force Press, Box 26477 Sunnyslope Station, 9635 N. 7th St., Phoenix, AZ 85020

Lip	J.B. Lippincott Co., East Washington Square, Philadelphia, PA 19105
Lit	Litton Educational Publishers, 7625 Empire Dr., Florence, KY 41042
LLC	Living Love Center, 1730 La Loma Ave., Berkeley, CA 94709
LLL	La Leche League, 9616 Minneapolis Ave., Franklin Park, IL 60131
LlP	Llewellyn Publications, P.O. Box 3383, St. Paul, MN 55165
Lon	Longman Inc., 19 West 44th St., New York, NY 10036
LPC	Lucis Publishing Co., 866 United Nations Plaza, Suite 566 New York, NY 10017
LtA	Littlefield Adams, 8 Adams Dr., Totowa, NJ 07512
LTP	Lawton-Teague Publications, P.O. Box 656, Oakland, CA 94604
Lus	Lust Enterprises, Inc., 490 Easy St. (P.O. Box 777), Simi, CA 93065
M&H	Medicine & Health Publishing Co., 17 Gough St., G/F, Hong Kong
MAP	Middle Atlantic Press, Box 263, Wallingford, PA 19086
MAr	Medical Arts Press, P.O. Box 536, Summerland, CA 93067
May	Mayflower Books, 4 Upper James St., London W1R 4BP England
MCD	MacDonald Publishing Services, Ltd., Nr. Briston, Avon, England
MCh	Mason Charter, 641 Lexington Ave., New York, NY 10022
McK	David McKay Co., 750 Third Ave., New York, NY 10017
McM	Macmillan Company, 866 Third Ave., New York, NY 10022
McN	McNaughton Foundation, P.O. Box B-17, San Ysidro, CA 92073
Mer	MERCO, 620 Wyandotte East, Windsor, Ontario, Canada N9A 3J2
Mey	Norman Meyer, 115 Dover Rd., Wellesley, MA 02181
MGH	McGraw Hill Book Co., Princeton Rd., Hightstown, NJ 08520
MiP	Mineral Perspectives, 8915 N.E. 4th Rd., Miami Shores, FL 33138
MIT	MIT Press, 28 Carleton St., Cambridge, MA 02142
MNS	Movement Notation Society, % Dr. Annelis S. Hoyman, 117 Freer Gymnasium, University of Illinois, Urbana, IL 61801
MNT	Montana Books, 1716 North 45th St., Seattle, WA 98103
Mor	Wm. Morrow & Co., Wilmor Warehouse, 6 Henderson Dr., West Caldwell, NJ 07006
MPC	Mayfield Publishing Co., 285 Hamilton Ave., Palo Alto, CA 94301
MRG	Metaphysical Research Group, Archers Ct., The Ridge, Hastings, Sussex, England
NAF	New Age Foods, 1122 Pearl St., Boulder, CO 80302
NAL	New American Library, P.O. Box 120, Bergenfield, NJ 07621
NAP	New Age Press, 4636 Vineta Ave., La Canada, CA 91011
NAS	National Academy of Sciences, Printing & Publishing Office, 2101 Constitution Ave., Washington, D.C. 20418
Nas	Nash Publishing Corp., One Dupont St., Plainview, NY 11803
Nat	Naturegraph Publishers, P.O. Box 1075, Happy Camp, CA 96039
NHP	Natural Hygiene Press, 1920 Irving Park Rd., Chicago, IL 60613
Nil	Nilgiri Press, Box 381, Berkeley, CA 94701
Nit	Nitty Gritty Productions, P.O. Box 5457, Concord, CA 94522
NKB	New Knowledge Books, P.O. Box 9, Horsham, Sussex RH12 2LB England
NoP	Norwalk Press, P.O. Box 13266, Phoenix, AZ 85002
Nor	W.W. Norton & Co., Inc., 500 Fifth Ave., New York, NY 10036
NPC	Newcastle Publishing Co., P.O. Box 7589, Van Nuys, CA 91409
Nsw	Newsweek Books, 444 Madison Avenue, New York, NY 10022.
NuB	Nutri-Books Corp., P.O. Box 5793, Denver, CO 80217
NuS	Nutritional Science Research Inst., Mulberry Tree Hall, Brookthorpe, Gloucester, England GL4 0UU
NUY	N.U. Yoga Trust and Ashrama, Gylling, Denmark
NYA	New York Astrology Center, 127 Madison Ave., NY, NY 10016
NYT	Qudrangle/New York Times Book Co., Three Park Ave., NY, NY 10016

OLL   Orient Longman Ltd., Nicol Rd., Ballard Estate, Bombay 400038 India
Oma   Omangod Press, P.O. Box 255, Wethersfield, CT 06109
One   101 Productions, 834 Mission St., San Francisco, CA 94103
OvP   Overlook Press, Lewis Hollow Rd., Woodstock, NY 12498
Owe   Peter Owen, 12 Kendrick Mews, Kendrick Place, London SW7, England
Oxf   Oxford University Press, 16-00 Pollitt Dr., Fair Lawn, NJ 07410

PaR   Para Research, Rockport Whistlestop Mall, Rockport, MA 01966
Pau   Paulist Press, 400 Sette Dr., Paramus, NJ 07652
PAV   Philosophisch-Anthroposophischer Verlag am Goetheanum,
      4143 Dornach/Sol., Switzerland
Php   Henry Phillips Publishing Co., 519 N.E. 83rd St., Seattle, WA 98115
Pin   Pinnacle Books, 275 Madison Ave., New York, NY 10016
PjP   Panjandrum Press, 99 Sanchez St., San Francisco, CA 94114
Pop   Popular Library, 600 Third Ave., New York, NY 10016
PPF   Price Pottenger Nutrition Foundation, Inc., 2901 Wilshire Blvd.,
      Suite 345, Santa Monica, CA 90403
PPr   Popular Prakasham, 35C Tardeo Rd., Bombay 34 WB India
PrH   Prentice-Hall, Inc., Box 500, Englewood Cliffs, NJ 07632
PRS   Philosophical Research Society, Inc., 3341 Griffith Park Blvd.,
      Los Angeles, CA 90027
Prv   Provoker Press, Lakeshore Rd., St. Catherines, Ontario, Canada
PTF   Police Training Foundation, 3412 Ruby St., Franklin Park, IL 60131
Pyr   Pyramid Publications, 757 Third Ave., New York, NY 10017

QFx   Quick Fox, Inc., 33 West 60th St., New York, NY 10023

RaH   Random House, 457 Hahn Rd., Westminster, MD 21157
Rai   Rainbow Bridge, P.O. Box 40208, San Francisco, CA 94140
Reg   Henry Regnery Co., 180 N. Michigan Ave., Chicago, IL 60601
RHI   Rams Head Inc., P.O. Box 2949, San Francisco, CA 94126
Rin   C. Ringer & Co., 23 Lallbazar St., Calcutta 1, India
RMN   Rand McNally, P.O. Box 7600, Chicago, IL 60680
RMP   Red Moon Press, 12 Orpheus St., London SE5 England
Rod   Rodale Press, 33 E. Minor St., Emmaus, PA 18049
Ros   Rosicrucian Fellowship, Oceanside, CA 92054
RPP   Real People Press, Box F, Moab, UT 84532
RSP   Rudolf Steiner Press, 35 Park Rd., London NW1 6XT England
Ruk   Ruka Publications, P.O. Box 1072, Santa Cruz, CA 95060
RuP   Running Press, 38 S. 19th St., Philadelphia, PA 19103

S&B   Science & Behavior Books, P.O. Box A.J., Cupertino, CA 95014
S&D   Stein & Day, Inc., Scarborough House, Briarcliff Manor, NY 10510
S&S   Simon & Schuster, 1 W. 39th St., New York, NY 10018
SAM   Sheed, Andrews & McMeel, Inc., 6700 Squibb Rd., Mission, KS 66202
Sar   Saraswati Studio, 12429 Cedar Rd., Cleveland Heights, OH 44106
SBL   Sphere Books Ltd., 30/32 Gray's Inn Rd., London WCiX 8JL England
ScB   Schocken Books, 200 Madison Ave., New York, NY 10016
SCR   Society for Cancer Research, Arlesheim, Switzerland
Scr   Charles Scribners Sons, 597 Fifth Ave., New York, NY 10017
Sea   The Seabury Press, 815 Second Ave., New York, NY 10017
SeD   Sett Dey & Co., 40A Strand Rd., P.O. Box 563, Calcutta 700001 India
Shl   Dr. Shelton, P.O. Box 1277, San Antonio, TX 78206
ShM   Shala-Min of New Mexico, Inc., 1605 Coal Ave., SE, Albuquerque,
      NM 87106.
ShP   Shambhala, P.O. Box 271, Boulder, CO 80302
SHS   Spiritual Healing Sanctuary, Burrows Lea, Shere, Guildford, Surrey,
      England
SIU   Southern Illinois University Press, P.O. Box 3697, Carbondale, IL 62901

SLB   Science of Life Books, 4-12 Tattersall Ln., Melbourne, Victoria 3000
       Australia
SMP   St. Martin's Press, 175 Fifth Ave., New York, NY 10010
SnB   Sun Publishing Co., P.O. Box 4383, Albuquerque, NM 87106
SPC   Sufi Publishing Co., 53 West Ham Ln., London E15 4PH England
Spe   Neville Spearman, Ltd., 112 Whitfield St., London W1 England
Srm   Starmast Publications, P.O. Box 704, Berkeley, CA 94701
SSk   South Sky Book Co., 107-115 Hennessy Rd., Hong Kong
SSP   76 Press, P.O. Box 2686, Seal Beach, CA 90740
Str   Sterling Publishing Co., 419 Park Ave. South, New York, NY 10016
Stu   Lyle Stuart, 120 Enterprise Ave., Secaucus, NJ 07094
Swa   Swallow Press, Inc., 811 W. Junior Terr., Chicago, IL 60613
SwH   Swan House, P.O. Box 170, Brooklyn, NY 11223

Tar   Tarnhelm Press, Lakemont, GA 30552
Tho   Charles C. Thomas, Publishers, 301-327 E. Lawrence Ave.,
       Springfield, IL 62703
Top   Top-Ecol Press, 3025 Highridge Rd., La Crescenta, CA 91214
TPH   Theosophical Publishing House, P.O. Box 270, Wheaton, IL 60187
TPL   Thorson's Publishers Ltd., Denington Estate, Wellingborough,
       Northants. NN8 2RQ England
Tro   Troubador Press, 126 Foulshom St., San Francisco, CA 94105
TSC   Taraporevala Sons & Co., 210 Dr. Dadabhai Naoroji Rd., Bombay, India
Tut   Charles E. Tuttle Co., Inc., Rutland, VT 05701

UCa   University of California Press, 2223 Fulton St., Berkeley, CA 94720
UnB   Universe Books, 381 4th Ave., New York, NY 10016
UnC   United Communications, P.O. Box 320, Woodmere, NY 11598
UOk   University of Oklahoma Press, 1005 Asp Ave., Norman, OK 73019
UPP   Univ. Park Press, Chamber of Commerce Bldg., Baltimore, MD 21202
USP   Univ. of Science & Philosophy, Swannanoa, Waynesboro, VA 22980
UTP   Univ. of the Trees Press, Box 644, Boulder Creek, CA 95006

VCh   Vita Chart, P.O. Box 478, Riverdale Station, Bronx, NY 10471
VdC   Vedanta Centre, 130 Beechwood St., Cohasset, MA
Vik   Viking Penguin Inc., 625 Madison Ave., New York, NY 10022
VNR   Van Nostrand Reinhold Co., 300 Pike St., Cincinnati, OH 45202

War   Warner Paperback Library, 75 Rockefeller Plaza, New York, NY 10019
Wat   Watkins, 45 Lower Belgrave St., London SW1W 0LT England
Wdf   Weidenfeld Publishers Ltd., 11 St. John's Hill, London SW11 England
Wea   Weatherhill, 149 Madison Ave., New York, NY 10016
Wei   Samuel Weiser, Inc., 625 Broadway, New York, NY 10012
Whi   H.G. White, 166 Geary St., No. 1105, San Francisco, CA 94108
Wil   Wilshire Book Co., 12015 Sherman Rd., North Hollywood, CA 91605
Wld   World Publications, Box 366, Mountain View, CA 94040
WoP   Woodbridge Press, P.O. Box 6189, Santa Barbara, CA 93111
WPC   Workman Publishing Co., 231 E. 51st St., New York, NY 10022
WRP   Writers & Readers Publishing Cooperative, 14 Talacre Rd., London
       NW5 3PE England
Wte   H.C. White Publications, P.O. Box 8014, Riverside, CA 92505
Wyd   Peter H. Wyden, Publisher, 750 Third Ave., New York, NY 10017

YFH   Yoga For Health, P.O. Box 475, Carmel, CA 93921
YPS   Yoga Publication Society, P.O. Box 8885, Jacksonville, FL 32211

Acknowledgements

I would like to thank the following people who helped make this book possible:

Kathleen Hintz, who did the typesetting on our IBM electronic composer; Daniel Friedman, who designed the book and did much of the layout and pasteup; Lloyd Wolf, who finished up the pasteup; and Wayne Hagood, who prepared the author index. And special thanks to my husband Ollie, who first interested me in holistic healing and who provided a loving and supportive environment while I worked on the book.

I would also like to thank the authors and publishers of the following books from which I have taken excerpts and condensed material to use as introductions to chapters:

East/West Exercise Book by David Smith, copyright 1976 by the author, and published by McGraw-Hill Book Co.; *Color and the Edgar Cayce Readings* by Roger Lewis, copyright 1973 by the Edgar Cayce Foundation, and published by A.R.E. Press; *Laurel's Kitchen* by Laurel Robertson, Carol Flinders and Bronwen Godfrey, copyright 1976 by Nilgiri Press, and published by them; *Death, the Final Stage of Growth* by Elisabeth Kubler-Ross, copyright 1975 by the author, and published by Prentice-Hall, Inc.; *The Well Body Book* by Michael Samuels, M.D. and Harold Zina Bennett, copyright 1973 by the authors, and published by Random House, Inc.; *The Herb Book* by John Lust, copyright 1974 by Benedict Lust Publications, and published by them; *New Light on Therapeutic Energies* by James Gallert, copyright 1966 by the author, and published by James Clarke Ltd.; *Commonsense Childbirth* by Lester Dessez Hazell, copyright 1969, 1976 by the author, and published by G.P. Putnam's Sons; *Nutrition and Your Body* by Benjamin and Sarah Stewart Colimore, copyright 1974 by Light Wave Enterprises, and published by them; and *Shiatsu: Japanese Finger Pressure. . .* by Yukiko Irwin and James Wagenvoord, copyright 1976 by Lippincott, and published by them.

The illustrations used in *Wellness* are from the following sources:

p. 8, *A Pattern of Herbs,* Doubleday; p. 10, *The Well Body Book,* Random House; p. 12, *Man's Body,* Paddington Press; p. 16, *The Well Body Book,* Random House; p. 22, *What Is Aikido?,* Japan; p. 28, *Aches and Pains,* Random House; p. 31, *Learning Through Dance,* Paulist; p. 37, *Zen Combat,* Random House; p. 40, *The*

Massage Book, Random House; p. 41, *The Massage Book*, Random House; p. 46, *Running for Health and Beauty*, Bobbs Merrill; p. 49, *Japanese Archery: Zen in Action*, Weatherhill; p.52, *Mensendieck: Your Posture and Your Pains*, Doubleday; p. 54, *Introduction to Yoga*, Lyle Stuart; p. 56, *Easy Does It Yoga*, Saraswati; p. 60, *Light of Yoga Beginner's Manual*, Simon & Schuster; p. 64, *Light of Yoga Beginner's Manual*, Simon & Schuster; p. 67, *Light of Yoga Beginner's Manual*, Simon & Schuster; p. 73, *Principles of Color*, Litton; p. 79, *The Well Body Book*, Random House; p. 83, *Color Psychology and Color Therapy*, Lyle Stuart; p. 88, *Cooking for Consciousness*, Ananda Marga; p. 89, *Chinese Vegetarian Cooking*, Random House; p. 92, *The Classic Wheat for Man Cookbook*, Woodbridge; p. 95, *Chinese Vegetarian Cooking*, Random House; p. 98, *Chinese Vegetarian Cooking*, Random House; p. 102, *Chinese Vegetarian Cooking*, Random House; p. 103, *Laurel's Kitchen*, Nilgiri Press; p. 105, *Egyptian Book of the Dead*, Dover; p. 112, *Fabric of the Universe*, Crown; p. 115, *The American Book of the Dead*, And/Or Press; p. 119, *The Well Body Book*, Random House; p. 122, *Lifearts*, St. Martin's Press; p. 125, *Goldenseal, etc.*, Ruka; p. 129, *The Handbook of Alternatives to Chemical Medicine*, Lawton Teague; p. 135, *Man's Body*, Paddington Press; p. 143, *Maggie's Back Book*, Houghton-Mifflin; p. 147, *Diet for a Small Planet*, Random House; p. 152, *The Handbook of Alternatives to Chemical Medicine*, Lawton Teague; p. 158, *Making Your Own Baby Food*, Bantam; p. 161, *Laurel's Kitchen*, Nilgiri Press; p. 166, *Bee's*, Cornell University Press; p. 172, *The Handbook for Alternatives to Chemical Medicine*, Lawton Teague; p. 177, *The Well Body Book*, Random House; p. 181, *Man's Body*, Paddington Press; p.189, *Survival Into the 21st Century*, Omangod; p. 193, *Be Well*, Random House; p. 199, *The Well Body Book*, Random House; p. 205, *Unsweetened Truth About Sugar*, Double Tree; p. 208, *Diet for a Small Planet*, Random House; p. 211, *Man's Body*, Paddington Press; p. 217, *A Pattern of Herbs*, Doubleday; p. 223, *A Pattern of Herbs*, Doubleday; p. 227, *A Guide to the Medicinal Plants of the United States*, Times Books; p. 230, *Secrets of the Chinese Herbalists*, Prentice-Hall; p. 235, *A Guide to the Medicinal Plants of the United States*, Times Books; p. 241, *A Pattern of Herbs*, Doubleday; p. 244, *A Pattern of Herbs*, Doubleday; p. 248, *A Pattern of Herbs*, Doubleday; p. 252, *Common Herbs for Health*, Schocken; p. 257, *Common Herbs for Health*, Schocken; p. 261, *Common Herbs for Health*, Schocken; p. 265, *Common Herbs for Health*, Schocken; p. 270, *Common Herbs for Health*, Schocken; p. 276, *Authentic Indian Designs*, Dover; p. 279, *Dowsing—Techniques and Applications*, Warner; p. 283, *Pyramid Power*, DeVorss; p. 288, *Alive to the Universe*, University of the Trees Press; p. 292, *The Wizard from Vienna*, G.P. Putnam's Sons; p. 299, *Wilhelm Reich*, Viking-Penguin;

p. 311, *Nine Months, One Day, One Year,* Harper & Row; p. 313, *Motherlove,* Running Press; p. 317, *Inside Mom,* St. Martin's Press; p. 321, *Inside Mom,* St. Martin's Press; p. 326, *Mothering,* Volume III, Mothering; p. 332, *How to Feel Younger Longer,* Rodale Press; p. 336, *The Book of Miso,* Autumn Press; p. 338, *The Book of Miso,* Autumn Press; p. 343, *Laurel's Kitchen,* Nilgiri Press; p. 359, *Laurel's Kitchen,* Nilgiri Press; p. 363, *Laurel's Kitchen,* Nilgiri Press; p. 365, *The Well Body Book,* Random House; p. 366, *The Book of Miso,* Autumn Press; p. 374, *Laurel's Kitchen,* Nilgiri Press; p. 377, *Step-by-Step to Organic Vegetable Gardening,* Rodale Press; p. 381, *Cosmic Cookery,* Starmast; p. 383, *Step-by-Step to Organic Vegetable Gardening,* Rodale Press; p. 388, *Acupuncture: Cure of Many Diseases,* Random House; p. 392, *Finger Acupressure,* Random House; p. 399, *Acupuncture: Cure of Many Diseases,* Random House; p. 403, *Shiatzu,* Lippincott.

Author Index

Abehsera, M. 100
Abraham, D. 375
Abraham, G. 375
Abrahamson, E.M. 203
Abramowski, O.L.M. 358
Abrams, A. 276
Acharya, P. 54
Adams, R. 183, 203, 330, 366, 367
Agarwal, J. 210
Agarwal, R.S. 210, 211
Agran, L. 132
Airola, P. 119, 120, 121, 133, 145, 155, 203, 330, 331
Allen, H.C. 248
Allen, J.H. 248
Allen, T.F. 248
Alph, T. 248
Alth, M. 88
Altman, N. 363
Amber, R. 120
Anderson, M. 74
Andrews, S. 358
Aoyagi, A. 102
Archdale, F.A. 276
Arms, S. 309
Asimov, I. 11
Askew, S. 276
Austin, M. 386

Bach, E. 125, 126
Back, P. 235
Bagnall, O. 74
Bailey, A. 127
Bailey, H. 127, 344, 367
Baker, D. 11, 127
Baker, E. 295
Banik, A. 338
Banks, J. 121

Barkas, J. 364
Barlow, W. 23
Barrett, W. 276
Bartal, L. 24
Bates, W.H. 211
Bean, C. 310
Bean, R. 400
Bearne, A. 276
Beasley, V. 277
Beasse, P. 277
Becker, E. 106
Beckett, S. 121, 223, 224
Beesley, R.P. 75
Behanan, K. 54
Bendit, L. 277
Bendit, P. 277
Benjamin, H. 127, 212
Bennett, H. 116, 193
Berglund, B. 224
Bergson, A. 397, 400
Berjeau, J. 249
Berland, T. 406
Bernard, T. 54
Besant, A. 75
Besterman, T. 276
Bethel, M. 224
Bhattacharjee 249
Bianchini, F. 224
Bieler, H. 331, 332
Bing, E. 310
Bircher-Benner 121, 147, 332, 358
Bird, C. 305
Birren, F. 75, 76
Blackie, M. 249
Blackwood, A.L. 249
Blaine, T. 128, 183
Blair, L. 277
Blate, M. 401
Block, J. 324

Blythe, P. 128
Boadella, D. 295, 296
Bock, R. 367
Boenninghausen, C. 249
Boericke, W. 249, 250, 253
Boger, C.M. 250
Boos-Hamburger, H. 76
Borland, D. 250, 251
Bose, S.K. 251, 313
Boulding, E. 90
Bowers, E. 391
Boyd, D. 128
Boyle, J. 278
Bradley, R. 313
Brady, M. 313
Bragg, P. 155
Brainard, B. 9
Brandt, J. 155
Braue, J. 91
Brena, S. 55, 128
Brennan, B. 313
Brennan, R.O. 303
Bressler, H. 401
Bricklin, A. 313
Bricklin, M. 128
Bristow, R. 28
Brod, R.H. 192
Brook, D. 313
Brooks, C. 29
Brown, B. 130
Brown, E. 91, 92
Brown, J. 279
Buchman, D. 351
Budge, E.A.W. 106
Bullen, V. 126
Buranelli, V. 290
Burang, T. 130
Burnett, C.W.F. 314
Burnett, J.C. 252
Burr, H.S. 279
Butler, W.E. 76

Cadwallader, S. 92, 93
Caldwell, G. 338
Cameron, V. 279, 280
Campbell, G. 121
Campbell, S. 375, 376
Carlson, R. 139
Carmen, R. 139
Carper, J. 335, 343
Carr, R. 55
Carrington, H. 156
Carter, M. 397, 398
Carter, M.E. 140
Cassell, E. 140
Castleton, V. 350, 351
Cave, F. 280
Cayce, E. 76, 140
Cayce, J.G. 140
Ceres 224, 225
Cerney, J.V. 141, 401
Chaitow, L. 141, 388
Challoner, H.K. 141
Champdor, A. 106
Chan, P. 388, 389, 401
Chancellor, P. 126
Chang, I.L. 405
Chang, S. 389
Chapman, E. 253
Chapman, J.B. 253
Chavanon, P. 254
Chen, P. 332
Cheng Man-Ch'ing 51
Cheraskin, E. 141, 142, 183
Chesser, E. 296
Chrapowicki, M. 280
Christensen, A. 55, 56
Christopher, J. 142, 147,
    157, 225
Clark, J.W. 142
Clark, L. 77, 142, 143,
    252, 333, 338, 351
Clarke, J.H. 254, 255
Clausen, T. 390

Cleave, T.L. 203
Clemence, R. 382
Clements, H. 121, 143, 144
Clyne, D. 314
Coca, A. 144
Colimore, B. 326, 333
Colimore, S. 326, 333
Collins, J. 340
Colville, W.J. 77
Coon, N. 225
Cooper-Hunt, C.L. 280
Corbett, M. 212
Corbetta, F. 224
Cornish, J. 106
Cott, A. 157
Coulter, H. 256
Courter, G. 93
Cowen, K. 77
Cowperthwaite, A.C. 256
Cox, D. 257
Cox, J. 257
Crabb, J. 144
Crabb, R. 78, 137, 144,
    145, 280, 281
Crenshaw, M.A. 352
Crisp, T. 56, 314
Crouch, J. 11
Crow, W.B. 226
Culbert, M. 133
Culpeper, N. 226
Cyan, E.D. 367, 368

Da Liu 29, 390
Dakin, H.S. 281
Dalton, R. 379
Davis, A. 93, 144, 281,
    282, 334
Davis, R.E. 144
Day, L. 283
De La Warr, G. 283
Dechanet, J.M. 56

Decker, N. 145
Deimel, D. 212
Dempsey, D. 106
DeSola, C. 29, 30
Devi, I. 57
Dewey, W. 253, 257
Dextreit, R. 145
Dick-Read, G. 314
Dickinson, A. 344
Dimond, E.G. 390
Dintenfass, J. 150
Diskin, E. 57
Dobson, T. 20
Dong, C.H. 121
Dooley, A. 150
Douglas, M. 63, 187
Downing, G. 39, 40
Doyle, R. 334
Drake, S. 107
Dresser, H. 150
Duffy, W. 204
Duke, M. 391
Dumont, T. 11
Dunne, D. 57
Duquette, S. 93
Durrell, L.W. 230
Duz, M. 151
Dworkin, F. 91, 93
Dworkin, S. 91, 93
Dychtwald, K. 32

Ebon, M. 283
Eden, J. 283, 291, 296
Edmonds, A. 302
Edmunds, H.T. 151
Edwards, H. 151, 153
Eeman, L.E. 284
Egami, S. 36, 37
Ehrenreich, B. 153
Ehret, A. 156
Eichenlaub, J. 153
Eiger, M. 311

Eisenberg, H. 195
Elbert, G. 226
Elbert, V. 226
Elliot, J.S. 284
Eloesser, L. 314
Elwood, C. 334
Emboden, W. 226
English, D. 153
Eshkol, N. 32, 33
Evans, J. 126
Evans-Wentz, W.Y. 107
Ewald, E. 93
Ewart, C. 391
Ewy, D. 311, 315
Ewy, R. 311, 315

Farrington, E.A. 257
Feifel, H. 107
Feingold, B. 162
Feldenkrais, M. 33
Feldzamen, A.N. 368
Fell, D. 376
Fere, M. 133
Fergie-Woods, H. 257
Finch, E. 78
Finch, W.J. 78, 284
Fisher, R. 162
Fisher, S. 34
Fitzgerald, D. 315
Fitzgerald, W. 391
Flack, D. 91
Flammonde, P. 162
Flanagan, G.P. 284, 285
Flath, C. 148
Fleming, A. 315
Flinders, C. 84, 90, 101
Fluck, H. 227
Flugelman, A. 34
Foley, D. 227
Foothorap, M. 41
Ford, M. 94
Fortune, D. 108

Foster, C. 376
Foster, G. 227
Fredericks, C. 145, 148,
    184, 204, 344
Fremantle, F. 108
Friedlander, B. 94, 344
Friedmann, L. 162
Fryer, L. 344
Fulder, S. 228
Fuller, J. 163
Furlong, M. 227
Fyfe, A. 134

Gabriel, I. 227
Gallert, M. 273, 285
Gallwey, W.T. 34, 35
Galt, E. 314
Galton, L. 148, 162
Gammon, M. 360
Garde, R.K. 58
Garrison, O. 338
Garten, M.O. 163
George, K. 285
Gerrard, D. 244
Gerras, C. 94
Gerson, M. 134
Ghazzali, A. 156
Gibson, D.M. 258
Glas, N. 315
Glasser, R. 134, 163
Glick, J. 164, 324
Gluck, J. 35
Godfrey, B. 84, 90
Godfrey, G. 101
Goethe, J. 78
Goggin, K. 287
Gold, E.J. 108
Goodavage, J. 286
Goodman, H. 204
Goodwin, M. 94
Gosling, N. 229
Goswami, S.S. 58

Goulart, F. 94
Grant, D. 338
Graves, T. 286
Gray, H. 12
Graziano, J. 398
Greene, J. 95
Gregg, R. 379
Gregory, D. 344
Grieve, M. 229
Griffin, E. 134
Griffith, R. 376
Grof, S. 108
Grollman, E. 109
Gross, L. 43
Guernsey, H.H. 258
Guernsey, J. 258
Guernsey, W. 258, 259
Guirdham, A. 164
Gunther, B. 35
Gyorbiro, Z. 49

Haehl, R. 259
Hahnemann, S. 259, 261
Haich, E. 53, 67, 216
Haines, B. 37
Halifax, J. 108
Hall, G. 164
Hall, M.P. 12, 78, 164, 392
Hall, R. 339
Halsell, G. 345
Hammond, S. 165
Hampton, C. 109
Hand, W. 165
Haney, E. 58
Hannaford, K. 95
Hansen, O. 261
Harding, A.R. 228
Harper-Shove, F. 229
Harriman, S. 228
Harrington, H.D. 230
Harris, B. 230, 345

Harris, L. 230
Hartman, R. 316
Hartmann, F. 165
Harwood, C. 31
Hashimoto, M. 392
Hauck, J.A. 355
Haught, S.J. 135
Hauschka, R. 345
Hauser, G. 346
Hawksey, H. 346
Hazell, L. 317
Heckel, A. 377
Heffern, R. 231
Heidenstam, D. 12
Heilman, J. 313
Heindel, M. 13, 95, 165, 166
Heline, C. 13, 78
Hemingway, I. 314
Henderson, J. 45, 109
Hering, C. 261, 262
Herrern, R. 228
Hertzberg, R. 95
Hewitt, J. 95
Hewlett-Parsons, J. 166, 231
Hick, J. 109
Hightower, J. 339
Hilgard, E. 166
Hilgard, J. 166
Hill, R. 148, 166
Hills, C. 79, 286
Hillyard, S. 94
Hittleman, R. 58, 59, 60, 96, 346
Hobhouse, R. 262
Hobson, P. 96
Hodson, G. 317
Hofer, J. 41
Hoffer, A. 184
Hoffman, E. 287
Holzer, H. 167
Homola, S. 167

Hooker, A. 96
Hornbacher, F. 361
Houston, F.M. 402
Howard, A. 377
Howard, B. 30
Huang, A.B. 51
Huang, H. 392
Huang, W. 51
Huard, P. 392
Hunt, R. 79
Hunter, B. 91, 96, 339, 340, 346
Hur, R. 364
Hurd, F. 96
Hurd, R. 96
Hurdle, J.F. 167, 204
Huson, P. 231
Hutchens, A. 232
Huxley, A. 209, 212
Hylton, W. 232

Ichazo, O. 35
Illich, I 168
Ilstrup, C. 360
Ingham, E. 398, 399
Inkeles, G. 41
Irwin, Y. 383, 399, 402
Ismael, C. 171
Issels, J. 130, 136
Itten, J. 80
Iyengar, B.K.S. 60

Jackson, J. 212
Jackson, M. 171
Jacobs, B. 232
Jacobson, M. 340, 346
Jaegers, B. 80
Jahr, G.H.G. 262
Jain, K.K. 392
Jansky, R. 253
Jarvis, D.C. 122, 171
Jeavons, J. 377

Jensen, B. 97, 122, 169, 173, 347
Johari, H. 173
John, B.F. 61
Johnson, D. 35
Johnson, K. 80
Johnson, L. 25
Johnson, T. 36
Jones, F. 23
Jordan, J. 97
Jury, D. 109
Jury, M. 109

Kadans, J. 233, 347
Kapleau, P. 110
Kapp, M.W. 13
Karmel, M. 317
Kaufman, M. 262
Kauz, H. 52
Keleman, S. 25, 110
Kelley, W. 136
Kelso, I. 174
Kenda, M. 89
Kent, H. 61
Kent, J.T. 262, 263
Kerr, R. 233
Kerrell, B. 287
Kervran, L. 174
Keyes, K. 347
Keys, J. 233
Khan, H.I. 174
Kiev, A. 174
Kilner, W. 80
Kimmens, A. 228
Kincaid-Smith, M. 266
Kinderlehrer, J. 97, 348
King, S. 288
Kipnis, C. 38
Kippley, S. 311
Kirban, S. 157, 175
Kirschner, H.E. 157
Kirschner, M.J. 61

Kiss, M. 61
Kittler, G. 136
Kitzinger, S. 317
Kloss, J. 233
Koepf, H. 378
Koestenbaum, P. 110
Koock, M. 94
Korth, L. 175, 288
Kostrubala, T. 45
Krebs, E. 137
Kriege, T. 170
Krippner, S. 80, 175, 288
Kriyananda, S. 62
Krochmal, A. 233
Krochmal, C. 233
Kroeger, H. 176
Krok, M. 358, 359
Kruger, H. 176
Kubler-Ross, E. 104, 110,
    111
Kugler, H. 348
Kulvinskas, V. 176, 359
Kuppers, H. 81
Kurland, H. 176
Kurtz, R. 26
Kushi, M. 100, 392
Kutumbiah, P. 177
Kuvalayananda, S. 62

Lakhovsky, G. 288
Lamaze, F. 317
Lance, K. 46
Lane, E. 81, 288
Lang, R. 318
Langerwerff, E. 42
Langre, J.D. 393, 403
Lanson, L. 177
Lappe, F.M. 97, 340, 364
Lavier, J. 393
Law, D. 178, 233, 234
Laws, P. 178
Lawson-Wood, D. 178, 393,

394, 403
Layne, M. 288
Layne, N.M. 137
Leadbeater, C.W. 13, 75, 81
Leboyer, F. 318
Lee, G. 98
Leftwich, R. 289
Leonard, G. 38
Leong, L. 394
Lerner, I. 38
Leroi, A. 137
Lerza, C. 340
Leshan E. 111
Leslie, C. 178
Lettvin, M. 179
Levannier, R. 254
Levy, J. 234, 235
Lewis, R. 68, 82
Li, C.P. 235
Lifton, J. 111
Lighthall, J.I. 235
Lilienthal, S. 263
Lilliston, L. 184
Linden, W.Z. 318
Lindlahr, H. 170
Liu Zhaoyuan 394
Livingston, V. 137
Lo, K. 98
Loewenfeld, B. 99
Loewenfeld, C. 99, 235
Long, J.W. 179
Long, M.F. 289
Loomis, E. 179
Lorusso, J. 164
Lovell, P. 319
Lowen, A. 24, 26, 27
Lowenkopf, A. 179
Lucas, R. 229, 236
Luk, C. 39
Lundgren, M. 31
Luscher, M. 82
Lust, J. 158, 218, 236

Lysebeth, A.V. 62

Macfarlane, A. 319
Macfarlane, H. 193
Mackarness, R. 180
Macon, N. 405
Mae, E. 137
Maisel, E. 23
Majno, G. 181
Majumdar, S.K. 63
Manaka, Y. 395, 403
Mann, F. 395, 396
Mann, W.E. 296
Maple, E. 181
Marine, G. 341
Marks, M. 206
Martin, C. 205
Martine, Y. 77
Marzollo, J. 319
Massy, R. 289
Matson, A. 112
Matsumoto, T. 396
Maury, E.A. 264
May, I. 320
Mayer, G. 82
Mayer, P. 101
McCamy, J. 349
McGarey, W. 140, 180, 394
McGinnis, T. 180
McGrath, W. 348
McGuire, T. 180
McKillip, B. 378
Meares, A. 182
Medexport, V.O. 138
Medsger, O. 237
Medvin, J. 63, 320
Meek, G. 289
Mellor, C. 182
Mensendieck, B. 42
Mercantante, A. 237
Mermet, A. 290

Meschter, J. 237
Messegue, M. 186, 352
Meyer, C. 186
Meyer, J. 237
Michele, A. 186
Milinaire, C. 321
Miller, D. 187
Miller, J.S. 307
Miller, L. 43
Miller, M. 91
Miller, R. 41
Miller, T. 36
Millspaugh, C. 238
Milner, D. 292
Milton, R.F. 349
Mitchell, I. 321
Montagu, A. 15
Montgomery, R. 187
Moody, R. 113
Moore, M. 63, 187
Morehouse, L. 43
Morella, J. 349
Morgan, W. 264
Morris, M. 31
Moyer, A. 149
Moyle, A. 149, 187, 349
Muir, A. 238
Muramoto, N. 187
Murphy, J. 188
Murray, F. 183, 203, 330,
    366, 367
Musashi, M. 43
Muzumdar, K.P. 264
Myles, M. 321

Nagai, H. 44
Nakatani, Y. 396
Namikoshi, T. 403, 404
Narayanananda, S. 63
Nash, E.B. 264, 265
Ne'eman, N. 24
Newbold, H.L. 184

Newman, L. 159
Nichols, J. 341
Nielsen, G. 292, 305
Nilsson, L. 13, 321
Nitobe, I. 44
Nittler, A. 188, 354
Noble, E. 321
Nogier 396
Nolen, W. 188
Norton, A.B. 265
Null, G. 188, 322, 341,
   352, 354, 365
Null, S. 322, 352, 354

O'Neill, J. 303, 304
Oakes, M. 109
Ohashi, W. 404
Ohr, J. 93
Ohsawa, L. 99, 100
Oki, M. 63, 64, 188
Olds, S. 311
Olkowski, H. 378
Olkowski, W. 378
Olson, E. 111
Osmond, H. 184
Ott, J. 292
Ouseley, S.G.J. 82
Oyle, I. 188

Page, M. 355
Page, N. 239
Palaiseul, J. 239
Palos, S. 397
Panchadasi, S. 82
Paramananda, S. 189
Parcells, H. 292
Passwater, R. 355
Pattison, E.M. 113
Pauling, L. 368
Paulson, J.S. 179
Pearce, E. 14
Pelgrin, M. 113

Pelikan, W. 265
Pelletier, K. 190
Pelstring, L. 355
Peppard, H. 213
Perlroth, K. 42
Perry, E. 265
Petrich, P. 379
Pettit, E. 301, 302
Pfeiffer, C. 185, 356
Pfeiffer, E. 379
Phelan, N. 64, 66
Philbrick, H. 379
Philbrick, J. 379
Pierrakos, J. 294
Pill, V. 227
Pincus, L. 113
Polansky, J. 292
Pollen, G. 94
Popov, I. 356
Porkert, M. 397
Powell, E. 190, 254, 265
Powell, M. 190
Prensky, J. 190
Presley, J. 341, 349
Prestera, H. 26
Price, W. 356
Proctor, W. 114
Pryor, K. 312
Puddephatt, N. 266

Quay, G.H. 266
Quick, C. 191

Raffe, M. 31
Rama, S. 65
Ramacharaka, Y. 191
Rankin, D. 55, 56
Raphael, D. 312
Ratti, O. 22
Rau, H. 239
Rawls, W. 281, 282
Raymond, D. 379

437

Rayner, C. 14
Read, A. 360
Rechung, R. 191
Redding, J. 334
Regardie, I. 192
Reich, P. 297
Reich, W. 138, 297, 298,
    299
Reichenbach, K. 300
Reilly, H.J. 192
Rendel, P. 14
Reuben, D. 149
Reyner, J.H. 192
Rezet, A.W. 203
Richards, R. 58
Richards, W.G. 300
Ringsdorf, W.M. 141, 142,
    183
Riotte, L. 379, 380, 381
Robbins, W. 342
Roberts, H. 266
Robertson, L. 84, 90, 101
Rodale, J.I. 360, 369,
    370, 381
Rodale, R. 381
Rodman, R. 113
Rohe, F. 46
Rosanes-Berrett, M. 213
Rose, J. 239, 240, 352
Rosen, M. 322
Rosenberg, H. 368
Rosenberg, J. 27
Rosenvall, V. 91
Ross, A.C.G. 267
Ross, S. 159
Rossiter, F. 192
Rottauscher, A.V. 406
Rowsell, H. 193
Royal, G. 267
Rubin, D. 80, 288
Ruddock, E.H. 267, 268
Rush, A.K. 47

Rusholm, P. 268
Russell, E. 301
Russell, W. 301
Rutherford, M. 240
Rycroft, C. 299

Sacharoff, S. 101
Salk, L. 322
Samuels, M. 116, 193
Sanecki, K. 241
Santa Maria, J. 102
Satchidananda, S. 65
Schindler, M. 83
Schlossberg, L. 15
Schneider, L.L. 194
Schoop, T. 31
Schroeder, H. 342
Schul, B. 301, 302
Schussler, W.H. 254
Schwantes, D. 205
Scofield, A.G. 194
Scott, C. 138
Segerberg, O. 114
Sehnert, K. 195
Selye, H. 195
Semple, D. 359
Serizawa, K. 404
Shackleton, B. 159
Shadman, A. 268
Sharma, C.H. 268
Sharpe, D. 83
Shealy, C.N. 196
Shears, C.C. 302, 360
Shelton, H. 159, 160, 361
Shepard, M. 114
Shepherd, D. 241, 268, 269
Sheppard, K. 269, 270
Sherman, H. 197
Shih-Chen, L. 241
Shioda, G. 21
Shurtleff, W. 102
Shute, W. 369

Si Chi Ko 51
Silverman, M. 241
Silverstein, M.E. 405
Simeons, A.T.W. 197
Simmons, A. 241
Simons, E. 65
Simpkins, B. 213
Siou, L. 47
Sivananda, S. 65
Slater, W. 65
Smart, E. 292
Smedt, E.D. 197
Smith, D. 17, 48, 270
Smith, F. 160
Smith, R.W. 48, 49, 51
Smith, W. 150, 241
Sneddon, J.R. 150, 198
So, D. 49
Sobel, D. 361
Sollier, A. 49
Sousa, M. 322
Soyka, F. 302
Spaulding, C.E. 198
Speight, P. 123
Spino, M. 44, 47
Stanford, R. 15, 83
Stark, N. 302
Stearn, J. 66, 199
Stebbing, L. 199
Steen, E. 15
Steiner, L. 185
Steiner, R. 200, 362, 381
Steinhart, L. 352
Stephenson, J. 270
Stoddard, A. 200
Stone, I. 370
Stone, R. 50, 200
Stout, R. 382
Sturzaker, J. 83
Subak-Sharpe, G. 150
Sullivan, G. 342
Sun, W.H. 138

Sweigard, L. 50
Swenson, A. 241
Szasz, T. 206
Szekely, E.B. 160, 161,
    206, 242, 359, 363,
    365, 370

Tan, L. 405
Tan, M.Y. 405
Tanaka, M. 52
Tansley, D. 303
Tanzer, D. 324
Taub, H. 342
Teague, T. 171
Terrell, J. 170
Terrell, M. 170
Tesla, N. 304
Thakkur, C. 206
Thie, J. 206
Thomas, A. 102
Thomas, L. 207
Thomas, V. 353
Thompson, J. 66, 323
Thompson, P. 207
Thompson, R.W. 207
Tilden, J. 207, 362
Tobe, J. 123, 242
Tobe, J.H. 138
Todd, M. 52
Toguchi, M. 242, 405
Tohei, K. 21
Tomilson, H. 305
Tompkins, P. 305
Toth, M. 305
Traven, B. 353
Trungpa, C. 108
Tuchack, V. 397
Turner, J. 89
Turner, M. 89
Turner, R.N. 208
Twitchell, P. 242
Tyler, M.L. 270, 271

Uchroeder, H. 369
Ullyot, J. 47
Urban, P. 38
Urbanowski, F. 66, 323
Urquhart, I. 395
Uyeshiba, K. 21

Valentine, T. 208
Valnet, J. 208
Van Allen, J. 341
Vannier, L. 271
Vaughan, B. 95
Veith, I. 405, 406
Veninga, L. 229, 242
Verma, S.P. 271
Verrett, J. 335, 343
Villoldo, A. 175
Vishnudevananda, S. 66
Voegeli, A. 271
Vogel, V. 213
Volin, M. 64, 66
Von Jeetze, H. 374

Wade, C. 123, 186, 214,
    371, 373, 406
Waerland, A. 214
Waerland, E. 139, 214
Wagenvoord, J. 383, 399,
    402
Walker, B. 16
Walker, N.W. 161, 215, 359
Wallnofer, H. 406
Walton, V. 323
Ward, C. 323
Ward, F. 323
Warmbrand, M. 123, 215
Warren, F. 406
Watson, G. 186
Watson, L. 114
Watt, B.K. 371
Wayland, B. 305
Wayland, S. 305

Weaver, R. 239
Webster, J. 371
Weeks, N. 126
Weiner, J. 103, 324
Weiner, M. 243
Weir, J. 271, 272
Weiss, J.E. 114
Weiss, P. 52
Welsh, P. 124
Wertheim, A. 343
Weslager, C.A. 243
Wesley, J. 243
Westbrook, A. 22
Westlake, A. 305, 343
Wethered, V. 306
Wexu, M. 407
Wheeler, C. 272
Wheeler, F.J. 126
White Eagle 215
White, G. 324
White, G.S. 83, 306
Whitehouse, G. 215
Whyte, K. 103
Wigmore, A. 216, 371, 372
Wilborn, R. 170
Willey, R. 306
Williams, P. 89
Williams, R. 372
Williamson, W. 272
Winter, R. 216, 343, 353
Wolf, R. 382
Wong, M. 392
Woods, H.G. 272
Worden, J.W. 114
Worrall, A. 216
Worrall, O. 216
Worsley, J.R. 407
Wosien, M. 32
Wren, R.W. 243
Wright, E. 324
Wu Wei-Ping 407
Wyckoff, J. 291

Wyschogrod, E. 115

Yaller, R. 216
Yau, P.S. 407
Yepsen, R. 382
Yesudian, S. 53, 66, 67,
    216
Yingling, W.A. 272
Yokochi, C. 16
Yudkin, J. 201, 205

Zanfagna, P. 338
Zaricor, B. 242
Zuidema, G. 15

About the Author

CRIS POPENOE, the author, has a BA in International Relations and History, and an MA in Latin American Studies. After spending three and a half years working for liberal political changes on Capitol Hill, she realized that the changes needed in the society around us weren't going to happen until changes first took place within us. In 1972 she started the Yes! Bookshop concentrating on the timeless books that can help bring about these changes. Today, the bookshop has probably the largest collection of such books of any bookshop in the world. This guide distills what Ms. Popenoe has learned from the books and from the many experts who have come to the bookshop. **Wellness** provides candid critical reviews of some 1500 books, plus introductory articles and brief summaries of the principal individuals, schools and ideas important to all aspects of holistic healing.